KU-784-550

OXFORD MEDICAL PUBLICATIONS

Emergencies in Obstetrics and Gynaecology

SECOND EDITION

EDITED BY

Stergios K. Doumouchtsis,
MPH, MSc, PhD, MRCOG
Consultant Obstetrician, Gynaecologist and
Urogynaecologist
Honorary Senior Lecturer, St George's University
Hospitals NHS Foundation Trust,
London, UK
Visiting Professor, University of Athens, Athens, Greece

Professor Sir S. Arulkumaran,
MD, PhD, FRCOG
Professor Emeritus in Obstetrics and Gynaecology
St George's University Hospitals NHS Foundation Trust,
London, UK
Visiting Professor, Imperial College, London, UK

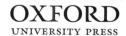

OXFORD
UNIVERSITY PRESS

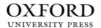

OXFORD
UNIVERSITY PRESS

Great Clarendon Street, Oxford, OX2 6DP,
United Kingdom

Oxford University Press is a department of the University of Oxford.
It furthers the University's objective of excellence in research, scholarship,
and education by publishing worldwide. Oxford is a registered trade mark of
Oxford University Press in the UK and in certain other countries

© Oxford University Press 2016

The moral rights of the authors have been asserted

First Edition published in 2006
Second Edition published in 2016

Impression: 1

All rights reserved. No part of this publication may be reproduced, stored in
a retrieval system, or transmitted, in any form or by any means, without the
prior permission in writing of Oxford University Press, or as expressly permitted
by law, by licence or under terms agreed with the appropriate reprographics
rights organization. Enquiries concerning reproduction outside the scope of the
above should be sent to the Rights Department, Oxford University Press, at the
address above

You must not circulate this work in any other form
and you must impose this same condition on any acquirer

Published in the United States of America by Oxford University Press
198 Madison Avenue, New York, NY 10016, United States of America

British Library Cataloguing in Publication Data

Data available

Library of Congress Control Number: 2015953378

ISBN 978–0–19–965138–2

Printed and bound in China by
C&C Offset Printing Co., Ltd.

Oxford University Press makes no representation, express or implied, that the
drug dosages in this book are correct. Readers must therefore always check
the product information and clinical procedures with the most up-to-date
published product information and data sheets provided by the manufacturers
and the most recent codes of conduct and safety regulations. The authors and
the publishers do not accept responsibility or legal liability for any errors in the
text or for the misuse or misapplication of material in this work. Except where
otherwise stated, drug dosages and recommendations are for the non-pregnant
adult who is not breast-feeding

Links to third party websites are provided by Oxford in good faith and
for information only. Oxford disclaims any responsibility for the materials
contained in any third party website referenced in this work.

Preface to second edition

The obstetrician and gynaecologist practises in a working environment where emergencies are common. Managing an emergency requires good knowledge of the condition and a systematic and logical approach. Preparation to manage emergencies requires planning and multidisciplinary teamwork. The first edition of the handbook provided succinct and easily accessible information to manage such emergencies and promote efficient management of emergencies at the point of care.

The second edition of this handbook serves the same vision and provides up-to-date knowledge and practical guidance in managing common emergencies in obstetrics and gynaecology. We aimed to keep the same format for ease of access and navigation and enriched the previous edition with symptom-based topics as well as updated information. New chapters have been added to cover new areas or topics not previously covered.

These chapters include obstetric complications associated with complex psychosocial needs, laparoscopy and emergencies following laparoscopic surgery, identifying sick patients and choosing monitoring, communication and handover, and preoperative assessment and consent.

We hope that this handbook will be a useful companion to students, doctors in training, as well as consultants, midwives, nurses, and other allied healthcare professionals in the triage areas, wards, theatres, and any clinical settings where rapid access to practical guidance may prove essential in the management of the acutely unwell woman.

Stergios K. Doumouchtsis
S. Arulkumaran

Preface to second edition

Acknowledgements

We wish to express our gratitude to our families for their selfless support, patience, and encouragement.

We are also grateful to the Editorial and Publishing Team at Oxford University Press for their assistance and support in completing this book.

Stergios K. Doumouchtsis

S. Arulkumaran

Acknowledgements

Contents

First edition contributors

Rukma Bhattacharya,
Specialist Registrar,
Torbay Hospital, Torquay, UK

Tom Bourne,
Consultant Gynaecologist, Early
Pregnancy Unit, St George's
Hospital, London, UK

James Clarke,
Consultant Anaesthetist, St
George's Hospital, London, UK

George Condous,
Clinical Fellow, Early Pregnancy
Unit, St George's Hospital,
London, UK

Kate Farrer,
Consultant Neonatologist, St
George's Hospital, London, UK

Michelle Fynes,
Consultant Urogynaecologist, St
George's Hospital, London, UK

Sarah Harper,
Specialist Registrar, Nottingham
City Hospital, Nottingham, UK

Emma Kirk,
Clinical Fellow, Early Pregnancy
Unit, St George's Hospital,
London, UK

Krishna Kumar,
Clinical Fellow in Maternal
Medicine, Espom and St Helier
University Hospitals NHS Trust,
Surrey, UK

Sandeep Mane,
Consultant Obstetrician and
Gynaecologist, Convenor of Basic
Surgical Skills Course, RCOG,
London, UK

Avidha Nejad,
SpR in Obstetrics & Gynaecology,
Espom and St Helier University
Hospitals NHS Trust, Surrey, UK

Nicholas Ngeh,
Specialist Registrar, Fetal Medicine
Unit, St George's Hospital,
London, UK

Penny Oakley,
Honorary Senior Lecturer in Family
Planning, St George's, University of
London, UK

Malini Prasad,
Specialist Registrar in Obstetrics
and Gynaecology, Norfolk &
Norwich University Hospital,
Norwich, UK

Jyothi Shenoy,
Specialist Registrar in Obstetrics
and Gynaecology, The Queen
Elizabeth Hospital, King's Lynn, UK

Abdul H. Sultan,
Consultant Obstetrician and
Gynaecologist, Honorary Senior
Lecturer, Mayday University
Hospital, Croydon, UK

Ranee Thakar,
Consultant Obstetrician and
Urogynaecology Subspecialist,
Mayday University Hospital,
Croydon, UK

Barry Whitlow,
Consultant Obstetrician &
Gynaecologist, Colchester General
Hospital, Colchester, UK

Second edition contributors

S. Arulkumaran,
Professor Emeritus in Obstetrics and Gynaecology, St George's University Hospitals NHS Foundation Trust, London, UK

Maya Basu,
Consultant Obstetrician and Gynaecologist, Medway NHS Foundation Trust, Kent, UK

Joanna Bécares Doumouchtsi,
Specialist Mental Health Midwife, Kingston Hospital NHS Foundation Trust, Kingston upon Thames, UK

Amar Bhide,
Consultant, St George's University Hospitals NHS Foundation Trust, London, UK

Hugh Byrne,
Consultant Gynaecologist, St George's University Hospitals NHS Foundation Trust, London, UK

Edwin Chandraharan,
Clinical Director for Women's Services , St George's University Hospitals NHS Foundation Trust, St George's Hospital, London, UK

Eleftheria L. Chrysanthopoulou,
Specialty Registrar, King's College Hospital NHS Foundation Trust, London, UK

Christina Coroyannakis,
Senior Registrar, St George's University Hospitals NHS Foundation Trust, London, UK

Deepika Deshpande,
Clinical Fellow in Obstetrics & Gynaecology, St George's University Hospitals NHS Foundation Trust, London, UK

Jonathan Dominguez-Hernandez,
Specialist Midwife, University College London Hospitals, London, UK

Claudine Domoney,
Consultant Obstetrician and Gynaecologist, Chelsea and Westminster Hospital, London, UK

Stergios K. Doumouchtsis,
Consultant Obstetrician, Gynaecologist and Urogynaecologist, Honorary Senior Lecturer, St George's University Hospitals NHS Foundation Trust, London, UK

Vishalli Ghai,
Specialist Registrar Obstetrics and Gynaecology, Kingston NHS Hospital Trust, Kingston, UK

Kevin Hayes,
Consultant Obstetrician and Gynaecologist, St George's University Hospitals NHS Foundation Trust, London, UK

Anna Haestier,
Consultant Obstetrician and Gynaecologist, The Norfolk and Norwich University Hospital NHS Foundation Trust, Norwich, UK

Claire Hordern,
Specialty Trainee in Obstetrics
and Gynaecology, Norfolk and
Norwich University Hospital,
Norwich, UK

George Iancu,
Assistant Professor, Filantropia
Clinical Hospital, Bucharest,
Romania

Olujimi Jibodu,
Consultant Obstetrician and
Gynaecologist, York Teaching
Hospital Foundation Trust,
York, UK

Emma Kirk,
Consultant Obstetrician and
Gynaecologist, North Middlesex
University Hospital, London, UK

Tahir Mahmood,
Consultant Gynaecologist, Victoria
Hospital, Kirkcaldy, UK

Edward Morris,
Consultant, Norfolk and Norwich
University Hospital, Norwich, UK

Sambit Mukhopadhyay,
Consultant Gynaecologist and
Clinical Director, Norfolk and
Norwich University Hospital
Foundation, Norwich, UK

Kostis I. Nikolopoulos,
Specialty Registrar in Obstetrics
and Gynaecology, Barking, Havering
and Redbridge University Hospitals
NHS Trust, Queen's Hospital,
London, UK

David Nunns,
Consultant Gynaecological
Oncologist, Nottingham University
Hospitals, Nottingham, UK

Christiana Nygaard,
Instructor of Urogynecology,
São Lucas Hospital, Pontificia
Universidade Católica do Rio
Grande do Sul, Brazil

Kamal Ojha,
Care Group Lead for Gynaecology,
St George's University Hospitals
NHS Foundation Trust,
London, UK

Astrid Osbourne,
Consultant Midwife and Supervisor
of Midwives, University College
London Hospitals, London, UK

Aris Papageorghiou,
Consultant in Fetal Medicine and
Obstetrics, St George's University
Hospitals NHS Foundation Trust,
London, UK

Leonie Penna,
Consultant in Obstetrics and Fetal
Medicine, King's College NHS
Foundation Trust, London, UK

Edward Prosser-Snelling,
National Medical Director's
Clinical Fellow (2014–15),
Royal College of Obstetricians and
Gynaecologists, London, UK

Sheila Radhakrishnan,
Consultant in Community
Gynaecology, Royal Free Hospital,
London, UK

Kanchan Rege,
Medical Director and Consultant
Haematologist, Peterborough City
Hospital, Peterborough, UK

Justin Richards,
Consultant Neonatologist,
Honorary Senior Lecturer,
St George's University Hospitals
NHS Foundation Trust,
London, UK

Vladimir Rivicky,
Specialty Registrar Obstetrics
and Gynaecology, Norfolk and
Norwich University Hospital NHS
Foundation Trust, Norwich, UK

Frank Schroeder,
Consultant in Anaesthesia and
Intensive Care, St George's
University Hospitals NHS
Foundation Trust, London, UK

Hassan Shehata,
Clinical Director, Women &
Children Services, and Consultant
and Lead for Obstetric Medicine
& Recurrent Miscarriages Units,
Epsom and St Helier University
Hospitals NHS Trust, Surrey,
UK; Honorary Senior Lecturer in
Obstetrics and Gynaecology, St
George's University Hospitals NHS
Foundation Trust, London, UK

Mishkat Shehata,
Clinical Fellow, Epsom and St Helier
University Hospitals NHS Trust,
Surrey, UK

Paul Simpson,
Clinical Research Fellow, Norfolk
and Norwich University Hospital,
Norwich, UK

Hannah Sims,
Associate Medical Director, PPD
Global Ltd, Cambridge, UK

Vikram S. Talaulikar,
Clinical Research Fellow, University
College London Hospital,
London, UK

Onnig Tamizian,
Consultant Obstetrician
Gynaecologist, Lead Colposcopy,
Royal Derby Hospital, Derby, UK

Eman Toeima,
Post CCT Speciality Doctor,
Colchester Hospital University
Foundation Trust, Colchester, UK

Hilary Turnbull,
Gynae-oncology Sub-specialty
Trainee, Norfolk and Norwich
University Hospital, Norwich, UK

Austin Ugwumadu,
Consultant Obstetrician and
Gynaecologist/Senior Lecturer, St
George's University Hospitals NHS
Foundation Trust, London, UK

Padma Vankayalapati,
Consultant Obstetrics &
Gynaecology, Medway NHS
Foundation Trust, Gillingham, UK

Dimuth Vinayagam,
Specialty Trainee in Obstetrics
and Gynaecology, St George's
University Hospitals NHS
Foundation Trust, London, UK

Ingrid Watt-Coote,
Consultant Obstetrician, Maternal
Medicine and Diabetes, St
George's University Hospitals NHS
Foundation Trust, London, UK;
Honorary Senior Lecturer, St
George's University of London, UK

Renate Wendler,
Consultant Anaesthetist, St
George's University Hospitals NHS
Foundation Trust, London, UK

Symbols and abbreviations

<	less than		EC	emergency contraception
>	greater than		ECG	electrocardiogram
↑	increased		EHC	emergency hormonal contraception
↓	decreased		EPU	early pregnancy unit
►	important		ERPC	evacuation of retained products of conception
►►	don't dawdle		EUA	examination under anaesthetic
~	approximately		FBC	full blood count
♠	controversial topic		FBS	fetal blood sampling
Δ	differential diagnosis		FHR	fetal heart rate
±	with/without		FMH	fetomaternal haemorrhage
°	degrees		FSH	follicle-stimulating hormone
ABC	airway, breathing, and circulation		G&S	group and save
ABG	arterial blood gas		GA	general anaesthetic
AC	abdominal circumference		GBS	group B *Streptococcus*
ADH	antidiuretic hormone		GI	gastrointestinal
AFI	amniotic fluid index		GIFT	gamete intrafallopian transfer
AFLP	acute fatty liver of pregnancy		GnRH	gonadotropin-releasing hormone
ALT	alanine aminotransferase		GnRHa	gonadotropin-releasing hormone agonist/analogue
ARM	artificial rupture of membranes (amniotomy)		GTD	gestational trophoblastic disease
AV	atrioventricular		GTN	glyceryl trinitrate
BMI	body mass index		GUM	genitourinary medicine
bpm	beats per minute		Hb	haemoglobin
BPP	biophysical profile		hCG	human chorionic gonadotrophin
CMV	*Cytomegalovirus*		HELLP	haemolysis, elevated liver enzymes, low platelet count
CNS	central nervous system		HIE	hypoxic ischaemic encephalopathy
COCP	combined oral contraceptive pill		HVS	high vaginal swab
CPR	cardiopulmonary resuscitation		ICSI	intracytoplasmic sperm injection
CRP	C-reactive protein		IHD	ischaemic heart disease
CS	caesarean section		IM	intramuscular
CT	computed tomography		ITP	idiopathic thrombocytopenic purpura
CTG	cardiotocography		IU	international unit
CTPA	computed tomography pulmonary angiography		IUCD	intrauterine contraceptive device
CXR	chest X-ray			
D&C	dilation and curettage			
DCDA	dichorionic diamniotic twins			
DIC	disseminated intravascular coagulation			
DUB	dysfunctional uterine bleeding			

IUD	intrauterine death or intrauterine device
IUFD	intrauterine fetal death
IUGR	intrauterine growth restriction
IUS	intrauterine system
IV	intravenous
IVC	inferior vena cava
IVF	*in vitro* fertilization
IVU	intravenous urogram
JVP	jugular venous pressure
LFT	liver function test
LH	luteinizing hormone
LMWH	low-molecular-weight heparin
LSCS	lower segment caesarean section
MAS	movement alarm signal
MBRRACE-UK	Mothers and Babies: Reducing Risks through Audits and Confidential Enquiries across the UK
MCDA	monochorionic diamniotic twins
MCMA	monochorionic monoamniotic twins
MI	myocardial infarction
MRI	magnetic resonance imaging
MSU	mid-stream urine
MVA	manual vacuum aspiration
NICE	National Institute for Health and Care Excellence
NSAID	non-steroidal anti-inflammatory drug
NST	non-stress test
OHSS	ovarian hyperstimulation syndrome
PCOS	polycystic ovary syndrome
PE	pulmonary embolism
PEP	post-exposure prophylaxis
PID	pelvic inflammatory disease
PP	placenta praevia
PPH	postpartum haemorrhage
PPROM	preterm, prelabour rupture of membranes

PR	per rectum
PROM	prelabour rupture of the membranes
PTE	pulmonary thromboembolism
PUL	pregnancy of unknown location
PVB	per vaginal bleeding
RCOG	Royal College of Obstetricians and Gynaecologists
RDS	respiratory distress syndrome
Rh	Rhesus
ROM	rupture of membranes
SABE	subacute bacterial endocarditis
SC	subcutaneous
SROM	spontaneous rupture of membranes
STI	sexually transmitted infection
STOP	suction termination of pregnancy
TEDS	thromboembolic deterrent stockings
TENS	transcutaneous electronic nerve stimulation
TOP	termination of pregnancy
TTP	thrombotic thrombocytopenic purpura
TTTS	twin–twin transfusion syndrome
TVS	transvaginal scan
U	units
U&E	urea and electrolytes
UNA	uterine nerve ablation
UPSI	unprotected sexual intercourse
US	ultrasound
UTI	urinary tract infection
V/Q	ventilation/perfusion
VTE	venous thromboembolism
vWD	von Willebrand disease
vWF	von Willebrand factor
WCC	white cell count
WHO	World Health Organization

:☻: —A true emergency, as outlined. Memorizing these conditions may help, rather than referring to this book when the patient is in the department! Call for immediate senior help. Try to remain calm and quickly assess the ABCs. Once the problem has been dealt with, remember to re-assess—other problems may have been forgotten or missed in the heat of the moment.

:☺: —These patients still need to be assessed very quickly, but you do not need to drop everything and run (so long as their ABCs have been managed). These patients can quickly shift into the emergency category if not sorted soon. Consider senior help/advice.

① —The majority of patients will fall into this and the last category. Although they do not need to be seen straight away, make sure you assess them thoroughly—some conditions can deteriorate if not treated properly. Think carefully of potential complications that may develop, such as atrioventricular block with inferior MIs or tamponade with pericardial effusions. Liaise with specialist help, if necessary.

⑦ —These are non-urgent conditions and general points of interest. Many of these patients, strictly speaking, should not come to casualty in the first place.

Part 1

Obstetrics

Pregnancy changes and early pregnancy complications

Contributors
S. Arulkumaran, Edwin Chandraharan,
Christina Coroyannakis, Kevin Hayes, and Emma Kirk

Contents

⑦ **Physiological changes in pregnancy**

Pregnancy is characterized by enormous physiological change in a short space of time mediated by the endocrine (progesterone, oestrogens, cortisol, catecholamines, and human placental lactogen), paracrine (prostaglandins and cytokines), and the physical effects of the utero-placental unit. They are well tolerated by the vast majority of women. Understanding the normal changes can help to:

- Differentiate normality from the minority of women who experience pathological changes
- Explain the development of common pathophysiological conditions, e.g. gestational diabetes and pre-eclampsia
- Explain why some women with pre-existing medical conditions decompensate in pregnancy, e.g. cardiac + renal disease
- Explain the multitude of symptoms described in 'normal' pregnancy
- Explain the altered reference ranges in pregnancy for laboratory investigations and their subsequent interpretation
- Explain the different responses to some emergencies in pregnancy and why pharmacological action can be altered in women on medication.

Cardiovascular changes

- Cardiac output increases by 40–50% (1500–2000 mL/min) by 10 weeks due to a large increase in stroke volume and a smaller increase in heart rate (overt tachycardia is not considered normal).
- There is a marked reduction in total peripheral resistance (systemic vasodilatation) resulting in reduced blood pressure (BP; diastolic > systolic) in the first two trimesters returning to pre-pregnancy levels by the third trimester.
- It is a failure of vasodilatation and overt vasoconstriction that leads to hypertension in pre-eclampsia.
- Venous pressure increases as uterine size increases (mass effect) explaining why up to 80% of women develop some leg oedema.

Haematological changes

- Plasma volume increases relatively more than red cell volume.
- Dilutional reduction in haemoglobin (Hb) concentration and haematocrit (maximal at 28–30 weeks).
- The term 'physiological anaemia of pregnancy' is erroneous.
- The World Health Organization (WHO) definition of anaemia is Hb <10.5 g/dL and this requires investigation for underlying causes.
- Other changes in full blood count (FBC) include:
  - raised white count (neutrophilia)
  - 10–15% reduction in platelets by term
  - reduction in cell-mediated (lymphocytic) immunity and altered T:B-cell ratio.
- Commonest cause of anaemia in pregnancy is iron deficiency (increased haematinic demand for iron around 4 mg/day unmasking underlying depletion or deficiency in iron stores).

- Iron absorption increases from 5–10% to 40% to meet demand (this relies on adequate intake).
- Most women do not require iron supplementation.
- Folate deficiency is unusual and B_{12} deficiency very rare (demand for both increased).
- Marked increases in coagulation factors VII, VIII, IX, X, XII, and particularly fibrinogen and a decrease in antithrombin III leading to a hypercoagulable state.

Respiratory changes

- Overall increase in ventilation (increased depth of ventilation more than respiratory rate). Mild respiratory alkalosis (CO_2 loss).
- Reduced diaphragmatic mobility in late pregnancy (especially in recumbent position).

Renal and urinary tract changes

- 40–50% increase in renal blood flow and glomerular filtration rate (by first trimester). Urea and creatinine concentrations are lower in normal pregnancy (larger excretion). Small reduction in serum sodium.
- Overall net gain in fluid balance (mineralocorticoid effect).
- Proximal tubular glucose reabsorption may be exceeded leading to glycosuria (this may be physiological).
- Dilatation of ureters and pelvicalyceal systems (progesterone and mass effect).

Gastrointestinal changes

- Gastro-oesophageal reflux is almost universal (reduced lower oesophageal tone).
- Gastric and intestinal motility reduced: 'bloatedness' and constipation common.
- Liver function changes:
  - increased placental alkaline phosphatase
  - reduction in serum albumin
  - reduction in alanine aminotransferase (ALT).

Metabolic changes

- 17β-oestradiol (E_2), human placental lactogen, and cortisol all induce insulin resistance.
- Hyperinsulinaemia leads to anabolism and storing of carbohydrate and fats.
- Susceptible individuals (e.g. those who are obese) may develop glucose intolerance or sometimes frank gestational diabetes.

Clinical significance

- Large circulating volumes enable pregnant women to cope with hypovolaemia well and there may be minimal haemodynamic response to losses of up to 1000–1500 mL giving a false sense of security in the management of obstetric haemorrhage.
- Overall net fluid gains mean excessive use of oxytocin (antidiuretic hormone (ADH)-like effect) can lead to fluid overload.

- The initial reduction in BP is less marked and the latter increase is exaggerated in pre-eclampsia due to poor initial vasodilatation and later vasoconstriction.
- The procoagulant state and pelvic mass effect are additive in increasing the risk of thromboembolic disease throughout the whole pregnancy and the puerperium.
- Hb <10.5 g/dL needs investigation and antenatal correction to reduce risk at delivery from postpartum haemorrhage (PPH).
- Some women describe tachypnoea and this may need to be differentiated from underlying causes such as cardiorespiratory disease or symptomatic anaemia.
- Repeated glycosuria is often physiological but may be an indicator of gestational diabetes and needs investigation.
- Physiological reductions in baseline serum levels of urea, creatinine, albumin, ALT, and platelets all need to be borne in mind when assessing blood results in women with pre-eclampsia.
- There is an overall degree of immunosuppression predisposing to sepsis (urinary tract infections (UTIs) and genital tract sepsis, community-acquired group A streptococcal infection, influenza, and more worldwide malaria are the most significant issues).

☺ Pain/bleeding in early pregnancy

All women who present with lower abdominal pain and/or bleeding per vagina (PVB) in the reproductive age group must have a pregnancy test. If pregnant and in their first trimester, ideally they must have a clinical assessment and transvaginal scan (TVS). This confirms viability, gestation, and, most importantly, the location of the pregnancy.

Causes:
- Miscarriage
- Ectopic pregnancy
- Pregnancy of unknown location (PUL)
- Gestational trophoblastic disease (GTD)
- Genital tract pathology
- Unexplained.

Miscarriage

Bleeding in the first trimester affects over 20–30% of pregnancies. Up to 50% of those who bleed will go on to have a miscarriage. 10–15% of clinically recognized pregnancies will miscarry.

Causes
- In the majority there is no demonstrable cause.
- Known causes include chromosomal abnormality, abnormal placental development, multiple pregnancy, uterine abnormality, corpus luteum failure, and infection.

Symptoms and signs
- PVB: may only be spotting or can be heavy with clots.
- Pain or cramping in lower abdomen, possibly radiating to back.
- Weakness, dizziness, collapse: vasovagal attacks may occur if products of conception are in the cervical os.

Investigations
- Physical examination: including speculum and bimanual pelvic examination. The uterus may be smaller than expected for dates. The cervical os may be open or closed. There may be products of conception within the cervical os that need to be removed.
- TVS is essential for ultrasound (US) classification of miscarriage: may demonstrate a sac with or without a fetal pole, retained products of conception, or an empty uterus.
- Serial serum human chorionic gonadotrophin (hCG): needed and case should be managed as a PUL (see 'Other causes of bleeding in early pregnancy', pp. 12–13) if TVS shows an empty uterus with no previous TVS confirming an intrauterine pregnancy, in order to exclude an ectopic pregnancy.
- FBC and sample for group and save (G&S).

Classification
Clinical classification of miscarriage is misleading and not helpful. A threatened miscarriage is a clinical diagnosis and always requires US follow-up. Classification should therefore be US based as this confirms a diagnosis:

1. *Viable intrauterine pregnancy*: fetal pole with cardiac activity.
2. *Early intrauterine pregnancy*: gestational sac with mean diameter <25 mm or fetal pole <7 mm without cardiac activity—rescan > 10 days to confirm viability.[1]
3. *Incomplete miscarriage*: heterogeneous tissue within the uterine cavity.
4. *Anembryonic pregnancy or blighted ovum* (early embryonic demise): empty gestational sac with mean diameter >25 mm.
5. *Missed or delayed miscarriage* (early fetal demise): fetal pole >7 mm with no cardiac activity.
6. *PUL—empty uterus*: needs serial hCG to confirm whether complete miscarriage, an early pregnancy too early to visualize, or ectopic pregnancy.

Management
Depends on the clinical state of the woman and the presenting symptoms and signs. As with an ectopic pregnancy, resuscitation in an emergency situation may be necessary. Immediate removal of products from the cervical os for pain relief and vagal response may be helpful.

Surgical
Surgical management of miscarriage or evacuation of retained products of conception (ERPC) may be performed as an elective day case procedure or as an emergency if needed, usually under general anaesthetic. A manual vacuum aspiration (MVA) may be performed in the outpatient setting with or without local anaesthetic.

Expectant
Highest success rates are in women with incomplete miscarriages. The majority of women in this group will complete their miscarriage within 2 weeks. Women with a missed miscarriage or an anembryonic pregnancy have only a 50% chance of resolving their pregnancy within 2 weeks.

Medical
Usually in the form of prostaglandin analogues (misoprostol or gemeprost), with or without antiprogesterone priming (mifepristone). High success rates. Again success depends on type of miscarriage, with highest success rates in incomplete miscarriage.

Anti-D immunoglobulin
Needed in rhesus-negative women over 12 weeks with any bleeding and in any women having surgical intervention.

Psychological
Pregnancy loss can be an extremely distressing time for both the woman and her partner so it is important that there are resources available to offer counselling and support as necessary.

Ectopic pregnancy
- A diagnosis of ectopic pregnancy should be considered in any woman of reproductive age presenting with abdominal pain ± PVB who has a positive pregnancy test.
- Incidence is 11.3/1000 pregnancies in the United Kingdom (UK).[2]

- Mortality is 16.9/100,000 ectopic pregnancies.[2]
- Over 10,000 ectopic pregnancies are diagnosed annually in the UK.
- The majority of ectopic pregnancies are tubal but other types include interstitial, cornual, cervical, ovarian, caesarean section (CS) scar, intramural, and abdominal.
- A heterotopic pregnancy occurs when there is an intrauterine pregnancy in conjunction with an ectopic pregnancy.
- Although collapse of a woman in the reproductive age group is uncommon, this should be considered to be due to an ectopic pregnancy until proven otherwise.

Risk factors
- Previous ectopic pregnancy
- Previous tubal surgery (including tubal ligation)
- History of pelvic inflammatory disease (PID), chlamydia or gonorrhoea infection
- Past or current smoking
- Increased maternal age
- History of infertility
- Assisted conception (e.g. *in vitro* fertilization (IVF), gamete intrafallopian transfer (GIFT), or intracytoplasmic sperm injection (ICSI))
- Intrauterine contraceptive device *in situ*
- The use of emergency contraception in this pregnancy.

Symptoms and signs
The following 'classical triad of symptoms' may be present:
- Amenorrhoea
- Lower abdominal pain (unilateral or bilateral)
- PVB.

However, most women with an ectopic pregnancy in modern practice are clinically stable at presentation and have non-specific symptoms. Gastrointestinal (GI) symptoms, particularly diarrhoea, and dizziness are common. The earliest symptom is usually brown vaginal discharge that often starts after the missed menstrual period. Other symptoms may include shoulder tip pain, which is a reflection of significant haemo-peritoneum with blood irritating the diaphragm.
- Abdominal palpation may be unremarkable or, less commonly, confirms an acute abdomen with rebound tenderness, and in some cases guarding.
- Vaginal examination may be unremarkable or, less commonly, confirms cervical excitation, adnexal tenderness, or, very rarely, an adnexal mass.

Investigations
- Qualitative urinary hCG is almost always positive in an ectopic pregnancy.
- Quantitative serum hCG is useful if urinary test is equivocal. It is important to quantify hCG levels in order to decide management strategy or confirm successful resolution of trophoblastic tissue after treatment.

- Serum progesterone <20 nmol/L indicates a probable failing pregnancy.
- FBC, G&S—transfusion may be required, rhesus-negative women should receive anti-D immunoglobulin 250 IU.
- TVS is the diagnostic tool of choice.

Management

Depends on the clinical state of the woman. If a woman is haemodynamically compromised, resuscitation (Airway, Breathing, Circulation) is essential with concurrent transfer to the operating theatre for emergency surgery (usually a laparotomy). If a woman is stable, a TVS should be performed and this will confirm the diagnosis in >90% of women with an ectopic pregnancy. This is based upon the positive visualization of an adnexal mass, rather than the absence of an intrauterine sac (Fig. 1.1).

The combination of TVS with quantitative serum hCG levels are well-described diagnostic tools. Laparoscopy should be used to confirm TVS findings and treat tubal ectopic pregnancies rather than as a diagnostic tool.

TVS should not be performed in a clinically unstable woman, thus delaying theatre.

Surgical treatment

- Indications: haemodynamic instability, pain, an ectopic pregnancy with fetal cardiac activity on TVS, significant haemoperitoneum on TVS, hCG >5000 U/L.
- Laparoscopy preferable to laparotomy: decreased admission time, shorter postoperative recovery, and reduced analgesic requirements.
- Whether salpingectomy or linear salpingotomy should be performed is uncertain. If a salpingotomy is performed there is a significant increased risk of residual trophoblast tissue so follow-up with serial serum hCG measurements is necessary. RCOG guidelines state that if the contralateral tube is diseased, a salpingotomy should be attempted to preserve fertility.[3]

Medical treatment (methotrexate) in selected patients

- Indications: asymptomatic, hCG <3000 U/L,[3] no fetal cardiac activity on TVS, no haemoperitoneum on TVS, non-tubal ectopic pregnancies.
- Most commonly given as a single intramuscular (IM) dose of 50 mg/m^2 of body surface area. Treatment successful if hCG decreased >15% between days 4–7 post injection. Success rates are between 65% and 95%.[4] May also be given intra-amniotically under TVS guidance or locally at the time of laparoscopy but this has no advantage over a systemic approach.

Expectant treatment—'wait and see' approach in selected patients

- Indications: asymptomatic, low hCG levels, decreasing hCG level, no fetal cardiac activity on TVS.
- Successful in 48–70% cases, especially if low hCG and progesterone levels.[4]

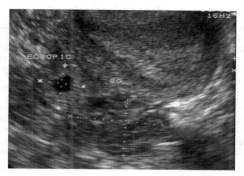

Fig. 1.1 Transvaginal scan image of a tubal ectopic pregnancy.

Other causes of pain in early pregnancy

Some pain or lower abdominal discomfort is very common in early pregnancy. The over-riding clinical principle is always:

'*This is due to an ectopic pregnancy till proved otherwise.*'

Ovarian cyst: haemorrhagic, rupture with bleeding, or torsion

Acute pain from an ovarian cyst accident (usually a corpus luteum) is relatively common. Haemorrhage into the cyst is commonest followed by rupture with intraperitoneal bleeding and then torsion. Torsion is much more likely to be associated with a coincidental dermoid cyst or fimbrial tubal cyst.

It can be very difficult to distinguish from an ectopic pregnancy, particularly with a ruptured cyst.

All cases need TVS as this will identify the presence of an intrauterine pregnancy, and the characteristic appearances of haemorrhagic cysts or free fluid and a 'blown out' cyst wall associated with a ruptured cyst.

There may rarely be a tender discrete mass in the lower abdomen or adnexal mass on vaginal examination (vast majority of ovarian cysts in the first trimester are, however, small and non-palpable).

The vast majority of acute cyst accidents will resolve with analgesia and observation but operative intervention will usually be required if:
- The patient is haemodynamically unstable
- Torsion is the likely clinical diagnosis
- The diagnosis of ectopic pregnancy cannot be ruled out (e.g. no intrauterine pregnancy seen on TVS)
- Where pain symptoms do not resolve and diagnosis is unclear
- In the very rare presence of a heterotopic pregnancy.

Urinary tract infection

Dysuria, increased frequency, urgency of micturition, and suprapubic pain. Proven UTIs are actually rare in early pregnancy and unless the clinical history and urine dipstick is highly suggestive (nitrite, leucocytes, and blood) it should be a diagnosis of exclusion of the other above causes—do *not* blame a UTI for pain in early pregnancy until you have excluded an ectopic pregnancy!

Appendicitis

Low-grade pyrexia, nausea/vomiting, anorexia, paralytic ileus, pain worse on right side, rebound tenderness, and guarding. This is rare in early pregnancy and is a clinical diagnosis once an intrauterine pregnancy has been confirmed and no other more likely cause seen, e.g. corpus luteum cyst accident—if suspected, a surgical opinion should be sought as morbidity and mortality are higher in pregnancy.

Miscellaneous causes

All other causes of abdominal pain that affect young women can coincide with pregnancy including constipation, irritable bowel syndrome, ureteric/renal colic, pancreatitis, reflux, gastritis, etc. The same principle applies as mentioned earlier: exclude an ectopic first before considering other causes.

Acute PID is actually very rare in early pregnancy and is therefore highly unlikely.

It is not uncommon for many women to have unexplained pain—this is a diagnosis of exclusion and requires nothing more than reassurance and analgesia as long as she is systemically well and the location of the pregnancy is confirmed to be intrauterine.

Other causes of bleeding in early pregnancy

Ectopic pregnancy

See 'Ectopic pregnancy', pp. 8–10.

Pregnancy of unknown location

Defined with TVS as there being no signs of either an intra- or extra-uterine pregnancy or retained products of conception in a woman with a positive urinary pregnancy test. 8–31% of women attending for US assessment in early pregnancy will have an inconclusive scan and be classified as having a PUL. Management is expectant and based upon serum measurements of hCG and progesterone. All must be followed up until the final clinical outcome is known: intrauterine pregnancy, failing PUL, or ectopic pregnancy. The majority will have early intrauterine pregnancies or a failing PUL. Only 10–15% will have an underlying ectopic pregnancy.

Molar pregnancy (gestational trophoblastic disease)

Most often diagnosed following histological assessment of products of conception and should be referred to a tertiary trophoblastic unit (Charing Cross, Sheffield, or Dundee) (see 'Gestational trophoblastic disease', pp. 14–15).

Cervical pathology
Cervical polyps, ectropion, infective cervicitis, carcinoma.

Infection
Vaginal candidiasis, chlamydia.

Implantation bleeding
Small amount of bleeding associated with the normal implantation of the embryo. Frequently on day period would have been due.

References

1. Royal College of Obstetricians and Gynaecologists. *The Management of Early Pregnancy Loss* (Green Top Guideline No. 25). London: RCOG Press, 2006.
2. Saving Mothers' Lives: Reviewing maternal deaths to make motherhood safer: 2006–2008. *BJOG* 2011; 118(Suppl. 1):1–203.
3. Royal College of Obstetricians and Gynaecologists. *The Management of Tubal Pregnancy* (Green Top Guideline No. 21). London: RCOG Press, 2004.
4. Kirk E, Condous G, Bourne T. The non-surgical management of ectopic pregnancy. *Ultrasound Obstet Gynecol* 2006; 27:91–100.

Further reading

Condous G, Okaro E, Bourne T. The conservative management of early pregnancy complications: a review of the literature. *Ultrasound Obstet Gynecol* 2003; 22:420–30.
Jurkovic D, Wilkinson H. Diagnosis and management of ectopic pregnancy. *BMJ* 2011; 342:d3397.

Gestational trophoblastic disease

Gestational trophoblastic disease (GTD) is a spectrum of disorders characterized by excessive proliferation and abnormal morphological features in trophoblastic (placental) tissue. They occur in ~1–2/1000 pregnancies, are more common at the extremes of reproductive life, in the Far East, and with previous molar pregnancy and comprise:

- Hydatidiform mole (partial or complete)
- Invasive mole/persistent trophoblastic disease
- Choriocarcinoma
- Placental site tumours
- Non-gestational trophoblastic tumours.

Types of disease

- *Complete moles* are diploid and androgenetic (i.e. dispermic) and have characteristic hyperplastic trophoblastic tissue with hydropic villi with no fetal tissue.
- *Partial moles* are triploid gestations with abnormal and some normal villi and fetal tissues may be present. Histological features are often less clear than complete moles.
- *Invasive moles* refer to when a molar pregnancy has invaded the uterine wall and indeed may have spread to extrauterine sites. Choriocarcinomas are highly malignant tumours of both syncitio- and cytotrophoblast. They invade the uterus and spread widely by vascular dissemination.
- *Persistent trophoblastic disease* (PTD) is a general term for persistently elevated β-hCG and can occur with moles, invasive moles, and choriocarcinoma—there is considerable overlap and little attempt is made to distinguish them as management is similar and driven by β-hCG and evidence of metastases.

Clinical presentation and diagnosis of moles

- Irregular bleeding with a positive pregnancy test is invariably present (>90%). Heavy bleeding can occur but is unusual. They may have pain (usually mild) and the classic symptoms of hyperemesis, hyperthyroidism, and severe early-onset pre-eclampsia are very rare nowadays.
- Though the uterus may be larger than expected for gestation this is a poor clinical sign as most present early to early pregnancy units.
- Examination will usually be normal and classic vesicular PV loss is very rare.
- ~60–70% of molar pregnancies are suspected on TVS (complete > partial) by large-volume retained products of conception with a cystic and highly vascular appearance—the rest are discovered incidentally on histology following 'miscarriage'.
- A severely IUGR fetus in a partial mole is extremely rare as they present early.
- If suspected, β-hCG is usually very high but there is considerable overlap between moles and normal gestations and β-hCG is best reserved for monitoring rather than diagnosis per se.

Management of GTD

Both partial and complete moles are managed by uterine suction evacuation (ERPC) if suspected on TVS. The following should be considered:

- Heavier bleeding more likely with moles (a 20–50 mL catheter balloon may be useful to tamponade the cavity)
- Oxytocics should be used (risk of dissemination low)
- Experienced surgeon required as perforation rates slightly higher
- Tissue must be sent for histology
- Repeat ERPC usually inadvisable (consider referral)
- Rarely uterine artery embolization or hysterectomy is required for intractable uterine bleeding.

Follow-up of GTD

All molar pregnancies need to be referred to one of three regional follow-up centres (Charing Cross, Sheffield, and Dundee) to detect the risk of PTD requiring chemotherapy (0.5% and 10–15% risks for partial and complete moles respectively). Partial and complete moles have 6–12 monthly urinary hCG assays and are discharged if still negative.

Indications for chemotherapy on monitoring

- Static or rising hCG post ERPC
- hCG >20000 IU > 4 weeks after ERPC
- Evidence of metastases or persistent bleeding
- Proven choriocarcinoma.

Chemotherapy

- PTD following molar pregnancies is treated with single-agent chemotherapy with methotrexate (MTX) with 98–100% cure rates. Subsequent pregnancy rates are normal and can be pursued after 6 months of negative hCG.
- Invasive mole, choriocarcinoma, and high-risk PTD require specialist evaluation and formal staging as distant spread by the time of diagnosis is usual (particularly pulmonary).
- Chemotherapy includes MTX for lower-grade disease or sequential EMA-CO (etoposide/MTX/dactinomycin—cyclophosphamide/vincristine) therapy.
- Rarely salvage surgery with hysterectomy (useful for placental site tumours and persistent bleeding), lobectomy, or craniotomy is required.
- Prognosis is still excellent with >90% survival and unaffected future fertility.

:O: Vomiting in pregnancy

Emesis gravidarum refers to nausea and vomiting in pregnancy and these are common early symptoms of pregnancy, believed to be due to physiological hormonal changes of the pregnant state.

However, hyperemesis gravidarum or excessive vomiting may result in dehydration and electrolyte and metabolic derangements that can compromise maternal and fetal well-being. Many medical and surgical emergencies may present with vomiting during pregnancy and thus pose a diagnostic difficulty. It is essential to identify the underlying cause early so that appropriate treatment can be instituted.

Causes

Physiological

Emesis gravidarum: this refers to the nausea and vomiting of pregnancy that normally occurs around 8–10 weeks, with the peak of serum hCG levels. There is no electrolyte or metabolic derangements and the condition often settles by 12 weeks.

Pathological

Any vomiting that is excessive or continuing beyond 20 weeks should be considered pathological unless proven otherwise.

- Hyperemesis gravidarum: refers to any nausea and vomiting of pregnancy that is severe enough to cause dehydration and electrolyte and metabolic derangements that may endanger the life of the patient. This normally occurs around 8–10 weeks, may continue beyond 12 weeks, but rarely after 20 weeks. Multiple pregnancy and GTD (hydatidiform mole, choriocarcinoma) need to be excluded.
- Obstetric: severe pre-eclampsia/obstetric cholestasis/acute polyhydramnios
- Gynaecological: torsion of ovarian cyst/pedunculated fibroid. Acute red degeneration of fibroid.
- Infections: UTIs (pyelonephritis), chorioamnionitis, hepatitis, acute pancreatitis, GI (including acute appendicitis), central nervous system (CNS) infections (meningitis, encephalitis, cerebral malaria—in developing countries), viral infections.
- Metabolic: diabetic ketoacidosis, hyperthyroidism.
- Others: CNS tumours (pituitary adenoma), GI tumours (e.g. gastric cancer), intestinal obstruction, gastro-oesophageal reflux.

Psychological

Attention seeking/lack of family support.

History

- Known metabolic disorders, assisted reproduction.
- Type of vomiting: projectile (raised intracranial pressure).

Associated factors

- Nausea: GI disorders, malignancies, metabolic disorders
- Dyspepsia: acute gastritis/gastric ulcer
- Fever: infections/red degeneration of fibroid
- Pain: infections/torsion/red degeneration/polyhydramnios

- Dysuria/pyuria/haematuria/loin to groin pain: UTI/pyelonephritis
- Jaundice/loss of appetite: hepatitis/cholestasis
- Headaches/visual disturbances: CNS tumours/pre-eclampsia
- Tremors/sweating/anxiety/palpitations: hyperthyroidism
- Confusion/delirium/acetone breath: diabetic ketoacidosis
- Constitutional symptoms: viral infections
- Haematemesis: gastro-oesophageal reflux, gastric cancer, lower oesophageal tears due to excessive vomiting (Malory–Weiss syndrome).

Examination

General condition
- Level of consciousness (?delirious/comatose, abnormal behaviour)
- Deep breathing (Kussmaul's breathing), ?acetone breath
- Level of hydration
- ?Icterus/?in pain.

Vital signs
Pulse/BP/temperature/respiration.

Systemic examination
Cardiovascular system/respiratory system/CNS if pathology is suspected.

Abdominal examination
- Abdominal distension (if more than the uterine distension—?fluid or flatus due to intestinal obstruction)
- Guarding/rebound tenderness (peritonitis)
- Tenderness: suprapubic/renal angle/epigastric/right hypochondrial/uterine/iliac fossae/McBurney's point
- Abdominal masses (e.g. lump in epigastric region with gastric cancer)
- Fluid thrill.

Investigations
- Urine dipstick: to exclude UTI, ketonuria
- Exclude infections: FBC, C-reactive protein (CRP)
- Severity of vomiting: blood urea and serum electrolytes, serum creatinine, packed cell volume (haematocrit)
- US scan: to exclude multiple pregnancy, GTD, or adnexal masses.

Additional investigations—depending on the suspected aetiology
- Midstream sample of urine for microscopy & culture (*UTI*)
- Blood gases (*diabetic ketoacidosis*)
- Thyroid function tests (*hyperthyroidism*)
- Fasting/random blood glucose (*diabetic ketoacidosis*)
- Serum amylase (*pancreatitis*)
- Liver function tests (LFTs) (*hepatitis, severe pre-eclampsia, cholestasis*)
- Hepatitis serology (*hepatitis*)
- Abdominal US (*pyelonephritis, hepatitis, cholestasis*)
- Blood cultures (*chorioamnionitis, pyelonephritis*)
- Blood for malarial parasites (*malaria endemic areas*)
- Visual field testing/magnetic resonance imaging (MRI) scan (*CNS tumours*)
- Lumbar puncture (*CNS infection*).

Sequelae
- Maternal and fetal compromise due to electrolyte and metabolic derangements
- Metabolic acidosis with multi-organ failure
- Wernicke's encephalopathy and Korsakoff's psychosis due to severe intractable vomiting
- Maternal collapse and death in severe cases, if untreated.

Management
All patients with severe or intractable vomiting and/or with ketonuria need to be admitted. The principles of management of severe vomiting in pregnancy are given as follows:
- Immediate correction of dehydration (hypovolaemia), and electrolyte and metabolic derangements
- Medications to stop further vomiting
- Specific management of the aetiology—may require a 'multi-disciplinary' approach
- Counselling and improving the psychological well-being.

Immediate correction of dehydration (hypovolaemia) and electrolyte and metabolic derangements
- Rapid intravenous (IV) infusion of 1 L of normal saline or 5% dextrose solution.
- Addition of 20–40 mmol/L of potassium based on the serum electrolyte result.
- Continuation of IV fluids until the patient is able to tolerate oral fluids and there is a clinical improvement in the degree of dehydration, disappearance of ketones in the urine, and decrease in the haematocrit.
- If diabetic ketoacidosis is confirmed, insulin needs to be administered via a separate infusion pump (with potassium), usually at a rate of 1 unit/hour—in conjunction with a diabetic physician. A sliding scale is mandatory. Patient may need sodium bicarbonate infusion to neutralize the metabolic acidosis.

Medications to stop further vomiting
- Metoclopramide 10 mg (IV/IM/oral) 8-hourly—patient needs to be counselled regarding extra-pyramidal side effects.
- Cyclizine 50 mg (IV/IM/oral) 8-hourly.
- Domperidone 10 mg (oral) 8-hourly or 60 mg twice daily (per rectum (PR)).
- Pyridoxine (vitamin B_1) 10 mg—may help to reduce severe nausea.
- Antacids (ranitidine 50 mg IV/IM or cimetidine 200 mg IV/IM) may help reduce acute gastritis secondary to severe vomiting or if peptic ulcer disease is suspected. Can be continued orally after vomiting has resolved (ranitidine 150 mg twice daily).
- Thiamine 50 mg to prevent the development of Wernicke's encephalopathy and Korsakoff 's psychosis, which are the dreaded complications of severe vomiting in pregnancy.

In intractable vomiting, the following drugs may be administered:
- Ondansetron 4 mg (IV/oral)—not licensed in pregnancy
- Methyl prednisolone.

Alternative therapies have been proven to reduce the sensation of nausea and the number of episodes of vomiting. These include:
- Ginger (either in tablet/syrup form)
- Acupressure wristbands on P6 point on wrist (3 fingerbreadths from wrist on volar aspect of forearm).

Flowchart of management
Fig. 1.2 presents a management algorithm for hyperemesis gravidarum.

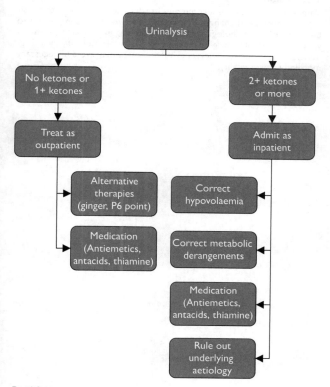

Fig. 1.2 Management algorithm for hyperemesis gravidarum.

Specific management of the aetiology—may require a 'multi-disciplinary' approach

- Antibiotics—for UTI, chorioamnionitis
- Evacuation of the hydatidiform mole when the condition is stable
- Bromocriptine/cabergoline (pituitary adenoma) or surgery for CNS tumours
- Medical management of hepatitis, pancreatitis, degenerating fibroid, cerebral malaria
- Surgical management of acute appendicitis, intestinal obstruction, and torsion of ovarian cysts or pedunculated fibroids.

Conclusion

Vomiting in pregnancy is a common disorder and is often due to physiological (hormonal) changes of pregnancy. However, it is important to be aware of the pathological causes of vomiting in pregnancy, some of which are medical or surgical emergencies. Clinical suspicion, early diagnosis, and appropriate emergency management may avoid unnecessary morbidity and mortality.

Medical emergencies in pregnancy

Contributors

Stergios K. Doumouchtsis, Claire Hordern, Sambit Mukhopadhyay, Aris Papageorghiou, Onnig Tamizian, and Ingrid Watt-Coote

Contents

:skull: **ABC of resuscitation in pregnancy**

- Cardiac arrest occurs in about 1/30,000 pregnancies.
- The survival of the mother and fetus depends on the management in the first critical minutes.
- All obstetricians should be able to diagnose cardiac arrest and start basic cardiopulmonary resuscitation (CPR) (Fig. 2.1 and Box 2.1).
- All obstetricians should be able to recognize impending cardio-respiratory arrest and institute appropriate measures to prevent deterioration into an arrest.

Airway

- Clear airway of debris/dentures/vomit.
- Tilt head back and thrust lower jaw forward, moving base of tongue from posterior pharyngeal wall creating clear passage from lips to larynx.

Breathing

- If patient is breathing, place in coma position
- If patient is not breathing, commence artificial ventilation immediately:
  - mouth to mouth
  - mouth to nose
  - face-mask and self-inflating bag (100% oxygen)
  - laryngeal mask with self-inflating bag (100% oxygen)
  - once expert help is available the patient's trachea should be intubated as soon as possible to prevent possible aspiration of gastric contents.

Ventilation should be at a rate of 2 breaths to 30 chest compressions.

Box 2.1 ABC of resuscitation (basic life support)

A. Airway: is the airway clear?
B. Breathing: is chest moving or air movement at lips?
C. Circulation: can you feel a carotid or femoral pulse?

If there is no circulation:
- Start CPR resuscitation immediately.
- Call cardiac arrest team.
- For pregnant women > 24 weeks, two further important actions must be undertaken:
  - D. Displacement of the gravid uterus to decrease effect of aortocaval compression on venous return
  - E. Emergency caesarean section within 5–10 minutes of arrest if initial resuscitation is unsuccessful.

Based on the The ABCDE approach (Resuscitation Council, UK; https://www.resus.org.uk/resuscitation-guidelines/abcde-approach/).

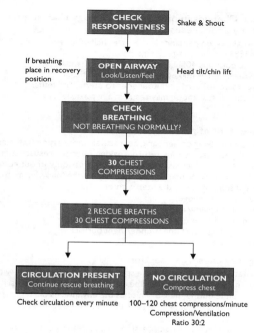

Fig. 2.1 ABC algorithm. Based on Adult Basic Life Support algorithm (Resuscitation Council, UK).

Circulation

- To be effective, cardiac massage must be carried out on a firm surface. If necessary, place patient on the floor.
- Cardiac massage is more difficult in the pregnant patient because of displacement of the diaphragm and rib cage by the gravid uterus (Box 2.2).
- Compression should be carried out mid sternum to avoid possible damage to the liver.

Chest compression should be carried out at a rate of 100/minute.

Box 2.2 Changes in maternal physiology that may adversely affect resuscitation
- Maternal oxygen demands in the latter half of pregnancy are 20% higher than in the non-pregnant state.
- Cardiac output is 40% higher than non-pregnant state.
- The gravid uterus makes ventilation more difficult.
- 10% of maternal cardiac output goes to uterus and fetus.
- Ineffective resuscitation may result in a hypoxic fetus.

Displacement of gravid uterus

With the patient lying on her back, aortocaval compression by the gravid uterus will decrease venous return, making effective resuscitation difficult (Box 2.2). To decrease aortocaval compression without compromising effective cardiac massage, employ one of the following methods:
- Manual displacement of the uterus anteriorly.
- Use of a Cardiff wedge.
- Place a folded pillow under the right buttock.
- Place inverted chair under right buttock.
- Whilst kneeling insert knees under right buttock.
- Emergency CS.

Emergency caesarean section

If resuscitation has not produced a spontaneous cardiac output within 5 minutes, an emergency CS should be carried out in situ. Full resuscitation should continue during the CS. This has the advantages of:
- Probably saving the baby's life (see Table 2.1) if performed in <10 minutes
- Decreasing aortocaval compression thus increasing chances of successful maternal resuscitation
- Improving chest wall compliance, thus improving maternal oxygenation.

Table 2.1 Fetal outcome following perimortem caesarean sections

Time from arrest (minutes)	Number of patients	Outcome
0–5	42	Normal infants
6–10	7	Normal infants
	1	Mild neurological damage
11–15	6	Normal infants
	1	Severe neurological damage
16–20	1	Severe neurological damage
21+	2	Severe neurological damage

Adapted from Katz V. et al, 'Perimortem Cesarean Delivery', *Obstetrics & Gynecology*, 68, 4, pp. 571–576, Copyright (1986) with permission from Wolters Kluwer Health, Inc.

Cardiopulmonary bypass

- There are a number of case reports of successful resuscitation using cardiopulmonary bypass in obstetric patients.
- If available, it should be considered.
- Is the method of choice in local anaesthetic toxicity, as drug is bound to myocardium for up to 2 hours, making resuscitation prolonged and difficult.

Training

There is some evidence that regular drills in cardiac arrest management in pregnancy can improve clinicians' confidence and possibly outcome.

Further reading

Morris S, Stacey M. Resuscitation in pregnancy. *BMJ* 2003; 327:1277–9.
Resuscitation Council (UK). *Quality Standards for Cardiopulmonary Resuscitation and Training.* [Online] https://www.resus.org.uk/quality-standards/

:O: **Abdominal pain in pregnancy**

Abdominal pain is a common complaint during pregnancy. Labour itself is a common cause and it is usually intermittent in nature with associated uterine contractions. The definition of labour is regular uterine contractions with cervical effacement or dilatation, and descent of the presenting part. However, cervical change may be preceded by a long latent phase of labour, and this may make the diagnosis more difficult. The fact that abdominal pain is common and often physiological in pregnancy can mean that pathological causes may be overlooked. Remember that pathological conditions can coexist with and even precipitate labour.

The causes can be divided into those caused by pregnancy, and those that are incidental to pregnancy.

Pregnancy-related causes

Physiological
- *Labour*: painful regular uterine contractions should be accompanied by cervical effacement or dilatation, and descent of the presenting part.
- *Musculoskeletal pain*, presumed to be due to ligament stretching: this affects as many as 30% of pregnancies, and is more common in early and late gestation. It is usually stabbing in nature and aggravated by movement.
- *Constipation*: this is a common condition, affecting up to a third of all pregnancies at some gestation. It is thought to be due to hormonal changes in pregnancy causing decreased bowel motility and increased absorption of water. Iron supplements can often worsen symptoms. The patient's history is usually sufficient to make the diagnosis, and there is frequently a history of pre-existing constipation. Conservative treatment and dietary advice usually improves the condition, but bulking agents and in some cases stool softeners or stimulant laxatives may become necessary.

Pathological
- *Ectopic pregnancy* (see pp. 8–10).
- *Miscarriage* (see pp. 7–8).
- *Placental abruption* (see p. 68).
- *Polyhydramnios*: both sudden- and gradual-onset polyhydramnios can be a cause of pain, though the former will usually present acutely. This can occur due to twin–twin transfusion syndrome (TTTS) in pregnancies with monochorionic twins, or in singleton pregnancies due to an underlying GI abnormality (e.g. oesophageal or duodenal atresia), fetal chromosomal abnormalities, renal anomalies causing over-production of urine, fetal anaemia or hydrops, neurological abnormalities which impair swallowing, or other congenital anomalies (such as congenital diaphragmatic hernia), other causes of extrinsic compression (such as a neck tumour), congenital infections or placental chorioangiomas. Maternal causes (such as diabetes) may also cause polyhydramnios but this is usually less severe. The condition is readily detected on US, although specialist assessment is required to establish the underlying cause. In TTTS, specialist

referral is indicated for possible laser ablation of intercommunicating placental vessels. For other causes, amniotic fluid drainage may be indicated to relieve maternal symptoms and to reduce the risk of preterm delivery.

- *Chorioamnionitis*: this may be accompanied by maternal vaginal discharge, pyrexia and tachycardia, uterine tenderness, leucocytosis or elevation of CRP, and fetal tachycardia. A history of prelabour rupture of the membranes (PROM) should raise the index of suspicion, but chorioamnionitis can also occur with no history of PROM. If there is evidence of chorioamnionitis, treatment with antibiotics should not delay the decision for delivery of the fetus regardless of gestational age, as the maternal condition can deteriorate rapidly.

- *Symphysis pubis dysfunction* (SPD): this common condition of unknown aetiology usually causes pain and tenderness over the symphysis pubis joint. Pain may radiate to the hips, groin, lower abdomen, and lower back. Walking and weight-bearing on one leg (e.g. climbing stairs, getting in and out of bed) are particularly painful. Apart from analgesia, the mainstay of treatment is specialist physiotherapy that can provide support belts, transcutaneous electronic nerve stimulation (TENS), and crutches to aid mobility.

- *Pre-eclampsia*: one of the symptoms of pre-eclampsia is epigastric pain, which is due to stretching of the liver capsule. The presence of this symptom in severe pre-eclampsia or haemolysis, elevated liver enzymes, low platelets (HELLP) syndrome is an ominous sign and must be taken seriously, as it increases the risk of subcapsular hepatic bleeding or liver rupture.

- *Acute fatty liver of pregnancy* (AFLP): this is a rare cause of acute severe liver disease of unknown cause, occurring in about 1/10,000 pregnancies. It usually presents in the late third trimester, with epigastric or right upper-quadrant abdominal pain, jaundice, nausea, and vomiting. Tiredness and confusion are often present, and can be signs of hepatic encephalopathy. Abnormal liver function or clotting may need to be followed by US of the liver for diagnosis. There are risks of maternal liver failure and coagulopathy, and fetal demise. Seek advice from a specialist liver unit early. Timely delivery will allow intensive care for the mother. In most cases the condition improves with supportive measures and liver function returns to normal within a few weeks. Rarely liver failure may ensue and transplantation becomes necessary. (Also see p. 54.)

- *Complications of uterine fibroids*: pain due to red degeneration or torsion of fibroids is usually localized, but can be very severe and may mimic placental abruption. Conservative management with analgesia (often opiates are required) and bedrest will usually allow spontaneous resolution of the symptoms. Laparotomy for both diagnosis and treatment is rarely required.

- *Uterine rupture or scar dehiscence*: this is an uncommon cause of pain, and can be difficult to diagnose as it is usually (but not always!) associated with labour. In most instances the pain occurs in the third trimester, and there is a history of previous CS. However, rupture of the uterus can occur in women without previous CS, and this is associated with multiparity, induction agents (prostaglandins and oxytocics), obstructed labour, or other previous uterine surgery, e.g. myomectomy. There is constant pain and scar tenderness even between uterine contractions, and this is often associated with vaginal bleeding that can be severe and can rapidly lead to maternal shock. Classically there is loss of the presenting part on vaginal examination. Abnormalities in the cardiotocograph (CTG) are often the first clue to impending rupture or ruptured uterus. The treatment is by aggressive resuscitation, prompt laparotomy and delivery, and subsequent repair of the uterine defect. Rarely hysterectomy may be necessary.

The condition can present, albeit rarely, in the immediate postnatal period. This will usually be with signs of vaginal or intra-abdominal bleeding and shock. Delay in performing laparotomy can have catastrophic consequences.

- *Uterine torsion*: this is a rare cause of pain, and is caused either by rapid rotation of the uterus, or by rotation of >90°. This will often be due to an associated uterine abnormality, uterine fibroids, or a large adnexal mass. Symptoms include abdominal pain, and a tender and firm uterus. Associated abnormalities in the CTG are often present, and this can make the condition difficult to distinguish from placental abruption. Clues are a more gradual onset of pain, urinary retention, and a lateral displacement of the urethra on catheterization. In severe cases CS may be necessary, but at earlier gestation expectant management with analgesia and altering of maternal position can be successful in prolonging pregnancy.

Causes unrelated to pregnancy

Gastrointestinal tract

- *Appendicitis*: a common cause of an acute abdomen. It affects about 1/1000 pregnancies. It can be a challenging diagnosis because:
  - the position of the appendix changes in pregnancy and is behind the broad ligament obscuring guarding and rebound tenderness
  - commonly there is absence of localization of pain
  - nausea and vomiting are common in pregnancy as it is with appendicitis
  - there is physiological leucocytosis in pregnancy.

Absence of leucocytosis may be reassuring. Pyrexia, nausea, vomiting, tachycardia, coated tongue, and right-sided abdominal pain should raise the index of suspicion. Tenderness over the caecal area on rectal examination suggests peritoneal inflammation. Delay in diagnosis can cause appendix rupture with resultant peritonitis (maternal mortality >10%) and premature labour or miscarriage. The risks of delayed diagnosis must be carefully balanced against the risks of surgical intervention on the mother and fetus. US can be useful to exclude other causes, and can be suggestive of appendicitis, especially in the first trimester. Early surgical referral is essential.

- *Acute cholecystitis*: it is not uncommon and occurs in around 1/1500 pregnancies. Symptoms include right upper-quadrant or epigastric pain with nausea, vomiting, and fever. Clinical jaundice is uncommon, but bilirubin and transaminases are usually elevated. The presence of cholelithiasis in most cases helps to differentiate it from obstetric cholestasis, acute fatty liver, and HELLP syndrome. Conservative management using antibiotics and analgesia is adequate in most cases. In more severe cases, cholecystectomy, which can be done using open laparoscopy in the first and early second trimester, may become necessary. (Also see p. 60.)

- *Acute pancreatitis*: this is rare in pregnancy (1/3000) and almost always occurs in the third trimester. Classical symptoms include epigastric pain radiating to the flanks, shoulders, or back. Serum amylase can be elevated in pregnancy, but a very high level will confirm the diagnosis. Most cases will resolve within a few days with conservative treatment: IV fluids, analgesia, antibiotics, nasogastric suction, and nil orally.

- *Intestinal obstruction*: uncommon and is about 1/3000 pregnancies. It can be due to adhesions or volvulus. It is usually characterized by short episodes of colicky pain, vomiting, and constipation. Clinical signs include abdominal tenderness and distention. Abdominal X-ray may be necessary if there is diagnostic difficulty. Treatment is by fluid/electrolyte replacement and nasogastric suction, with surgical intervention rarely necessary. Think of this diagnosis in women with ongoing unexplained hyperemesis into the second or third trimester.

- *Gastroenteritis*: this common condition has many causes and can range from mild to severe. Usual symptoms are those of abdominal pain, vomiting, and diarrhoea. Dietary and travel history should be sought as well and enquiry into symptoms in other family members. Examination reveals mild diffuse abdominal tenderness and borborygmi may be present. Bacterial and viral gastroenteritis is usually self-limiting. Dehydration can complicate the condition, and IV fluids and electrolyte supplementation may be necessary. If the condition does not resolve, consider other causes. Gastroenteritis may stimulate preterm labour. It is not known to cause any adverse perinatal outcomes.

- *Peptic ulcer disease*: this is rare in pregnancy, when the decreased gastric acid secretion is thought to reduce the incidence of this condition. Patients will often have a history of previous peptic ulceration or *Helicobacter pylori*, and typically present with epigastric or left upper-quadrant burning pain that can radiate to the back. It is frequently relieved by food, antacids, or vomiting. Sudden onset of symptoms may indicate perforation, although this is rare in pregnancy, as is gastrointestinal (GI) bleeding. Epigastric tenderness is usually mild, but if perforation has occurred, severe tenderness with signs of peritonitis may be present. H_2-receptor antagonists are usually sufficient to control symptoms, and testing and treatment for *H. pylori* should be performed after pregnancy.

- *Inflammatory bowel disease* (ulcerative colitis and Crohn's disease): this usually presents with abdominal pain and diarrhoea which can be accompanied by blood and mucus. Weight loss and anaemia are common. Exacerbations usually occur in the first and second trimesters, and are more common in women who have active disease at the time of conception. Diagnosis can be confirmed by sigmoidoscopy and biopsy if necessary. Treatment with sulfasalazine and corticosteroids is safe in pregnancy, but the use of azathioprine should be avoided if possible. Surgical management may sometimes become necessary for bowel obstruction, perforation, intractable haemorrhage, or toxic megacolon, and close liaison with the surgical team is essential.

- *Diverticulitis*: this is due to faecal material becoming trapped in the neck of diverticula allowing bacterial overgrowth. Although it is rare in pregnancy, up to a third of the population may have developed diverticula by the age of 45. Low left-sided pain is often accompanied by fever, nausea, and diarrhoea or constipation. Uncomplicated diverticulitis, will usually resolve with antibiotic treatment and food restriction. It can become complicated if perforation, abscesses, or peritonitis develop, and this will require surgery.

Urinary tract
- *Cystitis*: this is common (1–2% of pregnancies) and causes suprapubic discomfort and tenderness. Dysuria is often absent, and asymptomatic bacteriuria is a risk factor. A mid-stream urine (MSU) specimen culture will confirm the diagnosis. Treatment is with antibiotics. If untreated it may cause preterm labour or progress to pyelonephritis.
- *Acute pyelonephritis*: the patient feels unwell with fever, chills, nausea, vomiting, and dysuria. Uterine contractions may be present and if untreated the condition can lead to preterm labour. Maternal and fetal tachycardia may accompany the fever, and examination reveals renal angle tenderness. An MSU specimen should be collected for culture. Urinalysis should be taken and if it shows leucocytes, protein, and nitrites on dipstick examination, treatment is started with IV antibiotics, IV fluids, and analgesia. Recurrent episodes of pyelonephritis should be investigated with a renal US scan, and consideration given to prophylactic antibiotics.
- *Urolithiasis*: this occurs in about 1/500–2000 pregnancies. The symptoms of renal colic are severe intermittent flank pain, which may radiate to the groin, and this is associated with nausea, vomiting, dysuria, and haematuria. Patients may give a history of recent or recurrent UTI, or of previous renal stones. The patient is often restless and unable to get comfortable, and palpation reveals tenderness of the renal angle, lower abdomen, or flank. Discussion of imaging with a radiologist is advisable: renal US should be the first line of investigation, and may show hydronephrosis or areas of calcification. If US is equivocal, a limited IVU may be necessary. The risk of radiation must be balanced against the risks of renal damage, preterm labour, or inappropriate treatment. Conservative management with IV fluids, antibiotics and analgesia will allow passage of the calculus in most cases. Surgical intervention may be required if conservative measures fail.

Other causes

- *Sickle cell crises*: these occur in about a third of women with sickle cell disease during pregnancy. Often no exacerbating factors other than pregnancy may be present. Most patients will have a diagnosis of sickle cell disease established before pregnancy. Abdominal pain can be a feature of sickle cell crises accompanied by worsening anaemia. Treatment of a crisis is by keeping the patient well hydrated, warm, and well oxygenated with adequate analgesia (a patient-controlled morphine pump is often required). Early liaison with the haematology team is essential as blood transfusion and occasionally exchange transfusion are necessary. Delivery is for obstetric indications only, but if recurrent crises occur, near term early elective delivery may be considered.

- *Pleurisy*: pulmonary embolism or pneumonia can result in pleurisy that can occasionally present as upper abdominal pain. These are discussed on p. 47.

- *Splenic infarction*: this is a rare cause of abdominal pain and is usually associated with sickle cell disease. There is a large variation in symptomatology, with cases ranging from the clinically occult to severe left upper-quadrant pain and maternal shock. In the latter, surgical management with partial or complete splenectomy is required.

- *Malaria*: this can present with abdominal pain. A travel history should be taken and a history of typical symptoms of headache, nausea, vomiting, chills, sweating, fever, fatigue, and muscular pains should be sought. A peripheral blood smear will demonstrate the presence of parasites. If the diagnosis is confirmed, seek specialist advice for management of the condition and choice of antimalarial therapy as the condition can rapidly deteriorate and lead to convulsions and even death.

- *Acute intermittent porphyria*: this is a rare genetic disorder more frequently manifest in women. Attacks can be precipitated by infections as well as drugs. The attack involves the innervation to the gut leading to abdominal pain which can radiate to the back. Urinary porphobilinogen is elevated. Treatment is supportive.

- *Vascular complications*: very rarely abdominal pain can be due to spontaneous rupture of intra-abdominal vessels such as the uterine or ovarian veins, or splenic or aortic aneurysms. Such cases will present with symptoms and signs of intra-abdominal bleeding and require laparotomy. Rectus sheath haematoma can occur due to rupture of the superior or inferior epigastric vessels or their branches. It usually causes sudden and severe abdominal pain. While usually self-limiting it can rarely expand leading to hypovolaemic shock, and requiring surgical intervention.

☠ **Headache and feeling unwell**

Headaches or generally feeling unwell are common complaints in pregnancy. Women with pre-existing migraine often improve in pregnancy, but migraine may first present in pregnancy. Before dismissing symptoms as being benign, more serious causes should be excluded by careful history and examination, including neurological assessment.

Associations

Symptoms of headache, feeling generally unwell, nausea and vomiting, confusion, impaired consciousness, and irrational behaviour frequently overlap. Such symptoms can be warning signs before a convulsion; indeed, many causes of convulsions can also cause such symptoms, and there is some overlap in the list of differential diagnosis with that of convulsions (Table 2.2; also see pp. 35–40).

Table 2.2 Differential diagnosis of headache

Diagnosis	Comments
Migraine	Difficult to distinguish from tension headache. Usually throbbing, unilateral, intensify over minutes, and may last for hours. History of prodromal symptoms ('aura'). Nausea and vomiting are common
Cluster headaches	Unilateral. Nasal congestion and lacrimation are commonly associated. They occur in clusters, repeatedly every day, often for several weeks. The onset is sudden and typically during sleep. Can be triggered by smoking, alcohol use, glare, and stress
Tension headaches	These are due to muscular contractions of head and neck muscles. Dull, pressure-like headache which is usually worse at the scalp, temples, or back of the neck, are bilateral and described as 'a tight band on the head'. They are worsened or triggered by stress, fatigue, and noise, as well as by caffeine, alcohol, or tobacco use
Pre-eclampsia	Patients seeking medical attention in severe pre-eclampsia are frequently triggered to seek help by headache or generally feeling unwell. The diagnosis is established by the findings of hypertension and proteinuria
Infections: Meningitis Encephalitis Cerebral abscess	History of non-specific prodromal illness is often present, with headaches typically evolving over hours or days. Pyrexia, neck stiffness and photophobia are often present, but petechial rash is only seen in meningococcal meningitis

(Continued)

Table 2.2 (Contd.)

Diagnosis	Comments
Generalized sepsis	Frequently presents with headache and vague symptoms. Often accompanied by pyrexia. Efforts should be made to identify focus of infection before starting antibiotic treatment
Cerebrovascular accidents: Venous thrombosis Infarction Haemorrhage	Headache is severe and sudden in subarachnoid haemorrhage, and photophobia and altered consciousness is present in venous thrombosis. Focal neurological signs are often present. Imaging may not detect infarction in the first 24 hours. Venous sinus thrombosis is often due to underlying infection or pre-eclampsia
Space-occupying lesions: Cerebral tumours	Progressive and severe headaches that are 'bursting' in nature and develop over days or weeks. May be associated with gradually worsening neurological impairment
Metabolic/electrolyte imbalance: Hypoglycaemia Hyperglycaemia Hyponatraemia Hypocalcaemia	Causes of feeling unwell. Correction of the imbalance leads to improvement in symptoms. Can lead to convulsions if left untreated (see pp. 35–40 and Table 2.3)
Trauma	This will be evident from the history of head trauma
Drugs or drug withdrawal: Glyceryl trinitrate Nifedipine	Used for tocolytic and antihypertensive treatment, both are commonly associated with headaches due to severe vasodilatation
Cocaine Amphetamines Alcohol	History of drug overdose, withdrawal or poison ingestion. A toxicology screen (urine/blood) should be performed if this is thought to be the underlying cause

History

This should include onset (e.g. gradual in tension headaches and migraine, rapid in vascular accidents), severity (typically very severe in subarachnoid haemorrhage), character (e.g. throbbing in migraine, band-like in tension headache), and site (e.g. unilateral in migraine, retro-orbital in cluster headaches). Precipitating factors should be sought and may include glare or light in migraines, cluster headaches, and meningitis. Associated symptoms may include neck stiffness in meningitis and vascular accidents; flashing lights or epigastric pain in pre-eclampsia; visual loss in glaucoma and temporal arteritis (both very rare causes of headaches in this age group); and neurological signs which may be of rapid onset in infectious and vascular complications, or of slow and progressive nature in space-occupying lesions.

Examination

- *General*: BP will be elevated in pre-eclampsia and urine dipstick analysis will demonstrate proteinuria. Pyrexia may indicate cerebral or generalized infection. Formal assessment of consciousness (using the Glasgow Coma Scale) should be performed, and signs of impaired consciousness should alert the clinician to possible intracranial pathology such as infection, vascular accidents, or space-occupying lesions. Cerebral oedema may coexist secondary to these, but can also be a feature in pre-eclampsia.
- *Neurological*: detailed neurological examination should be performed and include fundoscopy which may reveal signs of raised intracranial pressure (papilloedema).

Investigations

These depend on the findings in the history and examination. A FBC may reveal leucocytosis in infection, and U&Es will reveal electrolyte imbalance and both are useful in pre-eclampsia. In the presence of pyrexia, blood cultures should be performed. Close liaison with neurology and radiology teams should be established to allow imaging of the brain using computed tomography (CT) or MRI if there are any neurological signs. Lumbar puncture for the diagnosis of suspected meningitis/encephalitis should be performed after exclusion of increased intracranial pressure.

Treatment

Treatment will depend on the underlying cause. For tension and cluster headaches, as well as migraines, the mainstay therapy is simple analgesia such as paracetamol and codeine phosphate. Ergotamine should be avoided, and avoidance of triggers, such as smoking, alcohol use, and specific foods should be advised. For cases with recurrent migraine resistant to treatment, consideration should be given to prophylactic aspirin therapy.

☀ Convulsions in pregnancy

Convulsions in pregnancy are most commonly caused by epilepsy and eclampsia, and details of their treatment are presented here. An unusual history, atypical symptoms and signs, or lack of response to treatment should alert one to the possibility of one of the rarer causes of convulsions in pregnancy, and these are listed in Table 2.3.

Apart from convulsions, these conditions can present with non-specific symptoms, such as confusion, impaired consciousness or irrational behaviour, headache, nausea, and vomiting. Accurate description of the convulsion will usually come from an observer. Careful examination, including a full neurological assessment is invaluable. Specialist input from the anaesthetic team, neurology, radiology, and microbiology is essential.

Table 2.3 Differential diagnosis of convulsions

Diagnosis	Comments
Eclampsia	Associated with hypertension and proteinuria
Epilepsy	Usually pre-existing history of epilepsy

Infections:
  Meningitis
  Encephalitis
  Cerebral malaria
  Cerebral abscess
	History of non-specific prodromal illness often present. Pyrexia, neck stiffness, and photophobia. Petechial rash in meningococcal meningitis only. Investigation: high inflammatory markers. In malaria positive blood film and anaemia. Lumbar puncture positive

Febrile convulsions	Identify focus of sepsis. IV antibiotics

Cerebrovascular accidents:
  Venous thrombosis
  Infarction
  Haemorrhage
	Most cases postnatal. May have focal neurological signs prior to convulsion. Headache common (severe and sudden in subarachnoid haemorrhage), photophobia, and altered consciousness in venous thrombosis. Urgent CT or MRI, but infarction may appear normal in first 24 hours. Sinus thrombosis can also occur as a complication of infection or pre-eclampsia, and is treated with anticoagulation

Space-occupying lesions: Cerebral tumours	Gradual, progressive neurological impairment. Imaging to identify lesion

(Continued)

Table 2.3 (Contd.)

Diagnosis	Comments
Metabolic/electrolyte imbalance: Hypoglycaemia	Low glucose, responds to glucose treatment Remember to seek cause for hypoglycaemia
Hyperglycaemia	High blood glucose, usually due to diabetic ketoacidosis. Responds to treatment
Hyponatraemia	Low serum sodium. Look for causes of SIADH (low serum osmolality, high urine osmolality). Specialist treatment as possible myelolysis if rapid increase in sodium. Fluid restriction
Hypocalcaemia	Causes include hypoparathyroidism and renal failure. Paraesthesia and tetany present. Serum calcium low, ECG abnormal (wide QT interval). Treat with calcium gluconate (cardiac monitoring)
Trauma	History of head trauma. Focal neurological findings. Imaging showing brain injury
Drugs or drug withdrawal: Cocaine Amphetamines Alcohol	History of drug overdose, withdrawal, or poison ingestion. Toxicology screen (urine/ blood) if suspicious of this
Movement disorders or chorea	Usually evident from history
Psychiatric disorders: Psychogenic seizures Pseudoseizures	Diagnosis of exclusion. Usually evident from history and clinical/negative laboratory findings

General management of seizures

The general management of seizures is given here. Subsequent management will depend on the underlying cause, as given in the earlier differential diagnosis section. As the majority of convulsions in pregnancy are caused by epilepsy and eclampsia, these are described in more detail here. Remember that unusual history, symptoms, or signs as well as failure of treatment may be due to a rarer cause of convulsions.

1. **Call for assistance**—senior obstetrician and anaesthetist.
2. **Protect the patient**—avoid maternal trauma by placing the patient in a safe environment.
3. **ABC**—assess Airway, Breathing, and Circulation. Measurement of BP and testing for proteinuria should exclude eclampsia.
4. **Respiratory support**—give oxygen.
5. **IV access.**
6. **Bloods**—draw blood for FBC, U&Es, liver function, glucose, clotting, G&S.
7. **Glucose**—give 50 mL of glucose (50%) if hypoglycaemia suspected.

8. **Assess fetal heart rate**
9. **Abolish seizures**—drugs used depend on the cause (see later). In summary:
- Epilepsy:
  - lorazepam 0.1 mg/kg IV (2 mg/min)
  - repeat at 10 minutes
    or
  - diazepam 10 mg IV bolus
  - repeat at 10 minutes 2 mg
  - 10–20 mg **rectally** if no IV access.
- Eclampsia:
  - loading dose magnesium sulfate 4 g/40 mL IV (over 10 minutes)
  - maintenance dose magnesium sulfate 1 g/10 mL/hr
  - if recurrent seizures, further boluses of magnesium sulfate 2 g IV
  - if magnesium contraindicated, give diazepam 10 mg IV bolus.
10. **Control BP**
11. **Consider delivery**—depending on the underlying cause, seizure activity, gestational age, and fetal well-being.
12. **Establish a cause**—if this is the first seizure, investigations are required after the acute event and should include specialist neurological assessment, FBC, U&E, LFTs, glucose and calcium, imaging (MRI or CT scan), and in some cases EEG or lumbar puncture.
13. **Debrief** prior to discharge—ensure that prior to discharge the patient understands their diagnosis, seizure safety, driving regulations, and that adequate follow-up is made.

Epilepsy

Background

Although epileptic convulsions during pregnancy carry a high risk to both mother and fetus, many women will discontinue their anticonvulsant treatment due to fears over fetal abnormalities. This, in addition to increased metabolism and excretion of anticonvulsants and changes in intravascular volume and binding proteins, means that seizure frequency increases in up to a third of cases. Suitable antenatal care should include careful management of anticonvulsant therapy in order to minimize the risk of seizures, using the lowest effective dose of anticonvulsants possible.

Apart from tailoring and modifying anticonvulsant medication, pregnancy care should include high-dose folic acid periconceptually, detailed US, and (in women taking enzyme-inducing antiepileptic drugs) oral vitamin K from around 36 weeks of gestation. Labour and delivery is best in a consultant-led maternity unit and seizure prophylaxis should be considered for high-risk cases. There is no contraindication to normal vaginal delivery. CS may be performed for obstetric reasons.

Most patients will have a pre-existing history of epilepsy but in some instances this may be their first seizure. In these cases a full work-up, including specialist neurological assessment, FBC, U&E, LFTs, glucose and calcium, imaging (MRI or CT scan), and EEG is required after the acute event.

Risks of seizures
- Maternal:
  - trauma
  - aspiration
  - abruption
  - status epilepticus.
- Fetal:
  - hypoxia
  - abruption.

Management
1–8. The first 8 steps are given previously under the general management of seizures (see pp. 36–7). Eclampsia should be excluded as a cause by checking BP and urine for proteinuria. Then steps 9 onwards are undertaken.
9. **Abolish seizures:**
- Lorazepam 0.1 mg/kg IV (2 mg/min)
  or
- Diazepam 10 mg IV bolus, followed by 2 mg boluses if required
  or
- Diazepam 10–20 mg can be given rectally if no IV access.
- If seizures continue:
  - phenytoin 15 mg/kg IV (maximum rate 50 mg/min) with ECG monitoring.
10. **If seizures continue** (refractory status epilepticus):
- Inform HDU/ITU (anticipate need for ventilation)
- Prepare for delivery (see step 11)
- Seek specialist advice
- Consider third-line drugs (some are unlicensed):
  - phenobarbital 10 mg/kg IV (maximum rate 100 mg/min)
  - propofol 1–2 mg/kg loading, then 3–10 mg/kg/hr
  - midazolam 0.2 mg/kg loading, then 0.06–1.1 mg/kg/hr
  - thiopental
- Consider other causes:
  - eclampsia
  - meningitis/encephalitis
  - trauma
  - drugs.
11. **When to deliver** depends on seizure activity, gestational age, and fetal well-being.
- If seizures are controlled, continue with appropriate pregnancy or labour care.
- Intractable/recurrent generalized seizures during labour or in the late third trimester may require CS under general anaesthetic.
12. Ensure **vitamin K** is given to the neonate.

Eclampsia

Background
Pre-eclampsia/eclampsia are multisystem disorders that can progress rapidly with high risks to mother and fetus. Women with eclampsia may have been known to have pre-eclampsia in their current pregnancy, and

there is little diagnostic difficulty. Frequently, it is symptoms of fulminant pre-eclampsia or eclampsia that triggers admission. Convulsions due to eclampsia with apparently mild or delayed onset of hypertension and proteinuria are widely reported. Predisposing factors include chronic hypertension, renal disease, or diabetes; multiple pregnancy; thrombophilia; or abnormal uterine artery Doppler in mid-gestation. Over a third of eclamptic fits occur postnatally.

The aims of management are:

- To arrest and prevent convulsions
- To control BP
- To effect planned, timely, and safe delivery.

Risks of seizures

- Maternal:
  - trauma
  - aspiration
  - HELLP syndrome
  - pulmonary oedema
  - cerebrovascular accidents
  - abruption
  - anaesthetic and surgical complications of delivery
- Fetal:
  - iatrogenic premature delivery
  - hypoxia
  - abruption.

Management

1–8. The first 8 steps are given previously under the general management of seizures (see pp. 36–7). Eclampsia should be confirmed as a cause by checking BP and urine for proteinuria. Then steps 9 onwards are undertaken.

9. Start HDU chart with 5-minutely BP and pulse until seizures arrested and BP controlled.

10. **Abolish seizures:**

- Loading dose magnesium sulfate 4 g/40 mL IV (over 10 minutes).
- Maintenance dose magnesium sulfate 1 g/10 mL/hr maintained for 24 hours.
- Recurrent seizures should be treated with further boluses of magnesium sulfate 2–4g IV given over 5 minutes.
- Or increase maintenance to 1.5–2 g/hr
- Other drugs such as diazepam, phenytoin, or lytic cocktail should not be used as an alternative to magnesium sulfate in women with eclampsia. However, if magnesium is contraindicated, diazepam 10 mg IV bolus should be given.

11. **Pre-load circulation** with colloid—250 mL Gelofusine® IV/20 min if hydralazine are given in step 12.

12. **Antihypertensive:**

- Labetalol 200 mg/100 mL IV at 20 mg/hr.
- Double every 30 minutes until target BP reached.
  or
- Hydralazine 5 mg IV (1 mg/min).

- Repeat after 15 minutes if systolic blood pressure (SBP) >160 mmHg; diastolic blood pressure (DBP) >110 mmHg or mean arterial pressure (MAP) >125 mmHg.
- If after three boluses SBP >160 mmHg; DBP >110 mmHg or MAP >125 mmHg start hydralazine infusion: hydralazine 40 mg/40 mL IV.
- Titrate to maternal BP:
  - Start: 2.4 mL/hr (40 mcg/min)
  - 30 minutes: 4.8 mL/hr (80 mcg/min)
  - 60 minutes: 7.2 mL/hr (120 mcg/min)
  - 90 minutes: 9.6 mL/hr (160 mcg/min)
  - reduce by 1.2 mL/hr if appropriate
  - if the pulse rate >140/min or there is a contraindication to hydralazine, give labetalol:
    or
  - oral treatment with nifedipine MR/retard 10 mg, swallowed whole, may be possible in certain cases

This can be repeated at 2 hours if needed.

13. **When to deliver**: delivery should be timed and well planned, after control of seizures and BP has been achieved. Uncontrolled hypertension or ongoing seizures make delivery inappropriate. Always ensure that:

- The maternal condition is stable.
- Senior personnel are present.
  In the presence of eclampsia, delivery is usually by CS, preferably with epidural or spinal anaesthetic. If thrombocytopenia or coagulation disorder is present, general anaesthesia may be necessary. After 34 weeks of gestation, and if the condition is well controlled, induction of labour may be considered if the cervix is favourable.

14. **Third stage**: oxytocin bolus. Avoid ergometrine or Syntometrine® as this can cause hypertension. If possible, avoid an oxytocin infusion as this can cause pulmonary oedema.

15. **After delivery**:

- HDU care, consider central venous pressure line early.
- Careful monitoring of pulse/BP/SpO$_2$.
- Continue seizure prophylaxis for 24 hours after last seizure or delivery.
- Antihypertensive as required.
- Fluid balance: fluid restriction to 85 mL/hr with hourly urine output measurement.

:◉: Chest pain in pregnancy

Chest pain is very common in pregnancy though most causes are benign. The evaluation of a pregnant patient with chest pain should be approached in a similar fashion as the non-pregnant patient. This is extremely important because of the increasing age of childbirth (late 30s and 40s) and hence increased morbidity (diabetes, hypertension, heart disease). There is also a significant increase in obesity, body mass index (BMI) >30kg/m². It is thus vital that those conditions having the potential to increase maternal morbidity or mortality are quickly diagnosed so that the appropriate treatment can be administered.

Aetiology

This may be divided into cardiac or non-cardiac:

Cardiac

- Angina (especially in the older, obese patient)
- Acute myocardial infarction/acute coronary syndrome *1/10,000 pregnancies*
- Aortic dissection (about half of all dissections in pregnancy < 40 years).

Non-cardiac

- Pulmonary:
  - pulmonary thromboembolism (PTE) (1:1600 pregnancies; *6–10 times more common in pregnancy than non-pregnant*)
  - pneumonia
  - pleurisy
  - pneumothorax
- Musculoskeletal/costochondritis
- Upper abdominal pathology, e.g. hepatic or biliary tree disorder; gastro-oesophageal reflux disease (GORD); complication of preeclampsia.
- Other, e.g. anxiety or panic disorder, shingles if rash, breast pathology, trauma.

Assessment

A detailed and complete history is essential as it helps to differentiate cardiac and non-cardiac. The onset, severity (scale 1–10), location, duration, type (sharp, dull, pressure, constricting etc.), radiation, and associated precipitating factors are all helpful in making a diagnosis.

- Chest pain of sudden onset, pleuritic, and associated with dyspnoea may indicate PTE or a pneumothorax.
- A central, crushing, dull pain radiating to either or both arms and lasting >20 minutes is suggestive of myocardial ischaemia/acute coronary syndrome; three to four times more common in pregnancy than non-pregnant.
- A sudden, severe, sharp substernal, 'tearing' pain that radiates towards the back (intercapsular) with jaw pain is the classic presentation of aortic dissection.
- Shoulder tip and anterior chest wall pain with a pleuritic component is suggestive of pericarditis. The history will also include a recent viral illness.

- Pain associated with a cough, dyspnoea, fever, productive sputum indicates a likely infective cause (e.g. pneumonia). Similar incidence and pathogens as the non-pregnant.

History should also include association with fatty food (biliary), sleep, relieving factors (e.g. antacids), recent travel, leg or pelvic pain (thrombosis). A past medical (Marfan's, thrombophilia, cardiac, lung disease), drug, allergies, smoking, and family history may all be useful in arriving at a diagnosis.

Physical examination
- A complete and thorough examination as with the non-pregnant patient. Starting with ABCs. BP (differential in both arms and or systolic hypertension indicate aortic dissection; oxygen saturation; temperature; heart and respiratory rate (tachycardia and tachypnoea may indicate PTE. A high index of suspicion is recommended).
- Chest examination to include inspection (rash, bruise), palpation (tenderness seen in musculoskeletal disorders); percussion and auscultation (crepitations, wheeze, reduced breath sounds), heart sounds, and cardiac murmur.
- Crepitations in one or both bases will suggest pneumonia.
- Abdominal examination to include epigastric and right-upper quadrant palpation. Abnormal examination will suggest a GI cause.
- The legs should be examined for swelling, tenderness, and erythema.

Investigations
- FBC to include differentials
- Troponin I (repeat at 6–8 hours if cardiac ischaemia suspected). *May be elevated in severe hypertension, PTE, sepsis, and pericarditis*
- Arterial blood gases (ABGs)
- D-dimer[1] is not useful in pregnancy because of the high false-positive rate. Objective testing is required
- Blood cultures if pyrexial (positive in <15% pneumonia)
- Sputum for culture and sensitivity
- Viral swabs for influenza
- Liver profile
- 12 lead ECG: may be normal initially in cardiac ischaemia hence serial studies
- Chest X-ray (CXR; must not be withheld); normal in cardiac ischaemia
- Echocardiogram
- Doppler US scan of the legs/pelvis
- Ventilation perfusion (V/Q) scan
- MRI
- Computed tomography pulmonary angiography (CTPA).

Management
- A multidisciplinary team approach to include the acute physician, anaesthetist, obstetrician, and neonatologist. Other relevant specialist as necessary, i.e. the respiratory physician, cardiologist, and haematologist.

- Acute chest pain must be immediately assessed to rule out life-threatening conditions such as PTE, myocardial ischaemia, and aortic dissection. Immediate pain relief with opiates usually morphine and correction of hypoxia.
- Fetal monitoring.
- Management plan to include the indication for delivery.
- Acute treatment:
  - Consider the need for transfer to the intensive treatment unit/ high dependency unit. This may need to take place to stabilize the patient prior to further imaging such as an echocardiogram, V/Q scan etc.
  - ABGs may reveal a reduced PaO_2 and/or $PaCO_2$
  - Nurse propped-up or in the left lateral position if in the third trimester.
  - If PTE is suspected, start high-dose low-molecular-weight heparin (LMWH) based on weight. In pregnancy this is administered 12-hourly for enoxaparin (1 mg/kg) and dalteparin (100 U/kg) and daily for tinzaparin (175 U/kg). Treatment may have to be started if the clinical suspicion is high prior to definitive investigations.
  - IV unfractionated heparin should be use if the need for urgent reversibility is anticipated
  - IVC filter may be used for recurrent or large pelvic/abdominal thrombus. Thrombolysis, pulmonary artery catheter, and thrombolectomy can be used in life-threatening cases.
  - If the diagnosis is made in the late third trimester, allow 2 weeks of therapy to ensure clot stabilization and reduction in clot burden prior to deliver if possible.
  - Myocardial infarction (MI) is becoming more common in pregnancy. It is associated with increased maternal and fetal mortality. The common cause is coronary artery dissection and embolus.
  - Presentation in pregnancy may be atypical such as abdominal and or epigastric pain, vomiting, and dizziness.
  - The risk is increased in patients who are older, obese, and are smokers.
  - Manage in a CCU (Coronary Care Unit). Nitrates, beta blockers, low-dose aspirin, LMWH, and opiates are all safe in pregnancy. Statins and angiotensin inhibitors are teratogenic.
  - The 2011 UK Confidential Enquiry reports eleven (11) deaths from myocardial ischaemia or chronic ischaemic heart disease.
  - Coronary angiography should **not** be withheld.
  - Pneumonia can be more severe in pregnancy because of suppressed cell-mediated immunity, especially for viral pathogens.
  - Management in hospital. Aim for oxygen saturation >95%.
  - General treatment to include tepid sponging and antipyretic agent (paracetamol). Antibiotic administration should be managed in conjunction with the microbiologist. A broad-spectrum agent to cover Gram negatives and Gram positives and community-acquired pathogens is recommended.
  - Encourage pregnant women to get vaccinated during the influenza season.

Differentiating signs and symptoms

For differentiating signs and symptoms of chest pain in pregnancy, see Table 2.4.

Differences in common investigations

For differences in common investigations of chest pain in pregnancy, see Table 2.5.

Table 2.4 Differentiating signs and symptoms

Symptoms/signs	MI	PTE	Pneumonia
Sputum	Dry	Dry	Productive
Abdominal pain	–	+	±
Lungs	Crepts	–	Rhonchi
Heart sounds	Quiet 1st, 3rd HS	3rd HS	N
BP	↓ or normal	↓ or Normal	N
Pulse Pulse rate	Thready, low volume	↑ or N	N ↑ or N

HS, heart sound; MI, myocardial infarction; N, no change; PTE, pulmonary thromboembolism.

Table 2.5 Differences in common investigations

Investigations	MI	PTE	Pneumonia
CXR	Normal	Usually normal/wedge-shaped infarction, pleural effusion, atelectasis, areas of translucency in underperfused lungs	Patchy/consolidation
ECG	Varied	Normal/right axis deviation, RBBB, peaked waves in lead 11, S1Q3T3 pattern	Normal
ECHO	Reduced function	Right-sided strain	Normal

RBBB, right bundle brunch block.

Further reading

Centre for Maternal and Child Enquiries (CMACE). Saving Lives, Improving Mothers' Care – Surveillance of maternal deaths in the UK 2011–13 and lessons learned to inform maternity care from the UK and Ireland Confidential Enquiries into Maternal Deaths and Morbidity 2009–13. MBRRACE-UK report 2015. Available at https://www.npeu.ox.ac.uk/downloads/files/mbrrace-uk/reports/MBRRACE-UK%20Maternal%20Report%202015.pdf.

Cook JV, Kyrion J. Radiation from CT and perfusion scanning in pregnancy. BMJ 2005; 331:350.

James AH, Jamison MG, Brancazio LR, et al. Venous thromboembolism during pregnancy and the postpartum period: incidence, risk factors, and mortality. Am J Obstet Gynecol 2006; 194:1311–15.

Knight M, Kenyon S, Brocklehurst P, et al. Saving Lives, Improving Mothers' Care – Lessons Learned to Inform Future Maternity Care from the UK and Ireland Confidential Enquiries into Maternal Deaths and Morbidity 2009–12. Oxford: National Perinatal Epidemiology Unit, University of Oxford; 2014.

Nelson-Piercy C (2015). Handbook of Obstetric Medicine (5th ed). Boca Raton, FL: CRC Press.

Powrie RA, Greene MF, William C. de Swiet's Medical Disorders in Medical Practice (5th ed), pp.42–43; 690–692. London: Wiley-Blackwell, 2010.

Royal College of Obstetricians and Gynaecologists. The Acute Management of Thrombosis and Embolism during Pregnancy and the Puerperium (Green-top Guideline No. 37b). London: RCOG, 2015.

☹ Breathlessness/difficulty in breathing/chest discomfort

Breathlessness, also known as shortness of breath (dyspnoea), is a subjective sensation of breathing discomfort. This is a very common symptom in pregnancy and reported by ~50% of women during the first half of pregnancy. This will increase to ~75% by the third trimester.[1]

Typically, breathlessness is noted at rest and does not interfere with daily activities. This subjective sensation is likely to be secondary to the increased awareness of the physiological hyperventilation of pregnancy. This should be a diagnosis of exclusion following a complete assessment with normal findings and no suggestion of cardiopulmonary disease.

The evaluation and management of breathlessness is directed by the clinical presentation, history, and physical examination along with preliminary investigation results (Fig. 2.2).

Diseases of the cardiopulmonary and neuromuscular systems are the most common aetiologies.

Symptoms of sudden onset, chest pain, cough, or wheezing should indicate likely pathology. Cough is a common symptom in PTE and pneumonia but mainly nocturnal in asthmatics and cardiac failure.

The presentation can be antenatal, intrapartum, or postnatal.

Associated symptoms: orthopnoea, paroxysmal nocturnal dyspnoea, exertional dyspnoea will indicate a cardiac pathology. Chills, rigors and fever will indicate an infective cause. Dizziness, lethargy, faint feeling may indicate anaemia or cardiac origin. Relieving factors, e.g. inhalers as in asthmatic. Haemoptysis, syncope.

Past medical and family history, recent travel, drug use. Consider acquired heart disease (rheumatic in the immigrant population).

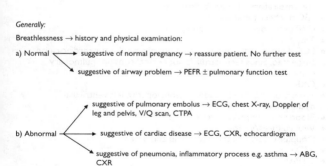

Generally:

Breathlessness → history and physical examination:

a) Normal ⟶ suggestive of normal pregnancy → reassure patient. No further test

⟶ suggestive of airway problem → PEFR ± pulmonary function test

b) Abnormal ⟶ suggestive of pulmonary embolus → ECG, chest X-ray, Doppler of leg and pelvis, V/Q scan, CTPA

⟶ suggestive of cardiac disease → ECG, CXR, echocardiogram

⟶ suggestive of pneumonia, inflammatory process e.g. asthma → ABG, CXR

Fig. 2.2 Assessing breathlessness.

Physical examination

- Complete assessment for mother and/or fetus. Inspection looking for evidence of distress and general posture: can the patient lie supine?; use of accessory muscles or abdominal retraction with inspiration (paradoxical breathing) as in severe asthma implies impending respiratory failure. Hyperventilation as in anxiety and asthma. They may have paraesthesiae of the hands and around the mouth.
- Peripheral oedema common in normal pregnancy or cardiac failure. Legs for DVT
- Inability to speak in complete sentences can be noted in severe cases.
- General examination to include respiratory rate, heart rate, temperature, BP, oxygen saturation, and blood gas. Peak expiratory flow rate (PEFR) should be undertaken if asthma is suspected.
- Hypotension can be a sign of pre-eclampsia, and in association with narrow pulse pressure can be signs of cardiac failure.
- Pyrexia may be a feature of underlying pneumonia, whereas hypoxia can be secondary to cardiac failure or pre-eclampsia.
- Oxygen saturation ≥95% with moderate exertion (e.g. stair climbing) is reassuring, indicating unlikely pathology but not impossible.
- Expiratory wheeze is an auscultation sign which disappears with treatment in patients with asthma, crepitations, reduced/ absent breath sounds, or cardiac murmur.
- Epigastric tenderness seen in reflux or upper abdominal pathology with associated breathlessness.

Investigations

- Oxygen saturation
- PEFR and compare to expected
- ABGs (reduced PaO_2 and $PaCO_2$ in pulmonary embolism. Hypercapnia and respiratory alkalosis in asthmatic)
- FBC to check for anaemia
- CRP (non-specific inflammatory marker)
- Troponin I
- ECG if tachycardia, hypoxic/pulmonary embolus, or cardiac cause suspected. Sinus tachycardia is not normal consider pulmonary embolus
- CXR
- Echocardiogram to exclude cardiomyopathy, left ventricular dysfunction or valvular disease
- Blood and sputum cultures
- Viral cultures/swabs
- Doppler US scan of the lower limb and pelvis
- V/Q scan[2]
- CTPA[3]
- MRI.

Causes of breathlessness

See Table 2.6 for causes of breathlessness.

Table 2.6 Causes of breathlessness

Acute	Subacute	Chronic
Hyperventilation/anxiety	Asthma	Physiological
Acute asthma	Pneumonia	Anaemia
Pulmonary embolus (thrombotic, amniotic fluid air)	(viral, bacterial, atypical)	Chronic lung disease, e.g. TB
Pneumothorax		Cardiac causes, e.g. cardiomyopathy,
Rhinitis/sinusitis		rheumatic heart disease,
Cardiomyopathy		e.g. mitral stenosis
Pulmonary oedema, e.g. secondary to nephrotic syndrome, MS, cardiac failure		Nephrotic syndrome
		Lung tumours

Management

- Rapid assessment to ensure a secure airway.
- Management should be multidisciplinary involving the acute and/or chest physician, anaesthetist, obstetrician along with other specialists i.e. cardiologist, haematologist, microbiologist ± neonatologist as is necessary.
- Consider delivery if this is necessary to optimize maternal care. Specific treatment will depend on the diagnosis and may necessitate intensive or high dependency care. *This must never be delayed.*
- Initial therapy would be to relieve symptoms i.e. nebulizer in an asthmatic, correct hypoxia and acid–base deficit by providing high-flow oxygen and fluid resuscitation, repositioning the patient etc.
- Pain relief with opiates.
- Fetal assessment/monitoring.
- Specific therapy will be based on initial suspicion and results of objective tests. *Radiological imaging must not be withheld.* The patient should be counselled about the risks and benefits.[2,3]

Some specific causes

- Asthma:
  - A chronic inflammatory reversible airway obstruction. Very common in pregnancy in varying severity. Breathlessness can be periodic with associated wheeze and chest tightness. Precipitating factors include cold, exercise, allergens, and poor patient compliance.
  - A detailed history of symptoms should include night-time awakenings, frequency of use of short-acting beta-agonists (e.g. salbutamol), interference with normal daily activity.
  - In acute exacerbations, assessment should be prompt and short-acting beta-agonist initiated via nebulizer giving up to three doses per hour ± oral steroids ± IV aminophylline depending on response.
  - Involve the chest team. Remember acute exacerbation can be life-threatening and may require admission to the intensive therapy unit (ITU).
  - Revert to beta-agonist and oral inhalers once stable.

- *Pulmonary embolus*:
  - Breathlessness and sudden-onset pleuritic chest pain will indicate PTE or pneumothorax. Examination will reveal tachycardia and tachypnoea. ECG will show sinus tachycardia. Blood gas may or may not show hypoxia and CXR may be normal or reveal a wedge-shaped infarct or an effusion.
  - Definitive diagnosis is made with a V/Q scan or a CTPA. Start high-dose LMWH based on weight if high suspicion or delay with objective testing.
  - In pregnancy this is administered 12-hourly for enoxaparin (1 mg/kg) and dalteparin (100 U/kg) and daily for tinzaparin (175 U/kg). IV unfractionated heparin is indicated for massive pulmonary embolus or if there will be a need for rapid reversibility. In cases of recurrent emboli or large clot burden then IVC filter maybe used. Thrombolysis, pulmonary artery catheter, and thrombolectomy can be used in life-threatening cases.[4]
- *Pneumonia*:
  - Supportive care. Antipyrexial agents.
  - Antibiotics following discussion with the microbiologist.
- *Cardiac*:
  - Manage in conjunction with the cardiologist.
  - Diuretics, beta blockers ± specific drugs, i.e. inotropes, digoxin, vasodilators, etc.
  - Cardiac surgery if needed, i.e. valve replacement in severe conditions if the risk is high.
- *Amniotic fluid embolism*:
  - Classically, occurs at the time of labour and delivery with a sudden onset of acute respiratory symptoms, shock, and collapse with associated disseminated intravascular coagulation (DIC) resulting in PPH.
  - Risk factors are advanced maternal age, multiparity, precipitous labour, uterine trauma, and induction of labour.
  - Management is early cardiorespiratory and haematological support. Admit to the ITU for ventilatory and supportive care. Mortality is high.
- Physiological cause secondary to pregnancy is a diagnosis of exclusion.

Differentiating signs and symptoms
See Table 2.7 differentiating signs and symptoms of breathlessness.

Differences in common investigations
See Table 2.8 for differences in common investigations in breathlessness.

Table 2.7 Differentiating signs and symptoms

Symptoms/ sign	Cardiac failure	Asthma	PTE	Pneumonia
Sputum	Nocturnal	Nocturnal	Dry	Productive
Abdominal pain	–	–	+	±
Lungs	Bi-basal crepts	Expiratory wheeze, ↓AE/ silent	–	rhonchi
Heart sounds	Gallop rhythm	N	3rd HS	N
BP	Low	N	↓/N	
Pulse character	↓ vol, pulsus alterans	Pulsus paradoxus	N	N
Pulse rate	↑	↑/N	↑/N	↑/N

AE, air entry; HS, heart sound; N, no change; PTE, pulmonary thromboembolism.

Table 2.8 Differences in common investigations

Investigations	Cardiac failure	Asthma	PTE	Pneumonia
CXR	Hilar shadowing, kerley B lines, cardiomegaly	Hyperinflated lungs	Normal/ wedge-shaped infarction, pleural effusion, atelectasis, area of translucency in underperfused lung	Patchy consolidation
ECG	Left ventricular strain/ enlargement	N	Normal/right axis deviation, RBBB, Peaked waves in lead 11	N
ECHO	Cardiomegaly, ↓ function ± valve abnormality	N	Right- sided strain	N

N, no change; RBBB, right bundle branch block.

References

1. Milne JA, Howie AD, Pack AL, et al. Dyspnoea during normal pregnancy. Br J Obstet Gynaecol 1978; 84:448.
2. Scarsbrook AF, Evans AL, Owen AR et al. Diagnosis of suspected venous thromboembolic disease in pregnancy. Clin Radiol 2006; 61(1):1-12.
3. Winer-Muram HT, Boone JM, Brown HL, et al. Pulmonary embolism in pregnant patients: fetal radiation dose with helical CT. Radiology 2002;224(2):487–92.
4. Royal College of Obstetricians and Gynaecologists. The Acute Management of Thrombosis and Embolism during Pregnancy and the Puerperium (Green-top Guideline No. 37b). London: RCOG, 2015.

Further reading

Nelson-Piercy C (2015). Handbook of Obstetric Medicine (5th ed). Boca Raton, FL: CRC Press.
Powrie RA, Greene MF, William C. de Swiet's Medical Disorders in Medical Practice (5th ed), pp.42–43; 690–692. London: Wiley-Blackwell, 2010.

⑦ Jaundice

Jaundice is the clinical manifestation of raised bilirubin levels in blood and becomes clinically detectable at bilirubin concentrations of 30 μmol/L or above. The haem component of spent red blood cells is normally broken down to bilirubin predominantly in the spleen and bone marrow and is transported to the liver bound to albumin. In the liver, bilirubin is conjugated making it water-soluble and then it is excreted in bile with the level of conjugated bilirubin in blood normally being very low. Bacterial action in the bowel converts conjugated bilirubin to urobilinogen, some of which is oxidized to stercobilin, giving faeces their characteristic brown colour. Some urobilinogen is reabsorbed, passing to the liver in the portal blood and re-excreted in the bile, completing the so-called enterohepatic recirculation. A small proportion of the urobilinogen having entered the systemic circulation is excreted in the urine.

Hyperbilirubinaemia may be a result of excessive production of bilirubin (usually through extrahepatic causes such as haemolysis) or a result of inadequate hepatic capacity (through liver injury, congenital deficiency of enzymes, or an obstruction in the elimination pathway from the liver—obstructive jaundice) to eliminate normal amounts of bilirubin.

Main causes of jaundice in pregnancy

- Causes unique to pregnancy:
  - intrahepatic cholestasis of pregnancy
  - AFLP
  - hyperemesis gravidarum
  - HELLP syndrome
- Causes coincidental to pregnancy:
  - viral hepatitis
  - gallstone disease (cholelithiasis)
  - congenital disorders of bilirubin metabolism
  - autoimmune hepatitis
  - cirrhosis
  - neoplasia.

Intrahepatic cholestasis of pregnancy

Also known as 'cholestasis of pregnancy' or 'obstetric cholestasis'. Commonly presents with itching in the third trimester of pregnancy.

Clinical features

- Severe itching/pruritus affecting trunk and limbs but no visible rash even if there are excoriations.
- There may be associated malaise and insomnia.
- On direct questioning there may be anorexia, dark urine, and steatorrhoea (fatty stools due to malabsorption of fat).
- A positive family history of obstetric cholestasis may be present in up to half the patients suggesting an autosomal dominant inheritance pattern.
- A previous history of a similar syndrome being precipitated by the administration of exogenous oestrogens such as the combined oral contraceptive pill (COCP) may be elicited.

Laboratory findings
- Raised bile acids (may represent the only biochemical abnormality)
- Moderate elevation in ALT
- Raised ALP (above that expected normally in pregnancy)
- Raised bilirubin
- Raised Gamma GT.
- Diagnosis of exclusion: causes of pruritus and abnormal LFTs should be sought. This may include carrying out a viral screen for hepatitis A, B, and C, Epstein–Barr virus and *Cytomegalovirus* (CMV), a liver autoimmune screen for chronic active hepatitis and primary biliary cirrhosis (antismooth muscle and antimitochondrial antibodies), and liver US. Pre-eclampsia and AFLP are pregnancy-specific causes of abnormal LFTs that might form part of the differential diagnosis in atypical or early cases.

Maternal risks
Vitamin K deficiency leading to abnormal coagulation and increased risk of PPH.

Fetal risks
Iatrogenic prematurity, spontaneous preterm delivery, intrapartum fetal distress, meconium-stained liquor. Increased risk of intrauterine fetal death—the risk of stillbirth increases towards term and is greatest after 40 weeks but is not correlated to severity of maternal symptoms.

Management
- Counselling about fetal risks and the rationale for close fetal surveillance and early delivery after 37 completed weeks balancing this against fetal and maternal morbidity from early delivery.
- Fetal surveillance by a combination of fetal activity monitoring by the mother as well as regular US scans to monitor fetal growth and amniotic fluid index appreciating that both US and CTG are not reliable methods for preventing fetal death in obstetric cholestasis.
- Maternal monitoring by symptoms, regular LFTs accepting that poor outcome cannot be predicted by biochemical results which therefore should not be relied upon in isolation to determine delivery decisions.
- Maternal supplementation with water-soluble vitamin K (menadiol sodium phosphate) at a dose 10 mg daily to reduce the risks of maternal and fetal bleeding.
- Ursodeoxycholic acid (UDCA) provides impressive relief of pruritus and improvement in both bile acid levels and LFTs. The dosage is 8–12 mg/kg per day in two divided doses but there is a lack of robust data concerning its protection against stillbirth and its safety to the fetus or the neonate. Symptomatic treatment of pruritus with antihistamines such as chlorphenamine or promethazine has also been used.

Postnatal management

Monitoring of biochemical resolution is essential, along with a full review of the results of the investigations performed antenatally. If the diagnosis is suspect or the condition appears to be progressive, further invasive investigation in the form of a liver biopsy may be indicated.

The recurrence in future pregnancies is 50%. Women should be counselled to avoid the combined oral contraceptive but HRT appears to be safe.

Acute fatty liver of pregnancy

This is a rare complication occurring in pregnancy, with an approximate incidence of 1/10,000. There appears to be an association with maternal obesity, a male fetus (three times more common), and multiple pregnancy. There is considerable overlap with HELLP syndrome and AFLP may be a variant of pre-eclampsia. A higher risk of AFLP is associated with patients who (1) have a genetic mutation that affects their mitochondrial fatty acid oxidation pathway or (2) carry a fetus with a long-chain 3-hydroxyacyl-coenzyme A dehydrogenase (LCHAD) deficiency.

Clinical features
- Gradual-onset malaise, nausea, and anorexia after 30 weeks' gestation and often approaching term.
- Severe nausea and vomiting for the first time in 70% of patients.
- Abdominal pain/right upper-quadrant pain.
- Jaundice within 2 weeks of onset of symptoms.
- Ascites and signs and symptoms of developing liver failure with hepatic encephalopathy, DIC, and renal failure.
- Hypertension and proteinuria in 50% of cases.
- Extreme polydipsia or pseudodiabetes insipidus.

Laboratory findings
- Abnormal LFTs with significant elevation in transaminases and alkaline phosphatase.
- Profound hypoglycaemia.
- Marked hyperuricaemia, out of proportion to other features of pre-eclampsia.
- Blood film is often leukaemoid or may show leucoerythroblastic change.
- Gold standard for diagnosis is liver biopsy with special fat stains (histology: microvesicular steatosis) but this is neither practical nor necessary in pregnancy.
- Liver imaging by US (increased echogenicity), CT (decreased or diffuse attenuation), or MRI may show evidence of fat infiltration but may also appear normal and therefore imaging cannot be used to exclude diagnosis.

Maternal risks

Fulminant hepatic failure, hepatic encephalopathy, coagulopathy, death (maternal mortality now estimated at 12–18%). Maternal complications include PPH, renal failure, hypoglycaemia, DIC, pancreatitis, and pulmonary oedema.

Fetal/neonatal risks

Intrauterine fetal death with a perinatal mortality rate of 15–65%. Neonatal risks include iatrogenic prematurity, transient derangement in LFTs, and hypoglycaemia.

Management

- Maternal resuscitation and stabilization.
- Continuous fetal monitoring.
- Urgent delivery.
- Admit to intensive care or high dependency area and multidisciplinary input from obstetrician, obstetric physician/gastroenterologist or hepatologist and anaesthetist/intensivist.
- Vaginal delivery probably better, if feasible, in view of potential to develop coagulation problems but urgency of situation may determine mode of delivery.
- GA may be safer than regional techniques for CS. Must have low threshold for drains.
- Parenteral glucose to maintain euglycaemia.
- Neomycin and lactulose to decolonize the bowel, reducing ammonia production and hepatic encephalopathy.
- Multivitamin supplementation.
- With fulminant hepatic failure, transfer to regional liver unit and possible liver transplantation may be required.

Postnatal

Gradual return to normal liver function. If abnormal LFTs persist beyond 6 weeks, consider alternative pathologies. Recurrence risk is in the region of 20% in a subsequent pregnancy. Close surveillance of LFTs with use of OCP is recommended.

Hyperemesis gravidarum

Severe or protracted vomiting, with onset in the first trimester, causing fluid and electrolyte imbalance, weight loss, and necessitating hospital admission. Occurs in 0.5–1% of pregnancies.

Investigations

Hyperemesis is a diagnosis of exclusion and investigations aim to identify if there is an underlying cause but also to guide treatment.

- FBC may reveal raised haematocrit (due to dehydration) and abnormally raised white cell count.
- U&Es. Hyperemesis is associated with hyponatraemia, hypokalaemia, and a hypochloraemic metabolic alkalosis. Serum urea is low due to low protein intake, but an elevated urea to creatinine ratio may be an indication of dehydration.
- LFTs serve as a marker of severity of the hyperemesis with deranged LFTs in the most severe cases (30–50%).
- Thyroid function tests may reveal a picture of biochemical thyrotoxicosis with a clinically euthyroid patient. Beware of a suppressed TSH with normal T_3 and T_4 as this may simply be due to hCG suppression of TSH and not due to hyperthyroidism.

- Urinalysis may reveal ketonuria (secondary to starvation and dehydration). A MSU needs to be sent to rule out UTI as cause for vomiting.
- Pelvic US scan, to confirm a viable singleton intrauterine pregnancy as both multiple pregnancy and molar pregnancy are associated with hyperemesis.

Maternal risks

- Deficiency of cyanocobalamin (vitamin B_{12}) and pyridoxine (vitamin B_6) causing anaemia and peripheral neuropathy.
- Wernicke's encephalopathy due to thiamine (vitamin B_1) deficiency, which can lead to maternal death. Symptoms of Wernicke's encephalopathy include diplopia, abnormal ocular movements, ataxia, and confusion. Typical ocular signs are nystagmus, gaze palsy, and sixth cranial nerve palsy. There is a higher incidence of abnormal LFTs in patients with hyperemesis gravidarum complicated by Wernicke's encephalopathy compared to patients with hyperemesis alone. Confirmation of the diagnosis is by detecting reduced red cell transketolase activity, or elevated thiamine pyrophosphate activity. There are characteristic lesions around the aqueduct and fourth ventricle on MRI scanning.
- Persistent prolonged vomiting may lead to haematemesis due to oesophageal Mallory–Weiss tears.
- Development of a catabolic state with weight loss, muscle wasting, and weakness.
- Hyponatraemia with plasma Na <120 mmol/L may lead to lethargy, seizures, and respiratory arrest along with risks of central pontine myelinolysis from rapid reversal of severe hyponatraemia.

Fetal risks

- No increase in congenital abnormalities.
- In severe hyperemesis in a mother with significant weight loss (>5%), infants are likely to have lower birth weights and birth weight percentiles therefore monitoring fetal growth by scans in the third trimester may be prudent.
- If maternal Wernicke's encephalopathy supervenes, significant risk (up to 40%) of fetal death.

Management

- Early aggressive rehydration: many early pregnancy units now run rapid rehydration day units to avoid unnecessary hospital admission with hyperemesis gravidarum.
- Avoid dextrose containing fluids as they may precipitate Wernicke's encephalopathy or worsen hyponatraemia. Titrate IV fluids against daily measurement of electrolytes.
- Regular urinalysis to monitor ketonuria, as symptoms of hyperemesis are worsened by ketosis. Breaking the cycle of nausea/vomiting, starvation, and ketosis is needed to prevent further exacerbation of nausea and vomiting.

- Antiemetics such as metoclopramide, prochlorperazine, promethazine. In intractable cases ondansetron has also been used. In its severest and most prolonged forms, hyperemesis gravidarum can be treated by a regimen of IV hydrocortisone. If response is obtained, follow on with oral prednisolone. Involvement of a dietician is helpful in these rare but challenging cases.
- Where LFTs are abnormal or hyperemesis has been protracted, supplementation with vitamins such as thiamine is recommended (25–50 mg three times a day PO, or 100 mg IV infusion in 100 mL saline).
- Antigastroesophageal reflux measures in the form of elevation of the head of the bed, small, frequent and bland meals, alginates and H_2 receptor antagonists such as ranitidine may also help.
- Psychological support and reassurance is essential.
- Total parenteral nutrition may be needed in very rare cases.
- In intractable cases termination of pregnancy may need to be considered.

Viral hepatitis

Viral hepatitis is the commonest cause of hepatic dysfunction in pregnancy.

Hepatitis A

- Faecal–oral transmission, inversely related to levels of sanitation.
- Short incubation period of 14–50 days.
- Clinical features: abrupt but non-specific clinical features of flu-like illness, nausea, anorexia, vomiting, diarrhoea, fatigue. Cholestatic jaundice with pale stools, dark urine and pruritus follows prodromal illness. Usually it is a self-limiting illness.
- Management and prognosis are similar to non-pregnant women with recovery expected within 1–2 months.
- Post-exposure immunoprophylaxis may not prevent viral shedding. Potentially infected individuals should be isolated.
- Asymptomatic women in the third trimester of pregnancy in contact with an index case should be given immunoglobulin (increased risks of preterm labour).
- Consider immunoglobulin prophylaxis to women about to travel to high-prevalence areas.

Hepatitis B

- Causative organism is a DNA virus with incubation period of 2–6 months but detectable in circulation from 1 month post infection.
- Transmission through blood and blood products, IV drug abuse, sexual activity. Vertical transmission is the predominant route in developing world.
- Clinical features: in acute HBV infection, approximately two-thirds of cases are asymptomatic, subclinical, or associated with minimal, influenza-like symptoms. There may be upper GI symptoms such as nausea, vomiting, anorexia, right hypochondrial discomfort but no evidence of jaundice in almost half the cases. The acute illness may, however, be followed by a protracted period of malaise and anorexia.

- Prognosis: complete resolution in 90% of cases within 6 months. Remaining 10% become chronic carriers where HBsAg persists for >6 months with symptoms (chronic active hepatitis—CAH) or without symptoms but deranged LFTs (chronic persistent hepatitis—CPH). Rarely infection may progress to fulminant infection, hepatic failure and death.
- Diagnosis: detection of viral specific antigens and antibodies. HBsAg is an antigen from the viral capsule and indicates infectivity. Anti HBsAb is an antibody to the surface antigen and a marker of immunological response and cure. HBeAg is the antigen from the core of the virus and indicates high infectivity and high risk of vertical transmission (90% risk). Presence of anti HBeAb, which is the antibody to core antigen, indicates partial immunological response and low risk of transmission (10%).
- Management: symptomatic and supportive to control nausea and vomiting. Advise total abstinence from alcohol. Monitor hydration, uterine activity, and LFTs. Offer counselling, testing, and vaccination of family members and sexual contacts. No congenital syndrome or risk of teratogenesis.
- Obstetric significance: vertical transmission carries a 90% risk of chronic active or chronic persistent hepatitis hence justification for universal antenatal screening. Majority of infants are infected at time of birth from blood and body fluids with a small proportion infected through transplacental bleeds *in utero*. Antenatal detection of HBsAg should be followed with a preventative programme of active and passive immunization at birth. This involves the newborn receiving hepatitis B immune globulin (HBIg) IM within 12 hours of birth along with the first of three doses of recombinant vaccine in the other thigh. The second and third doses should be administered at 1 and 6 months and immunity confirmed at 1 year. This regimen of vaccination can reduce the vertical transmission risk of 10–90% to the region of 0–3%.

Hepatitis C

- Commonest cause of post-transfusion hepatitis, with 50–90% of IV drug abusers in the UK being HCV infected.
- Significant risk (60–80%) of chronic infection, with detection of HCV antibody being a marker of persistent infection. Cirrhosis and primary hepatocellular cancer are associated with chronic HCV infection.
- Routes of transmission are blood and blood products, sexual activity, and IV drug use. Vertical transmission is affected by viral load and co-infection with HIV. Higher risk of vertical transmission if mother positive for HCV RNA but in chronic HCV infection, level of transaminases does not affect rates of transmission. Transmission through breast milk is uncommon. The risk of transmission to the infant is less (0–18%) if the mother is HIV negative and if she has no history of IV drug use or of blood transfusions. Transmission of the virus to the fetus is highest in women with hepatitis C RNA titre >1 million copies/mL. Mothers without detectable HCV RNA levels did not transmit HCV infection to their infants.

- There are no vaccines to prevent HCV infection and HCV immune globulin is not recommended to infants of HCV-positive mothers.
- Treatment with interferon alfa may lead to biochemical, histological, and virological improvement in 25% of patients after 6–12 months of therapy but interferons are contraindicated in pregnancy. Similarly patients on Rebetron® medication (combination therapy of interferon and ribavirin) are advised to avoid pregnancy for 6 months after completion of treatment.
- It is recommended that a baby born to a mother with hepatitis C, especially where the mother is HCV RNA positive, is screened for hepatitis C at 6 weeks and 6 months after birth.

Hepatitis E
- Predominantly waterborne, non-A, non-B form of enteric hepatitis.
- Epidemics associated with contaminated water in India, Southeast Asia (Nepal, Burma), North Africa (Ethiopia), and Middle East.
- Antibody immunoassays available in reference centres and can distinguish acute infection (IgM positive) from previous exposure (IgG positive).
- Not reported in UK except in travellers returning from high-prevalence areas.
- Clinical features are similar to hepatitis A and are self-limiting with case fatality of <1% in non-pregnant individuals, so care is supportive.
- The obstetric significance is that the virus appears to have a predilection for pregnant women—reason unknown.
- Infection in pregnancy, especially if acquired in the third trimester, is associated with increased maternal mortality especially with genotype 1 isolated in Asia, Middle East, and North Africa.
- No immunoprophylaxis available.

Hepatitis—other viral causes

Epstein–Barr virus (EBV)
- Common transmission routes include sexual contact and via body fluids such as saliva.
- Blood-borne transmission is uncommon.
- Commonest form is in young adults and children—infectious mononucleosis (glandular fever).
- No special predilection for pregnancy.
- <5% of cases develop hepatitis.

Cytomegalovirus (CMV)
- May account for up to 10% of mental retardation in children up to 6 years of age.
- Risk of primary infection in pregnancy is 1–2%.
- Amongst women of childbearing age, 50–80% are seropositive for CMV.
- Routes of transmission are sexual contact, through transfused blood and perinatally (transplacentally or from exposure to the virus from the cervix or birth canal).
- After primary infection, the virus persists and latent virus reactivation may occur in 3–5% of women during pregnancy.
- Majority of infections are asymptomatic or associated with malaise, fever, atypical lymphocytosis, and lymphopenia with hepatitis being a rare complication.

- Diagnosis of primary infection is by detecting a significant rise in IgM levels (persists for 4–8 months) with a recurrent infection heralded by a rise in IgG levels.
- Primary maternal infection carries up to 40% risk of fetal infection. If contracted early in pregnancy, it may be associated with stillbirth, the latter accounting for ~10 stillbirths a year in England and Wales.
- CMV is found in 1% of newborns of whom 5–10% are clinically affected at birth and a further 5–10% develop long-term sequelae, therefore 85–95% of infected infants are asymptomatic at birth and 70–80% will not develop sequelae of CMV infection either at birth or thereafter. Approximately 180 children born in England and Wales each year will develop severe mental retardation due to CMV infection. ~85% of babies born to women with CMV in pregnancy, ~75% of infected infants therefore have no CMV-related problems at birth or thereafter.
- Confirmation of CMV infection in pregnancy has to be accompanied by careful counselling regarding the risks to the fetus and consideration of invasive tests to detect fetal infection. Fetal risks include deafness, blindness, mental retardation, growth restriction, and intrauterine fetal death.

Herpes simplex virus

- Very rarely causes hepatitis but may do so in third trimester or in the immunocompromised patient.
- Non-specific features—mucocutaneous stigmata may be absent and jaundice is not invariable.
- Prognosis for herpes simplex hepatitis is grave—mortality exceeding 90% even with treatment.

Gilbert's disease

- Affects 1–2% of population in Western world.
- Mild fluctuating jaundice.
- May be more noticeable with dehydration, exhaustion, and poor calorie intake.
- The increase in total bilirubin is a result of unconjugated hyperbilirubinaemia.
- LFTs are normal and the patient is constitutionally well.
- Gilbert's disease does not pose particular risks to pregnancy.

Autoimmune hepatitis

- Affects predominantly young women ultimately leading to amenorrhoea so only the earliest end of spectrum of disease is encountered in obstetrics.
- Clinical features include rash, arthralgia, fever, malaise, anorexia, and weight loss, and may often raise the possibility of systemic lupus erythematosus.
- Onset is insidious over weeks to months and often signs of chronic liver disease are present.
- LFTs are suggestive of hepatocellular injury but there may be associated derangements of haematological parameters (low platelets, low white cell count) and raised plasma globulins.
- Diagnosis is based on autoantibody studies showing the presence of antismooth muscle antibodies and antinuclear factor antibodies.

Cholecystitis

Decreased gallbladder motility and delayed emptying in pregnancy along with changes in bile salts lead to increased incidence of gallstone disease (cholelithiasis) in pregnancy. Asymptomatic gallstone disease is present in up to 6% of patients and the incidence of acute cholecystitis in pregnancy is 1/1000.

Clinical features
- Typically presents with severe epigastric and right upper-quadrant pain, often colicky in nature.
- Patient may be systemically unwell with fever, jaundice, nausea, and vomiting.
- There may be a previous history of gallstones.

Investigations
- LFTs may be deranged demonstrating a mixed hepatocellular/obstructive pattern. Serum amylase estimation should also be performed to exclude pancreatitis, as gallstones are a known predisposing factor for pancreatitis.
- A US scan of the upper abdomen may demonstrate gallstones and in cases of obstructive jaundice may show dilatation of the common bile duct. It may also exclude other causes of obstructive jaundice such as carcinoma of the head of pancreas or lymphadenopathy at the porta hepatis. Occasionally an MRCP (MRI retrogredade cholangiopancreatography) may be required to reach a diagnosis.

Management
For acute cholecystitis, management involves supportive treatment:
- Bed rest including appropriate consideration of thromboprophylaxis
- Analgesia
- Antiemetic
- IV antibiotics (co-amoxiclav or a combination of cephalosporin and metronidazole)
- IV fluids
- Period of resting the bowel: nil by mouth
- Where vomiting is a problem: nasogastric drainage may be required
- Dietary advice of avoidance of fatty foods is essential for secondary prevention.

Indications for surgical intervention
- Significant dilatation of the common bile duct suggestive of obstruction
- Empyema of gallbladder
- Recurrent attacks during pregnancy
- Recurrent pancreatitis.

Surgery during pregnancy carries a risk of preterm labour and hence this risk needs to be balanced and anticipated. The standard surgical approach of laparoscopic cholecystectomy may have to be replaced with an open technique with advancing pregnancy, dependent on the availability of local laparoscopic expertise.

① Diarrhoea in pregnancy

Diarrhoea is loosely defined as the passage of abnormally liquid or unformed stools at an increased frequency.

Normal physiological changes of pregnancy promote constipation, reported in up to one-third of women during pregnancy. In contrast, most cases of diarrhoea are not directly related to the pregnancy, but are due to the same disorders responsible for diarrhoea in non-pregnant women.

Causes
* Pregnancy related:
  * hormonal—increased prostaglandins (e.g. exacerbation of irritable bowel during pregnancy)
  * need to consider other symptoms/signs of ectopic pregnancy at early gestations
* Unrelated to pregnancy:
  * infections (gastroenteritis)—bacterial, viral, protozoan
  * medications—antibiotics, laxatives, prostaglandins
  * inflammatory bowel disease
  * malabsorption/maldigestion
  * secondary to systemic infections (e.g. listeriosis).

More than 90% of cases of acute diarrhoea are caused by infectious agents.

Management
* History:
  * onset of symptoms, relation to recent food intake including from public restaurants, anyone else in the family, or contacts with similar symptoms (food poisoning)
  * time interval—early onset (1–6 hours) suggests ingestion of preformed toxin (e.g. staph exotoxin)
  * duration of symptoms – acute suggests infective cause
  * fever, vomiting, abdominal pain
  * appearance of stool—bloody (*Escherichia coli* 0157, *Shigella* or *Campylobacter*, amoebiasis, and inflammatory bowel diseases), rice water (cholera)
  * recent exposure to antibiotics—side effect or due to pseudo-membranous colitis
  * recent travel (travellers' diarrhoea).
* Examination:
  * assess for signs of dehydration and hypovolaemia
  * any history and findings suggestive of preterm labour
  * assessment of fetal heart.

Investigations
* FBC, U&Es
* Blood culture
* Stool examination:
  * culture and antibiotic sensitivity for bacteria
  * analysis for ova and parasites

- faecal leucocytes—suggestive of intestinal inflammation
- stool assay for *Clostridium difficile* toxin—if history of recent exposure to antibiotics or contact with affected patients due to hospital admission or is a care worker
- flexible sigmoidoscopy—indicated in selected cases of prolonged diarrhoea not responding to usual conservative measures, studies in pregnant patients have shown lower GI endoscopy to present a low risk of complications in pregnancy.[1]

Complications
In addition to the usual complications of diarrhoea, pregnant patients are at increased risk of preterm labour, nosocomial spread to other hospitalized pregnant patients, and to babies if strict aseptic precautions are not followed.

Specific to organisms
- *Campylobacter* infection is associated with increased risk of spontaneous miscarriage, stillbirth, prematurity, and neonatal sepsis.
- *Salmonella typhi*—risk of intrauterine transmission.
- *E. coli*—infection with certain strains (e.g. 0157:H7) can lead to haemolytic uraemic syndrome, consisting of haemolytic anaemia, thrombocytopenia, and acute kidney injury.
- Listeria is associated with preterm birth, stillbirth, and neonatal infection.

Treatment
Conservative management with fluid replacement is the mainstay of treatment:
- Dietary changes
- Fluid replacement—oral rehydration and/or IV fluids depending upon the severity of dehydration
- Increased fibre intake for irritable bowel syndrome (IBS)
- Medications:
  - kaolin/calcium carbonate, no particular contraindication in pregnancy but not shown to be effective in adults
  - antibiotics—judicious use only if infectious aetiology is suspected, choice depending upon the aetiology
  - routine use of antimotility drugs is not recommended.

Prevention
- Hand hygiene and advice on food handling including cooking food thoroughly, care with re-heating.
- Taking care that correct standards are being met when eating out.
- Avoiding unpasteurized milk and products, certain soft cheeses, pâtés, raw fish, and raw or undercooked meat and eggs.

Reference
1. De Lima A, Galjart B, Wisse PH, *et al*. Does lower gastrointestinal endoscopy during pregnancy pose a risk for mother and child? A systematic review. *BMC Gastroenterol* 2015; 15:15.

Obstetric complications

Contributors

Edwin Chandraharan, Christina Coroyannakis, Vishalli Ghai, Claire Hordern, Edward Morris, Sambit Mukhopadhyay, Hassan Shehata, Mishkat Shehata, and Onnig Tamizian

Contents

⚠ **Leakage of fluid**

Vaginal leakage of fluid is the commonest presentation of spontaneous rupture of fetal membranes (SROM) occurring prelabour at term (4–18%) or preterm (2–3%). This is the diagnosis that needs to be confirmed or refuted when the patient complaining of 'leakage of fluid' is assessed by the midwife or obstetrician.

Maternal risks of ruptured membranes

- Infection: the risk of systemic maternal infection antenatally at term is low, especially with appropriate management, although the rate of subclinical or histopathological chorioamnionitis is higher.
- Higher risk of placental abruption.
- Higher incidence of obstetric intervention and associated risks if SROM occurs prelabour, including induction of labour, prolonged labour, and increased risk of operative delivery.
- Postnatally the risks of prolonged SROM include endometritis and pelvic infection.
- In cases of preterm prelabour rupture of membranes (PPROM), there are also the psychosocial sequelae of the birth of a preterm baby possibly needing an inpatient stay on the neonatal unit.

Fetal risks

The risks to the fetus increase significantly the lower the gestation at time of SROM:

- Infection including systemic sepsis, meningitis, and bronchopneumonia, especially where subclinical infection was the cause of underlying PPROM.
- With preterm SROM, fetal risks include prematurity and associated complications such as respiratory distress syndrome (RDS), necrotizing enterocolitis, bronchopulmonary dysplasia, and neurological problems.
- Fetal distress or fetal hypoxia due to cord compression, cord prolapse, abruption, infection, and difficulties of delivering a premature infant.
- With extreme prematurity and marked reduction in amniotic fluid levels, there may be long-term problems with pulmonary development and postural deformities, especially with SROM occurring before 24 weeks with persistent oligo- or anhydramnios.

Aetiology

Interaction of physical stresses with lack of resistance of fetal membranes:

- Cervical dilatation (during labour or silent cervical dilatation due to inherent weakness of the cervix—cervical incompetence) produces physical factors (lack of support) and biochemical factors (facilitated by infection of the exposed chorioamnion) which increase the probability of SROM.
- Weakness of the fetal membranes which may be congenital or acquired (deficiency of vitamin C, smoking, infection within the amniotic cavity or over the part of the membranes overlying the cervical os).

- Infection may act both by weakening the fetal membranes but also by a mechanism involving the release of prostaglandins with resultant increase in uterine activity.

Diagnosis of prelabour rupture of membranes (PROM)

- Meticulous assessment of patient history—timing of leakage and associated symptoms, amount of fluid lost (just dampness on underwear vs soaked trouser/bed clothes), colour (clear/yellow, bloodstained, thick/dark green, etc.), persistent loss after initial leak (needing to use pads/change underwear). Presence or not of any associated urinary symptoms.
- Diagnosis is based on visualization of either a pool of amniotic fluid in the posterior fornix or fluid draining through the cervix at the time of speculum examination. Confirmation of SROM may be difficult if loss of fluid has subsided, but may be helped by pressing on the uterine fundus, asking the patient to cough, or performing the Valsalva manoeuvre with the speculum *in situ*. An alternative approach if initial exam was inconclusive includes asking the patient to lie down for a couple of hours and repeating the speculum examination to see if a further pool of fluid has accumulated.
- Diagnostic aids include nitrazine paper/sticks (orange) or red litmus paper which turn blue by amniotic fluid due to its alkaline pH but these carry a false-positive rate of 25% as alkalinization of the vagina may be caused by blood, semen, antiseptic, infected urine, *Trichomonas* infection, or bacterial vaginosis. Alternatively, when a sample of amniotic fluid is allowed to dry on a microscope slide, a fern pattern will be formed. The fetal fibronectin isoenzyme test may also provide confirmation of ROM. *Generally, the diagnosis in clinical practice relies on visualization of pooling of amniotic fluid in the posterior fornix or leaking through the cervix.*
- The role of US in diagnosis of SROM is controversial, as a loss of significant volume of fluid is required to be detectable on US. In the absence of demonstrable loss of fluid at early gestations, a 'wait and see' approach with repeated dry pads and a normal liquor volume on scan may provide supportive evidence that PPROM has not occurred.
- Differential diagnosis includes urinary stress incontinence, UTI, and vaginal discharge. (Obtain MSU, genital swabs.)

Management

Management of the patient presenting with confirmed prelabour SROM is best considered by grouping the pregnancies based on gestational age.

PROM at term (36 or more completed weeks)

- Confirm diagnosis and obtain high vaginal swab (HVS) for culture (the main concern is group B streptococcal colonization/infection).
- Consider administration of steroids especially in diabetic mothers.
- If cephalic presentation and otherwise a low-risk pregnancy, expectant management for 24–48 hours to allow for onset of spontaneous labour (75–85% will labour in 24 hours and 90% by 48 hours).

- Patients are asked to report a fever or feeling unwell, the presence of bleeding, change in colour of liquor, and reduced fetal movements.
- If labour does not supervene, then induction of labour by prostaglandin tablets, pessary, or gel, oxytocin infusion, or forewater artificial rupture of membranes (if found to be present) should be recommended based on assessment of cervical favourability (Bishop score).
- When there is suspicion of meconium staining of liquor, maternal fever, bleeding, or any other non-reassuring features, the safest policy is to proceed with induction of labour at the earliest opportunity.

Preterm PROM

Before 24 weeks

- Individualized management after full and frank discussion with parents depending on gestation and parental wishes.
- If continuation of pregnancy is chosen, expectant management as an outpatient after an initial period of hospitalization is now becoming the norm.
- Baseline haematological (FBC, CRP), microbiological (swabs, MSU) screening, and US assessment of the fetus are performed.
- The mother is asked to monitor her own temperature, loss of fluid vaginally, other systemic symptoms, restrict activity, and report any concerns.
- The patient can be reviewed on a weekly basis on an obstetric day unit, monitoring re-accumulation of fluid, haematological and microbiological parameters, and scanned fortnightly for assessment of growth.
- The significance of the initial time invested in counselling about the risks and guarded prognosis cannot be overstated especially where SROM has occurred at very early gestations when even if the pregnancy continues for many more weeks, the outcome may remain grave for the baby due to pulmonary hypoplasia.
- The pregnancy is continued until such point that the risks (for mother and/or baby) of continuing the pregnancy outweigh the benefits.

Between 24 and 34 weeks

- Confirmation of diagnosis and presentation.
- Baseline investigations: FBC, CRP, genital swabs, and MSU. US assessment of fetal well-being.
- Administration of betamethasone or dexamethasone (24 mg IM in two doses over 12 hours apart) unless signs of overt sepsis.
- Commence patient on oral erythromycin 250 mg, four times a day for 10 days unless allergic to this antibiotic.
- If signs of preterm labour, a decision needs to be made on an individual basis regarding tocolysis to allow a window of opportunity for steroids to promote pulmonary maturity or transfer to a unit with appropriate neonatal facilities. The decision will depend on gestation, other complicating issues such as bleeding or signs of infection, both of which would be contraindications to considering tocolysis.

- Where PPROM is followed by onset of preterm labour a decision regarding mode of delivery needs to be made. In general, if cephalic presentation then a vaginal delivery would be aimed for in the absence of fetal distress, history of placenta praevia (PP), previous classical CS, or more than one previous lower segment CS (LSCS). In cases of breech presentation or non-longitudinal lie, a CS may be recommended dependent on other factors including gestation.
- Following PPROM, if labour does not supervene, then after a period of inpatient monitoring, the patient may be followed-up as an outpatient on a weekly basis on an obstetric day unit as above, until either 36–37 weeks of gestation is reached or maternal or fetal indications for delivery develop.

Between 34 and 36 weeks
- Similar to the 24–34 weeks' gestation group, though the benefit of steroids is smaller and therefore use should be individualized, i.e. may still be of greater value in women with diabetes.
- Antibiotics should be considered.
- Prolongation of pregnancy requires careful monitoring of maternal and fetal condition, using clinical (fetal movements), haematological, microbiological, and biophysical (US) parameters of fetal well-being.
- The main benefit of prolongation of pregnancy at this stage is to improve the chances of a successful induction of labour and vaginal delivery rather than improve fetal maturity; therefore the threshold to intervene is much lower than at earlier gestations.

:🔆: Bleeding in late pregnancy

Antepartum haemorrhage is bleeding from the genital tract in late pregnancy, occurring after viability (around 24 weeks' gestation) and through until the intrapartum period. It affects 2–5% of pregnancies and can be a significant cause of fetal and maternal morbidity and mortality.

Main causes of antepartum haemorrhage

- PP: bleeding from the margins of an abnormally sited placenta.
- Abruption: bleeding from premature separation of a normally sited placenta.
- Bleeding from cervical or vaginal lesions (cervicitis, trauma, infections, vulvovaginal varicosities, genital tumours).
- Unknown cause.

Management

- Initial management depends on the cause and severity of bleeding along with the stage of pregnancy (gestation).
- Maternal resuscitation if required based on amount of bleeding: IV access with two wide-bore cannulae, IV fluids, and blood transfusion in severe cases if maternal condition warrants.
- Continuous monitoring and ongoing evaluation of fetal and maternal condition.
- Reaching a diagnosis: history and examination—do not perform digital examination unless PP has been excluded by US scan. If examination has to be performed, this should be performed in theatre with set-up for delivery by CS should a PP be confirmed. Speculum examination after minimal bleeding and exclusion of PP may help in identifying local causes of bleeding.
- Investigations: FBC, G&S serum or cross-match blood according to need, coagulation screen where abruption is suspected, and Kleihauer test in Rh-negative women. A US scan will help with placental localization.
- Continuing antenatal care: treat as high risk for the remainder of the pregnancy with serial monitoring of fetal growth and aim to deliver at term.

Placental abruption

Premature separation of a normally sited placenta occurs in 0.5–2.0% of pregnancies. The abruption may be revealed (blood tracks between the membranes and appears as vaginal bleeding), concealed (no visible vaginal bleeding), or mixed haemorrhage (the vaginal bleeding that is detected does not reflect the true extent of the abruption and the amount of intrauterine bleeding).

Risk factors

In the majority of cases, there is no obvious cause. Increased risk of an abruption is associated with trauma and sudden uterine decompression such as with ROM in polyhydramnios. Other associations include maternal hypertension/pre-eclampsia, previous history of abruption (current or previous pregnancies), high parity, smoking, and substance abuse (especially cocaine).

Maternal complications

Anaemia, hypovolaemic shock, DIC, renal failure, postpartum haemorrhage (PPH), maternal morbidity, and maternal mortality.

Fetal complications

Prematurity, growth restriction, intrapartum asphyxia, perinatal morbidity, and perinatal mortality.

Clinical features

Variable amount of vaginal bleeding associated with abdominal pain, uterine activity, and tender uterus. In large abruptions, there may be fetal distress or intrauterine fetal death (IUFD) with cardiovascular collapse of the mother, along with increasing uterine fundal height/abdominal girth. The uterus feels 'woody' or 'hard', is irritable, and it may be difficult to palpate fetal parts. Backache may be an important symptom where the placenta is situated on the posterior uterine wall. Labour often supervenes in cases of significant abruptions.

Diagnosis

The clinical features are the most important clues to the diagnosis. Large abruptions may be visible on scanning. The main role of scanning is to subsequently monitor growth and well-being of the fetus in cases of conservative management.

Management

This depends on maternal and fetal condition, gestational age, severity of abruption, and presence of any other maternal complications.
- With large/severe abruption, stabilization of maternal haemodynamic status followed by delivery is needed. Maternal resuscitation and preparation for delivery need to occur concurrently.
- Mode of delivery will depend on whether the baby is alive/viable, the prospects of achieving a vaginal delivery, and the anticipated timeframe available before complications such DIC/fetal distress set in.
- If in labour, it may be appropriate to perform an amniotomy to expedite progress and where a decision to aim for a vaginal birth is made with a viable fetus, continuous fetal monitoring is recommended.
- After a major abruption, careful postnatal monitoring is required with respect to maternal cardiovascular, renal, and coagulation parameters.
- In cases of smaller abruptions, especially at earlier gestations, conservative approach with initial hospitalization followed by close surveillance of fetal growth and welfare is appropriate with a view to delivery at term. If <34 weeks' gestation, consider steroids.
- In Rh-negative patients, a Kleihauer test needs to be performed and appropriate dosage of anti-D immune globulin administered.

Placenta praevia

The placenta is partially or completely implanted in the lower uterine segment. This complicates ~0.5% of pregnancies. Classification is based on site of the placenta in relation to the lower uterine segment and cervical os. PP is defined as minor (grade one and two) and major (grades three and four):

- *Grade one*: placenta encroaching on lower segment but not reaching the os.
- *Grade two*: placenta reaching the internal os.
- *Grade three:* placenta covers the os but not centrally over it.
- *Grade four:* placenta centrally across the os.

The majority of cases of minor degrees of PP identified in late second and early third trimester resolve by term.

Predisposing factors

Cause is unknown, but associated features include previous PP (5–10% recurrence), multiple pregnancy, multiparity, previous CS/uterine surgery, smoking, and older mothers.

Clinical features

Unprovoked or postcoital, painless vaginal bleeding. Malpresentation, an unstable lie, or an unengaged presenting part at term may all be associated with PP. A significant proportion of PPs are picked up on routine scanning. In the absence of routine scanning, up to 15% may present in labour.

Diagnosis

US scanning is the most commonly utilized diagnostic modality. The risk of false-negative results is greater with a posterior PP as definition of the placental edge is harder in the absence of the contrast provided by the bladder when scanning an anterior placenta. Transvaginal scanning and more rarely an MRI may be useful in inconclusive cases. Occasionally, examination in theatre is required in the acute situation.

Management

This is determined in the acute situation by the mother's clinical condition, the fetal well-being, and the gestational age.

- Admit to hospital. The first bleed may be a small 'warning' bleed.
- Ensure mother is haemodynamically stable (IV access, FBC, G&S serum/cross-match as appropriate).
- Assess fetal well-being.
- If under 34 weeks' gestation, consider administration of steroids to promote pulmonary maturity.
- Where there is a major degree of PP, especially with a history of repeated antepartum bleeding, expectant management in hospital may be warranted with repeated scans to assess placental edge in relation to internal os and the presenting part (as the lower segment forms the leading placental edge may appear further from the internal os) and fetal growth/welfare (higher risk of IUGR with PP and recurrent bleeds).

- With minor degrees of PP examination in theatre, proceeding to amniotomy and induction of labour may be appropriate especially where the presenting part is below the placental leading edge.
- If evidence of maternal or fetal compromise with a bleeding PP, maternal stabilization and delivery is indicated.
- If CS is warranted, senior obstetrician involvement is required, with cross-matched blood being available in theatre.
- In the presence of a history of previous CS and anterior PP, there is a significant risk of placenta accreta and need for caesarean hysterectomy. At least 6 units of blood must be cross-matched. Senior obstetrician and anaesthetist should attend. Preoperative catheterization of internal iliac arteries, with the view to embolization to conserve the uterus or minimize bleeding to allow further surgery to be carried out more safely, should be considered where facilities permit in cases where preoperative investigations suggest placenta accreta.

Antepartum haemorrhage: miscellaneous causes

Bleeding in pregnancy may arise from any part of the lower genital tract and occasionally from the lower urinary and GI tract.

Bleeding from the lower genital tract

Causes
- Infections or inflammation of the cervix
- Cervical ectropion
- Cervical polyp
- Vulvovaginal trauma
- Vulval varicosities
- Cervical carcinoma.

Management
- Obtain history, especially of associated symptoms, including recent cervical cytology, pain, discharge, urinary, or bowel symptoms. Timing of recent intercourse in relation to vaginal bleeding.
- Clinical examination: inspection of vulva and a speculum examination when deemed to be safe (after placental localization by scan if required).
- Genital swabs may be appropriate to exclude infective causes of cervicitis.
- If the cervix looks abnormal, then an experienced review to decide whether colposcopy is warranted should be considered.
- In Rh-negative mothers, a Kleihauer test should be performed as a missed diagnosis of maternal isoimmunization can have disastrous implications for future pregnancies.
- If the bleeding is thought to be from the urinary tract or rectal in origin, referral to the appropriate specialties should be considered.

:O: **Leg pain and swelling in pregnancy**

Definition
As a physiological response to a gravid uterus, bilateral/unilateral oedema/ swelling is common. However pathological causes have to be ruled out.

Pathological causes
- Superficial thrombophlebitis
- Varicose veins
- Pre-eclampsia
- DVT
- Systemic disease, i.e. heart failure, venous insufficiency, nephritic syndrome, liver failure, malabsorption, and malnutrition
- Drugs such as nifedipine
- Pelvic mass/malignancy
- Trauma/arthritis/compartment syndrome
- Necrotizing fasciitis
- Cellulitis
- Ruptured Baker's cyst.

Association
Thromboembolism is a major and leading cause of maternal mortality and morbidity. In the UK, one-third of maternal deaths are due to DVT. DVT accounts for 85% of leg swelling events in pregnancy, with two-thirds occurring antenatally. Untreated DVT may result in pulmonary embolism (PE) in up to 24% of patients, bearing in mind that PE is the leading cause of maternal mortality in the developed world. Bilateral, swollen, pitting legs are associated with systemic disease i.e. right-sided heart failure, hypoalbuminaemia due to nephrotic syndrome, liver failure, malabsorption, and malnutrition. Necrotizing fasciitis is associated with diabetes, trauma, and malignancy. Non-pitting oedema (lymphoedema) is related to infection and Milroy's syndrome.

Risk factors
The risk of DVT and PE in pregnancy is increased by two- to fivefold in comparison to non-pregnant women due to physiological hypercoagulable state in pregnancy, venous stasis, and bed rest. After operative deliveries, the risk is increased to 10–20-fold and it increases even higher in those who had an emergency CS.
  Other risk factors for DVT are:
- Age >35 years
- Parity >5
- Oestrogen treatment to suppress lactation
- Sickle cell anaemia
- Obesity
- Blood group other than O
- Previous and family history of thromboembolism
- Prolonged immobility

- Malignancy
- Thrombophilia.
- Smoking (10–30 cigarettes per day)
- Hypertension
- Diabetes
- IVF
- PPH
- Infection
- Pre-eclampsia.

Presentation

- Varicose veins are common in pregnancy, occasionally associated with superficial thrombophlebitis.
- In DVT, calf swelling is 2–3 cm greater than the other calf, calf tenderness, calf redness, increased warmth and distended veins, mild fever, pitting oedema, Homan's sign (calf pain in response to squeezing or stretching the Achilles tendon).
- Usually iliofemoral (72% in pregnant vs 9% in non-pregnant)— abdominal pain may be the only presenting sign.
- Left-sided DVTs in pregnancy (85% left vs 15% right).
- 50% of patients who have classical DVT signs might not have DVT; therefore clinical assessment alone is not reliable in pregnancy.
- Bilateral pitting oedema, increased JVP, and hepatomegaly imply right-sided heart failure.
- Stiffness and knee swelling are related to Baker's cyst.
- Flu-like symptoms, increased temperature, unilateral swelling, redness, and pain are related to cellulites.
- Headache, epigastria pain, increased BP and usually bilateral oedema is related to preeclampsia.
- Skin changes, i.e. eczematous skin and ulcer, are related to venous insufficiency.
- Drug history, i.e. calcium channel blockers and vasodilators.
- Previous medical history (i.e. systemic disease).
- Personal or family history of thromboembolism.

Investigation

- Baseline assessment includes full thrombophilia screening, FBC, U&Es, and LFT.
- Urine for protein.

If DVT is suspected

- Compression ultrasonography (CUS) is the test of choice for suspected DVT in pregnancy, with a sensitivity of 97% and specificity of 94%.
- If CUS is negative, repeat the test in a few days.
- Magnetic resonance direct thrombus imaging (MRDTI) can be used when there is high suspicion of iliac vein thrombosis despite repeated negative CUS.
- MRI and CT scan (little reported evidence of its use in pregnancy).
- D-dimer (unreliable marker in pregnancy).
- If needed: ECG, CXR, Echo, and ABGs.

Management

- Anticoagulants are the cornerstone of treatment of DVT.
- Heparin does not cross the placenta and therefore is the drug of choice. Oral anticoagulants such as warfarin cross the placenta and may cause embryopathy in the first trimester and intracerebral haemorrhage in the second and third trimesters.
- Heparin regimens include continuous IV infusion of unfractionated heparin, subcutaneous injection of unfractionated heparin, or subcutaneous injections of LMWH.
- Subcutaneous LMWH is now considered an effective first-line method.
- Recommended doses: enoxaparin 1 mg/kg/twice daily, dalteparin 5000 U/twice daily up to a maximum of 10,000 U/twice daily, or tinzaparin 175 U/kg once daily.
- Peak anti-Xa activity (4 hours post injection) should be within the target therapeutic range. There is no need to repeat again if within range.
- Leg elevation and a graduated elastic compression stocking as well as mobilization. Compression stockings reduce the risk of post-thrombotic syndrome, which occurs in up to 60% of patients, by ~50%.
- Women should be taught to self-inject until delivery.
- Treatment should be continued for at least 6 months if the DVT was above knee or 3 months if below knee.
- If DVT occurs early in the pregnancy, the dose of heparin could be reduced after 3 or 6 months according to location of DVT to prophylactic levels until 6 weeks postpartum.
- Warfarin can be used in the postpartum period. INR should be checked according to local protocols.
- During labour and delivery, the dose of heparin should be reduced to an intermediate dose roughly halfway between prophylactic and therapeutic doses.
- Epidural and spinal anaesthesia can be sited usually 12 hours after the last prophylactic dose and 24 hours after the last therapeutic dose to avoid the risk of epidural haematoma.
- Surgical embolectomy or thrombolytic therapy if DVT threatens leg viability.
- A caval filter may be required if recurrent venous thromboembolism (VTE), despite satisfactory anticoagulation.

In systemic disease management is multidisciplinary

- Superficial thrombophlebitis: analgesia, compression stockings, AND leg elevation.
- Varicose veins: compression stockings.
- Necrotizing fasciitis: remove all dead tissue and give benzylpenicillin.
- Compartment syndrome: perform urgent fasciotomy.
- Baker's cyst: aspiration is the treatment of choice.
- Cellulites: treat with co-amoxiclav 375 mg/8 hours or erythromycin 500 mg/8 hours or phenoxymethylpenicillin 500 mg/4 hours PO or flucloxacillin 250 mg/6 hours PO.

Further reading

Chunilal SD, Bates SM. Venous thromboembolism in pregnancy: diagnosis, management and prevention. *Thromb Haemost* 2009; 101:428–38.

Grander MO, Monga M (eds). Management of the high-risk pregnancy. *Obstet Gynaecol Clin North Am* (Special Issue) 2004; 31(2):223–468.

Knight M, Kenyon S, Brocklehurst P, et al. *Saving Lives, Improving Mothers' Care – Lessons Learned to Inform Future Maternity Care from the UK and Ireland Confidential Enquiries into Maternal Deaths and Morbidity 2009–12*. Oxford: National Perinatal Epidemiology Unit, University of Oxford; 2014.

Marik PE, Plante LA. Venous thromboembolic disease and pregnancy. *N Engl J Med* 2008; 359:2025–33.

Nelson-Piercy C. Thromboembolic disease. In *Handbook of Obstetric Medicine* (5th ed), pp.45–62. Boca Raton, FL: CRC Press, 2015.

Shehata HA, Nelson-Piercy C. Medical diseases complicating pregnancy. *Anaes Inten Care Med* 2001; 2(6):225–33.

Royal College of Obstetricians and Gynaecologists. *Thromboembolic Disease in Pregnancy and the Puerperium: Acute Management* (Green-top Guideline No. 37b). London: RCOG, 2015.

⑦ **Fainting episodes in pregnancy**

Definition

Fainting or syncope is defined as transient loss of consciousness due to global cerebral hypoperfusion. Episodes are characterized by rapid onset, short duration, and complete recovery. A complaint of 'fainting' may not always imply actual loss of consciousness; some patients may mean no more than a feeling of unsteadiness or 'light-headedness'.

Associations

Convulsions, visual disturbances, vomiting, and sweating.

Causes

See Table 3.1 for different types of causes of fainting episodes in pregnancy.

Diagnostic steps

A thorough history is required from the patient and a witness history is valuable for an accurate diagnosis.
- What are the circumstances in which the attack occurs?
- Any associated symptoms such as palpitations, chest pain, shortness of breath?
- Is there any warning before the attack?
- During the attack is there a change in complexion, seizure activity?
- Duration of the event
- Any residual neurological deficit after the event?
- Any tongue biting, incontinence or post-ictal symptoms?
- Any previous episodes, frequency, and duration?
- Past medical history and drug history (insulin therapy, beta blockers).

Secure airway, breathing, and circulation (ABC). Obtain vital measurements: heart rate, BP, respiratory rate, saturations, and temperature. Assessment of cardiovascular and neurological systems is essential.

Table 3.1 Causes of fainting episodes in pregnancy

Vasomotor	Cardiac	Other causes
• Vasovagal attack: • emotion[1] • fatigue[1] • prolonged standing[1] • chronic illness[1] • haemorrhage (ectopic, placental abruption, postpartum)[3] internal bleeding[4] • Severe pain[2] • Postural hypotension[2] • Supine hypotension[2] • Carotid-sinus syncope[2]	• Arrythmia[3] • Aortic stenosis[3] • Hypertrophic cardiomyopathy[3] • Cyanotic attacks[3] • Ischaemic heart disease[3]	• Hyperventilation[1] • Anxiety/panic attack[1] • Eclampsia[3] • Epilepsy[2] • Hypoglycaemia[3] • Diabetic ketoacidosis[3] • Massive pulmonary embolism • Electrolyte imbalance[1] • Transient ischaemic attack (TIA)[2] • Carbon monoxide poisoning[3]

Vasovagal syncope is precipitated by pain, emotion, fear, and prolonged standing. This is due to a reflex bradycardia followed by peripheral vasodilatation. Prior to the event patients complain of nausea, sweating and visual disturbances. Episodes tend to last <2 minutes.

In contrast, Stoke–Adams attacks last seconds and have a sudden onset with no preceding symptoms. Patients are reported as pale and lose consciousness due to a transient bradycardia with a quick recovery seconds later. The pulse quickens, the patient flushes red and consciousness is regained.

In epilepsy, presenting as a loss of consciousness it is likely to be grand mal or partial. Attacks may be preceded by an aura comprising of a sense of déjà vu or change in smell. Associated features included tongue biting, incontinence (urine or faeces), and post-attack drowsiness.

Presence of cardiorespiratory symptoms such as palpitations, chest pain, and shortness of breath may indicate cardiac disease.

Pre-eclampsia is identified by symptoms such as a headache, visual symptoms, epigastric pain with evidence of hypertension, and proteinuria.

Investigations

- FBC
- U&Es
- CRP: suspected sepsis
- TFTs: in arrhythmia
- Troponin: in suspected acute coronary syndromes
- Plasma glucose
- ABGs: hypoxia, suspected diabetic ketoacidosis
- Urine dipstick: leucocytes and nitrites in infection, ketones in dehydration, and proteinuria in pre-eclampsia
- Septic screen: blood cultures/MSU/CXR
- ECG: identify the rate, if sinus rhythm, examine PR and QRS interval, identify ST segment abnormality
- Echocardiogram for left ventricular (LV) function and to exclude structural abnormality
- Electroencephalogram (EEG), sleep EEG: for seizures
- CT pulmonary angiogram: for PE
- CT and/or MRI if necessary.

Management

- In a haemodynamically unstable patient—manage with ABC.
- Involve relevant specialties accordingly (multidisciplinary management).

Vasomotor

Postural and supine hypotension are relieved by assuming lateral position to reduce pressure of the gravid uterus on the inferior vena cava.

Cardiac arrhythmia

- Identify the underlying rhythm and treat accordingly.
- Give oxygen and get IV access.

- In supraventricular tachycardia (SVT), try vagotonic manoeuvres (carotid sinus massage or Valsalva manoeuvre). If unsuccessful, treat with IV adenosine. Fetal monitoring should be performed at the time as fetal bradycardia has been reported. [5]
- Frequent symptomatic episodes of SVT need treatment with beta blockers, calcium channel blockers, digoxin, and quinidine.[5]
- Flecainide has been used for treatment of SVT in Wolff–Parkinson–White syndrome in pregnancy.
- Episodes of VT can be due to catecholamine sensitivity and are triggered by stress or exertion and suppressed with beta blockers.
- Direct current cardioversion is indicated for maternal and fetal haemodynamic instability.
- Amiodarone should be avoided if possible but can be used if benefit outweighs the risks of neonatal thyroid dysfunction, IUGR, and premature labour.[5]
- Anticoagulation requirements depend on the presence of additional risk factors, including LV function impairment identified by echocardiography.
- Low-dose aspirin 75 mg could be used when no additional risk factors are identified.

Diabetic ketoacidosis

- Calculate the fluid requirement (maintenance of 150 mL/kg normal saline).
- Add 20 mmol KCl to the fluid except the first litre if not oliguric or K >6.
- Replace the fluid aggressively with normal saline over 24 hours. 1 L stat, followed by 1 L over next hour, then 1 L over 2 hours, then 4 hours, then 6 hours.
- Sliding scale for insulin.
- Aim for blood glucose 4–8 mmol/L for the first 24 hours; maintain this with 5% glucose infusion.
- Septic screen and broad-spectrum antibiotics if suspected infection.
- Prophylactic LMWH.
- Monitor the patient closely for vital signs and urine output.
- Transfer patient to HDU or ITU if required.

Hypoglycaemia

- A plasma blood glucose <2.2 mmol/L is associated with a severe attack and coma occurs with levels <1.5 mmol/L.
- If conscious, treat with oral sugar and 50 g of oral glucose.
- If unconscious, if IV access give 200–300 mL of 5% glucose or 50–100 mL of 50% glucose followed by a 0.9% normal saline flush.
- If no IV access, glucagon 0.5–1 mg SC or IM. Repeat after 20 minutes following with carbohydrate.
- Do not give further IV bolus of glucose until repeat blood sugar is performed.
- If not conscious after 10 minutes, consider another cause, e.g. head injury.
- Recurrent hypoglycaemia may indicate diabetic nephropathy.

References

1. Shotan A, Ostrzega E, Mehra A, *et al.* Incidence of arrhythmias in normal pregnancy and relation to palpitations, dizziness, and syncope. *Am J Cardiol* 1997; 79(8):1061–4.
2. Arici A, Copel JA. Endocrinology of pregnancy. *Obstet Gynecol Clin North Am* 2004; 31(4):907–35.
3. Nelson-Piercy C. Respiratory disease. In: Nelson-Piercy C (ed.). *Handbook of Obstetric Medicine* (2nd ed), pp.59–81. London: Martin Dunitz, 2002.
4. Kniseley RM. Acute internal bleeding as a cause of syncope. *Am Fam Physician* 1995; 52(5):1278.
5. Trappe HJ. Emergency therapy of maternal and fetal arrhythmias during pregnancy. *J Emerg Trauma Shock* 2010; 3(2):153–9.

⑦ Pyrexia in pregnancy

Increased temperature or pyrexia during pregnancy may be due to inflammatory and non-inflammatory conditions. Fever is both a symptom and a sign which should be taken seriously during antepartum, intrapartum, and postpartum periods. Although it is often due to common bacterial and viral infections, other rare but potentially fatal causes like chorioamnionitis, DVT, and subacute bacterial endocarditis (SABE) need to be excluded during pregnancy. The risks to the fetus may be related to three different mechanisms: vertical transmission of infections leading to congenital infection, teratogenicity, or fetal death; direct effect of hyperpyrexia on developing fetal brain; and the possibility of preterm labour. The fetus may also be affected due to diagnostic investigations, and the treatment of the underlying cause of pyrexia.

It may be useful to consider the causes of pyrexia during antepartum, intrapartum, and postpartum periods separately.

Causes—antepartum period

Infections
- Organ specific:
  - urinary tract (cystitis, pyelonephritis)
  - respiratory tract (tracheo-bronchitis, basal pneumonia, tuberculosis)
  - uterine—chorioamnionitis
  - GI—hepatitis, pancreatitis, enteritis, appendicitis
  - cardiac—SABE
  - neurological—meningitis, encephalitis
- Systemic:
  - viral (including swine flu, rubella, varicella, CMV, herpes simplex infections)
  - bacterial—septicaemia
  - protozoal—toxoplasmosis, malaria, amoebiasis.

Dehydration
Severe hyperemesis gravidarum.

Adnexal accidents
- Torsion, haemorrhage into or rupture of ovarian cysts
- Torsion of pedunculated fibroid
- Red degeneration of fibroids.

Endocrine/metabolic
Diabetic ketoacidosis, phaeochromocytoma, hyperthyroidism.

Thrombosis
DVT, PE.

Malignancies
Lymphomas, leukaemias.

Pyrexia of unknown origin (PUO).
Others
Sickle cell crisis.

Causes—intrapartum period

- Chorioamnionitis: any of the antepartum causes can result in pyrexia during labour. It is important to exclude chorioamnionitis. If untreated, this can result in serious consequences to the mother (septicaemia, DIC, and death) and to the fetus (fetal compromise and death; neonatal sepsis including encephalitis and possible long-term neurological sequelae). The following risk factors should be considered:
  - prolonged ROM
  - prolonged labour, especially with repeated vaginal examinations
  - presence of vaginal discharge.
- Dehydration: due to prolonged labour/diabetic ketoacidosis.

Causes—postpartum period

Puerperal sepsis

This is the commonest cause of pyrexia following delivery. It is defined as any fever >38°C on two or more occasions, excluding the first 24 hours and up to 14 days after delivery or miscarriage. Causes are as follows:

- 90% are due to genital tract (endometritis, pelvic abscess) and urinary tract (cystitis, pyelonephritis) infections
- Breast engorgement/acute mastitis/breast abscess
- Respiratory tract infections including basal pneumonia
- DVT/septic thrombophlebitis secondary to pelvic infection.
- Wound infection—CS, episiotomy, perineal tears.

Other causes

Any systemic or organ-specific infections of the antepartum period may also occur during the postpartum period.

Associated clinical features

- Malaise, lethargy, myalgia, arthralgia, rash—systemic viral infections
- Chills and rigors—UTI, malaria
- Abdominal pain, nausea, vomiting, alteration in bowel habits—acute gastroenteritis, acute appendicitis
- Jaundice, loss of appetite, anorexia—hepatitis, pancreatitis
- Dysuria, haematuria, pyuria, loin to groin pain—UTI
- Ketone breath, 'Cheyne–Stokes' breathing—diabetic ketoacidosis
- Calf pain, swelling, redness—DVT
- Abdominal pain, vaginal discharge—chorioamnionitis, endometritis
- Pain, redness or engorgement of breasts, nipple discharge—acute mastitis, breast abscess
- Swinging temperatures, deterioration of clinical condition—pelvic abscess, septic thrombophlebitis
- Cough with sputum, haemoptysis—respiratory tract infections
- Onset of hypothermia and hypotension in a patient who has previously been pyrexial may indicate septicaemia.

Examination

A detailed and systematic clinical examination should be performed to identify the cause of pyrexia. The following approach may be useful:

General examination
- Level of consciousness, degree of pyrexia, hydration
- Rash
- Jaundice, cyanosis.

Head and neck
- Cervical lymphadenopathy
- Neck stiffness
- Thyroid gland, toxic nodular goitre.

Chest
- Cardiovascular system: vital signs/clubbing/changing murmurs
- Respiratory system: air entry, breath sounds, added sounds, evidence of consolidation
- Breasts: engorgement, redness, nipple discharge.

Abdominal examination
- Abdominal wall: tenderness, guarding, rigidity, rebound tenderness (signs of peritoneal irritation).
- Hepatic/epigastric tenderness (pancreatitis).
- Tenderness over McBurney's point is not a reliable sign to diagnose acute appendicitis in pregnancy due to the upward displacement of the caecum by the gravid uterus. Tenderness may be elicited right up to the right hypochondrium.
- Palpable liver (hepatitis), spleen (SABE, malaria).
- Iliac fossae—adnexal masses, tenderness.
- Uterus—tenderness (chorioamnionitis), masses (red degeneration of fibroids).

Wounds
Abdominal, perineal, genital tract for evidence of infection.

Calves
- Swelling, tenderness, red or blue discoloration
- Homan's sign and Moses's sign are best avoided to prevent the possible dislodgement of the clot.

Spine
Infection at the site of spinal and epidural anaesthesia.

Investigations

It is important to perform appropriate investigations based on the history and clinical examination findings to confirm the diagnosis and to monitor the response to treatment.
- FBC
- Blood urea and serum electrolytes
- LFTs
- MSU
- CRP—this is normally elevated during the immediate postpartum period

- Microbiology swabs—high vaginal/endocervical swabs/wound/nipple
- Virology swabs—throat
- Blood cultures (chorioamnionitis, septicaemia)
- CXR (with abdominal shield prior to delivery)
- Sputum for microscopy and culture
- Urine for ketones
- Blood gases (diabetic ketoacidosis, septicaemia)
- Abdominal US—to assist in the diagnosis of pelvic abscess, pyometra
- Doppler US scan—calf vein thrombosis, iliofemoral vein thrombosis. If PE is suspected, a ventilation/perfusion scan (V/Q scan) should be performed
- Blood for malarial parasites—if suspected
- Lumbar puncture—if meningitis or encephalitis is suspected.

Management

This depends on the cause and may require a 'multidisciplinary approach' in some situations (e.g. DVT, malignancies, diabetic ketoacidosis, and appendicitis). Antipyretics may be indicated to control pyrexia while specific treatment is essential to eradicate the underlying cause.

Infections

- Antibiotics—intravenously in severe cases
- Antivirals—if swine flu is suspected, a multidisciplinary approach and possibly admission to ITU may be indicated
- Antiprotozoal—for malaria, toxoplasmosis, amoebiasis.

Dehydration

IV fluids, insulin, and bicarbonate infusion in diabetic ketoacidosis.

Chorioamnionitis

- Induction of labour
- IV broad-spectrum antibiotics once the diagnosis is made. This should be continued during labour and in the immediate postpartum period.

Endometritis

Broad-spectrum antibiotics, monitoring of uterine involution, and exclusion of retained products of conception.

Deep vein thrombosis

Anticoagulants, TED stockings, involvement of a haematologist.

Surgical management

Acute appendicitis, adnexal accidents, and pelvic or breast abscess may warrant surgical intervention.

Fetal monitoring

Toxoplasmosis, rubella, CMV, herpes simplex virus, and syphilitic infections may be transmitted transplacentally, leading to fetal malformation or IUGR. If the mother is not immune to these infections and if one of these infections is suspected (or confirmed), she should be counselled regarding the possible detrimental effects and the plan of management.

A scan may be arranged after 5 weeks of infection to identify any structural defects. Serial US scans may be required to identify IUGR.

Conclusion

Pyrexia during pregnancy, labour, and puerperium needs to be investigated and treated appropriately. Although UTIs are one of the commonest causes of pyrexia in pregnancy, other more potentially serious causes need to be excluded (Box 3.1). A systematic approach to history taking and examination may help to decide on the most appropriate investigations to help in the diagnosis. The effects of pyrexia as well its underlying cause on the fetus should be recognized.

Box 3.1 In any case of pyrexia:

It is important to exclude swine flu.
  Then start the 'Sepsis Six':
1. High-flow O_2 via non-re-breathe bag
2. Take blood cultures (before starting antibiotics)
3. Give IV antibiotics
4. Start IV fluid resuscitation (Hartmann's/equivalent)
5. Check Hb and lactate
6. Monitor hourly urine output via catheter.

☼ Painful uterine contractions

Introduction

Braxton Hicks contractions are physiological uterine contractions during pregnancy and they are painless and intermittent. Pain arising from any smooth muscle organ, such as the uterus, may be due to ischaemia, irritation, or injury. It is important to distinguish physiological causes of painful uterine contractions (during labour and 'after-pains' following delivery) from pathological uterine contractions. As a general rule, physiological contractions are intermittent, whereas pathological contractions are often continuous or sustained. They may also be associated with other clinical features like vaginal bleeding, fever, and changes in fetal heart trace.

It may be useful to consider the pathological causes of painful uterine contractions during the first half of pregnancy, second half of pregnancy, during labour, and in the immediate puerperium separately.

First half of pregnancy

- Threatened miscarriage—mild pain and small amount of bleeding
- Inevitable and incomplete miscarriage—more severe pain/bleeding
- Septic miscarriage—continuous pain/fever/feeling unwell
- Pregnancy in a uterine horn/cornual pregnancy—colicky pain that may present with signs of intra-abdominal bleeding.

Second half of pregnancy

- Late miscarriage
- Preterm labour—idiopathic, uterine over-distension (multiple pregnancy, polyhydramnios, fibroids)
- Uterine irritability (abruption, chorioamnionitis, pyelonephritis and following procedures like amniocentesis or external cephalic version).

During labour

- Uterine hyperstimulation (injudicious use of oxytocin)
- Placental abruption
- Uterine scar dehiscence/rupture
- Intrapartum infections (chorioamnionitis, pyelonephritis).

After delivery

- Retained products of conception
- Acute inversion of the uterus.

Clinical approach

A detailed antenatal history should be taken and risk factors, if present, should be noted (e.g. augmentation of labour with oxytocin, multiple pregnancy, previous history of abruption, pre-eclampsia). It may be useful to identify the nature of pain and associated factors as follows:

Nature of pain

- Intermittent, progressive pain—preterm labour, late miscarriage
- Colicky abdominal pain—inevitable or incomplete miscarriage, cornual ectopic pregnancy, retained products after delivery

- Continuous sharp pain/breakthrough pain in between contractions—placental abruption, uterine scar dehiscence, or rupture
- Constant dull ache—uterine irritation (chorioamnionitis, septic miscarriage, pyelonephritis, red degeneration of a fibroid).

Associated features
- Vaginal bleeding—miscarriage, preterm labour, abruption, scar dehiscence or rupture, retained products of conception
- Vaginal discharge—septic miscarriage, chorioamnionitis
- Fever—pyelonephritis (with loin to groin pain, dysuria, haematuria, pyuria), chorioamnionitis, septic miscarriage.

Signs
General examination
- Shock/collapse—rupture of cornual pregnancy, placental abruption, uterine rupture, uterine inversion, severe sepsis, or severe haemorrhage
- Pallor
- Raised temperature—infection, irritation, inflammation
- Tachycardia/hypotension—severe bleeding, sepsis
- Bradycardia/hypotension—uterine inversion.

Abdominal examination
- Symphysio-fundal height—multiple pregnancy, polyhydramnios (tense abdomen, shiny skin)
- Uterine tenderness—placental abruption, chorioamnionitis, red degeneration of fibroid
- Frequency and duration of contractions
- Abdominal wall guarding, rigidity, tenderness or rebound tenderness—peritoneal irritation (chorioamnionitis, uterine rupture). Uterine 'scar tenderness' is a non-specific sign
- Fluid thrill—polyhydramnios
- Renal angle tenderness—pyelonephritis
- Epigastric/hypochondrial tenderness (if abruption is a part of pre-eclamptic process).

Cardiotocograph (CTG)
- Baseline fetal heart rate:
  - *tachycardia* (infections, fetal compromise, uterine rupture)
  - *bradycardia* (severe fetal compromise).
- Baseline variability: *poor variability* (0–5) fetal compromise—for >90 minutes.
- Decelerations: *late or prolonged decelerations are* ominous suggestive of acute fetal compromise secondary to placental abruption or scar rupture.
- Changes in uterine contractions ('TOCO'):

- *increased frequency* (>6/10 min)—uterine hyperstimulation/ irritability
- *increased baseline tone*—placental abruption, impending uterine rupture. After rupture, the contractions may not be recordable.

Examination of the lower genital tract
- To confirm vaginal bleeding (abruption, miscarriage, uterine rupture) or vaginal discharge or rupture of membranes (chorioamnionitis)
- To assess any cervical change (miscarriage/preterm labour)
- To take HVSs or to diagnose and correct uterine inversion.

Investigations (depending on the cause)
- FBC
- Blood urea and serum electrolytes
- CRP—infection/inflammation
- MSU for microscopy, culture, and sensitivity—pyelonephritis
- Blood cultures—for chorioamnionitis, severe pyelonephritis
- Kleihauer test—suspected abruption (possible feto-maternal haemorrhage)
- Clotting profile—abruption, severe sepsis
- US scan—not very useful in an acute clinical situation. It may be helpful in the diagnosis of multiple pregnancy, polyhydramnios, retained products, miscarriage, and cornual pregnancy. Fetal viability could be determined by US scan that may influence clinical decisions regarding further management.

Management
Depends on the cause of painful uterine contractions and may necessitate a multidisciplinary approach involving anaesthetists (fluid and pain management), haematologists (severe haemorrhage), microbiologists (sepsis), and neonatologists (see Table 3.2).

Key points
- Differentiate physiological from pathological causes of painful uterine contractions.
- Take relevant history, identify risk factors, and perform detailed clinical examination and appropriate investigations to diagnose the possible cause as well as complications.
- Consider multidisciplinary approach whenever necessary.
- Assess maternal and fetal condition prior to clinical decision-making.
- If appropriate, consider early:
  - anti-D (if Rh-negative)
  - antenatal corticosteroids
  - *in utero* transfer.

Table 3.2 Management of painful uterine contractions according to cause

Miscarriage/retained products of conception	Evacuation of retained products (ERPC)
Chorioamnionitis/ pyelonephritis/ septicaemia	IV antibiotics/IV fluids, pain relief, multiorgan support If fetus *in utero* consider delivering by induction or CS
Preterm labour	Tocolytics (if indicated) Betamethasone Plan for transfer or mode of delivery if no response to tocolytics
Uterine hyperstimulation	Stop oxytocin infusion, improve uterine perfusion (IV fluids, left lateral position) Consider—acute tocolysis (terbutaline 0.25 mg SC)
Placental abruption	Resuscitate, consider delivery if likely to cause fetal compromise (abnormal CTG, uterine irritability) or maternal compromise (haemodynamic disturbance)
Uterine rupture/cornual ectopic pregnancy	Emergency laparotomy
Uterine inversion	Replacement of uterine fundus under anaesthetic if immediate manual replacement was not undertaken Atropine if in neurogenic shock

⑦ Abnormal vaginal discharge in pregnancy

This is a common complaint among pregnant women. They should be informed that normal (physiological) discharge often increases in pregnancy due to increased oestrogen levels. The symptoms are often managed empirically, leading to inaccurate diagnosis and ineffective management.

Normal vaginal discharge is produced daily at the rate of 1–4 mL/day. It is typically white/clear and odourless. The discharge consists of vaginal transudate, epithelial cells, cervical mucus, and normal vaginal flora. The most common vaginal commensal is *Lactobacillus acidophilus*.

Causes
- Physiological: normal vaginal discharge can be excessive in some women although this may be subjective.
- Infective: candidiasis, bacterial vaginosis, chlamydia, gonorrhoea, trichomoniasis.
- Rare: malignancy, foreign body, douches, allergic reaction.

Also see Table 3.3.

Management
History
- Duration of symptoms:
  - recent
  - longstanding
  - intermittent
- Amount:
  - scanty
  - copious
- Colour:
  - greenish
  - white mucusy
  - blood stained
  - clear watery
- Itching: presence and severity
- Change in nature: becoming bloodstained from a clear or white mucusy discharge
- Odour:
  - hygiene problem
  - fishy smell
  - uriniferous odour
- Associated symptoms:
  - abdominal pain
  - dyspareunia (superficial/deep)
  - dysuria
  - vaginal bleeding.
- Sexual history—risk factors for STIs:
  - age <25 years
  - change of sexual partner in last year
  - >1 partner in last year.

Table 3.3 Common causes and treatment of vaginal discharge in pregnancy

Likely cause	Appearance	pH	Microscopy	When to treat	Treatment
Normal	Milky, white/clear, odourless,		Lactobacilli	Reassure	
Candidiasis	White, adherent (curd like), pain on examination	4.0–4.5	Hyphae present	Treat symptomatic women Avoid oral treatments	Clotrimazole pessary 500 mg stat. Use cream for 7 days to treat vulvitis
Bacterial vaginosis	Clear/thin, homoge-nous, fishy odour on addition of alkali	>4.5	Reduced lactobacilli, clue cells	Treat if symptomatic, consider if asymptomatic test of cure if still symptomatic at 1 month	Clindamycin 2%, 1 applicator a day × 7 days or Metronidazole 400 mg twice daily × 5–7 days
Chlamydia	Mucopurulent	Variable	Increased polymorphs. Gram's stain may show lactobacilli	Treat. Refer to GUM clinic for partner notification, treatment and contact tracing. Perform test of cure	Erythromycin 500 mg twice daily × 14 days
Gonorrhoea	Mucopurulent	Variable	As above. Gram-negative intracellular diplococci on culture	Treat. Refer to GUM clinic for partner notification, treatment, and contact tracing. Perform test for cure	Inj. Ceftriaxone 500 mg IM stat
Group B *Streptococcus*	Variable	Variable	Gram staining shows streptococci	Treat if symptomatic. Needs antibiotic prophylaxis in labour	Treat as per sensitivity. Usually sensitive to penicillin
Trichomoniasis	Greyish green, frothy discharge, *strawberry punctuation* of cervix	>4.9	Motile protozoa seen	Treat. Refer to GUM clinic for partner notification, treatment, and contact tracing	Metronidazole 400 mg twice daily × 5–7 days

Examination
- Local: look for signs of itching, erythema, oedema, fissures on the vulval skin.
- Speculum:
  - amount and nature of discharge
  - appearance of cervix
  - pain on examination
  - any obvious odour
  - take HVS from lateral vaginal walls and endocervical swabs for chlamydia and gonorrhoea (nucleic acid amplification test (NAAT)) testing.

Digital vaginal examination is not always necessary. It may be done when the cervix cannot be clearly seen and there is a chance the patient could be in labour.

Treatment

General

Local hygiene
- Keep area dry
- Avoid perfumed detergents locally
- Avoid douches.

Specific
See Table 3.3.

Differential diagnosis
- Ruptured membranes—clear, watery fluid
- Urinary incontinence—episodic, clear fluid, uriniferous odour.

Further reading

Bignell C, Fitzgerald M, Guideline Development Group, British Association for Sexual Health and HIV UK. UK national guideline for the management of gonorrhoea in adults. *Int J STD AIDS* 2011; 10:541–17.

British Association for Sexual Health and HIV Clinical Effectiveness Group. *2015 UK National Guideline for the Management of Infection with Chlamydia Trachomatis*. http://www.bashh.org/BASHH/Guidelines/Guidelines/BASHH/Guidelines/Guidelines.aspx

Faculty of Sexual and Reproductive Healthcare (FSRH), British Association for Sexual Health and HIV (BASHH). Management of vaginal discharge in non-genitourinary medicine settings. London: FSRH, 2012.

National Institute for Health and Care Excellence. *Clinical Knowledge Summary: Bacterial Vaginosis Scenario: Women who are Pregnant*. NICE, 2014. [Online] http://cks.nice.org.uk/bacterial-vaginosis#!scenario:1

⊙ **Frequency of micturition and acute retention of urine**

The anatomical and physiological changes in pregnancy are associated with significant changes in the function of the upper and lower urinary tract. The changes are so extensive that non-pregnant norms are inappropriate for pregnant patients. Awareness of this is essential to detect early signs of urinary tract dysfunction in order to prevent damage with potential long-term effects.

Antenatal problems

Frequency of micturition

Frequency is defined as more than seven daytime voids and one night-time void. One of the earliest symptoms of pregnancy is urinary frequency and this can even be noticed before the first missed period. Urinary frequency in pregnancy is secondary to the hyperdynamic circulation and increased urine production by the kidneys.

Urinary frequency increases as pregnancy progresses. Pressure from the enlarging uterus or the presenting part may directly irritate the bladder trigone and cause urinary frequency. Frequency is usually more common in nulliparous than multiparous mothers. Black nulliparous women are more prone to have increased frequency compared to white nulliparous women. Black parous women are more prone to increased nocturia compared to white parous women. The majority of women accept increased urinary frequency and nocturia as a normal part of pregnancy and will put up with it. Only a few (<4%) are actually distressed.

UTIs usually present with:
- Increased urinary frequency
- Dysuria
- Nocturia
- Urgency.

However, diagnosis on the basis of these symptoms alone is difficult as some or a combination of these symptoms could be considered a normal part of pregnancy. Therefore diagnosis must be based on urine testing or laboratory evidence: presence of leucocytes, proteins, and nitrites on dipstick examination suggests the possibility of UTI and the need to send a MSU sample for culture and antibiotic sensitivity test (ABST).

A count of >100,000 colony-forming units (CFU)/mL of urine is regarded as infection although a count of as low as 20,000 CFU may represent acute infection in pregnancy. Urinary white cell count also increases in pregnancy.

Escherichia coli is the commonest infective agent with *Proteus, Klebsiella,* and *Enterobacter* accounting for most of the remainder.

Management of antenatal urinary frequency
- Reassurance: once a urinary infection has been excluded, women can be reassured that increased urinary frequency is part of the normal physiological changes of pregnancy, is benign in nature, and will gradually resolve after pregnancy.

- Urine testing: in pregnancy, 5% of women will have asymptomatic bacteriuria, 30% of whom will develop a symptomatic infection if untreated. Urinary infection increases the risk of complications in pregnancy such as preterm labour and fetal growth restriction.
- An MSU sample should be taken for culture and ABST if urinary screening suggests infection. Additional screening (usually monthly) for infection is indicated in women with past history of UTIs and/ or renal disorders. Antimicrobials should be based on the culture and sensitivity report and continued for at least 7–10 days for initial infections and 21 days for recurrences.

Retention of urine

Urinary retention in pregnancy usually presents as an acute episode though its occurrence may have a slow onset and develop over several days or weeks. During the antenatal period, it presents most commonly during the first trimester.

The classic cause of retention during the first trimester is incarceration of the retroverted uterus. The mechanism of urinary obstruction has traditionally been thought to be due to pressure on the bladder neck from the uterus but as there is often no difficulty in passing a urinary catheter, the exact mechanism of obstruction remains unclear.

Clinical presentation is usually the inability to pass urine in association with pelvic pain. The bladder may or may not be palpable abdominally. Inspection of fluid charts may be falsely reassuring as the patient may be in chronic urinary retention with incomplete bladder emptying. It is therefore important to include assessment of post-void urinary residual volume estimation using either US estimation or passage of a urinary catheter.

Management of antenatal urinary retention

- Immediate insertion of a urinary catheter once urinary retention has been diagnosed will result in relief of pain.
- Measurement of the volume of urine within the bladder should be performed as sustained volumes >800 mL may be associated with longer-term urinary dysfunction (see 'Puerperium', p. 95).
- Urine should be tested for UTI.
- The catheter should be left *in situ* and when the patient is comfortable, a gentle vaginal examination should be performed to assess for uterine incarceration. The retention also could be due to compression of the bladder neck or elongation and compression of urethra. Occasionally the patient may be relieved lying prone or on all fours in a 'knee–chest' position. The catheter should remain *in situ* until the uterus remains reliably out of the pelvis. The patient should be warned that this may take several days.
- Once the catheter is removed, the patient should be observed for several hours to assess voided volumes and estimated urinary residuals using US. If the urinary residual is <100 mL the patient may be discharged.
- Several days later, further urinary residual estimation should be performed to ensure chronic retention does not persist.

Intrapartum problems

Retention of urine

During labour, retention of urine may be pathophysiological or iatrogenic. Part of the normal assessment of the healthy woman in labour should include recording of urine output. The commonest causes of low urine volumes are dehydration and retention of urine. Due to the compressive effects of the descending fetal head the likelihood of urinary retention increases as labour progresses. If the patient is unable to void then obstruction can be diagnosed by clinical inspection and palpation and confirmed by US assessment of urinary residual or with the use of intermittent catheterization.

Epidural analgesia is associated with loss of bladder sensation and although intermittent catheterization is an acceptable way of managing urine flow during the labour of a woman who wishes to remain mobile and has an epidural, it is important that attention is paid to the bladder, ensuring it is emptied at least every 2 hours. If the woman is less mobile and has an epidural, it may be appropriate to insert an indwelling catheter.

All women who have spinal anaesthesia for instrumental deliveries or CS should have an indwelling catheter inserted until sensation is fully restored.

Management of intrapartum urinary retention

This should be with the use of an indwelling urinary catheter, which should remain *in situ* until the patient is mobile following delivery or until the epidural is no longer functioning.

Puerperium

Frequency of micturition

Normal pregnancy is associated with an increase in extracellular fluid and puerperal diuresis is a reversal of this process. Increased urinary frequency between the 2nd and 5th postpartum day is primarily due to this diuresis. Thereafter urinary frequency gradually resolves although the presence of enlarged uterus could to some extent continue to give rise to frequency and urgency. Factors during labour such as haemorrhage or pre-eclampsia can influence the normal puerperal diuresis and frequency. Epidural analgesia in labour can alter bladder sensation leading to small volume frequency of micturition.

Retention of urine

One of the commonest causes of long-term bladder damage is an episode of acute urinary retention during the immediate postpartum period. Overdistension may be a consequence of either perineal trauma producing urethral oedema or a result of reduced bladder sensation following regional analgesia or anaesthesia.

The damage that can result from overdistension with sustained volumes >800 mL includes acute pain, and in severe cases bladder rupture and mucosal haemorrhage. If the retention goes unrecognized for long periods of time (>4 hours) damage to the neural network within the bladder may result in reduced bladder sensation and detrusor muscle hypocontractility. If overdistension goes unrecognized, it can lead to:

- Serious longstanding voiding difficulties
- Chronic infection
- Renal damage.

Management of postpartum urinary retention

It is particularly important that action is taken immediately if a woman is suspected of having urinary retention postnatally. The timely insertion of a urinary catheter may relieve the pain but if follow-up action is not taken over the next 2–4 hours, long-term damage may result as the bladder refills. It is therefore important to measure the urine volume upon catheterization and to leave an indwelling catheter for at least 24 hours if the volume is >800 mL. When the catheter is removed, post-void urinary residual volumes should be estimated after every void until they are reliably <100 mL. Bladder scanning is inaccurate in postnatal women and should not be used.

In some cases of missed or late diagnosis of bladder overdistension, the bladder may not show signs of recovery in the short term. This may indicate long-term management such as intermittent clean self-catheterization or long-term indwelling catheter. Such cases require close multidisciplinary follow-up by urogynaecologists, continence specialists, and specialist physiotherapists.

With the correct patient care pathways and guidelines in place for the management of urinary tract function during pregnancy, cases of severe bladder damage, with their accompanying high risk of litigation, can be avoided.

Concerns for the fetus and surveillance

Contributors

Amar Bhide, Deepika Deshpande, and Padma Vankayalapati

Contents

① **Absent fetal movements**

Normal pattern of fetal movements

Although fetal limb and body movements are visible on ultrasound from the 1st trimester, maternal perception starts only after 16–20 weeks of gestation. Typically the fetus demonstrates sleep–wake cycles every 40 minutes, where a period of active movements alternate with a period of quiescence. Towards the end of pregnancy the pattern of fetal movements often changes. Relative reduction in the available space and engagement of the head are some of the factors responsible for this change.

Significance of absent fetal movements

It was historically noted that in pregnancies complicated by intrauterine fetal death, fetal movements typically ceased 12–24 hours prior to disappearance of fetal heart activity. This sign was called the movement alarm signal (MAS). It was theorized that a hypoxic fetus saved energy by reducing fetal activity.

Application of this information to the general low-risk obstetric population, however, did not show benefit. In fact, there was a trend towards worse fetal outcome when interventions were carried out prompted by fetal movement reduction. Loss or a reduction of fetal movements generates considerable parental anxiety. Absence or reduction of fetal movements is a useful sign for monitoring pregnancies where ongoing fetal hypoxia is a likely possibility.

Clinical applications

- Placental insufficiency
- Post-term pregnancy
- Medical complications such as diabetes in pregnancy or obstetric cholestasis
- Fetal anaemia such as Rhesus disease
- Fetal cardiac failure
- Fetal hypoxia due to any cause.

Evaluation of the patient

Evaluation is aimed at establishing the risk status of the pregnancy.

History—present and past

- The history of reduction or loss of fetal movements should be explored in greater detail. The previous pattern should be established.
- Essentially, the history forms a part of risk assessment.
- Placental insufficiency is more common in the first pregnancy. It is extremely uncommon in subsequent pregnancies if the first baby was well-grown, as long as the pregnancy is by the same father.
- Pregnancy complications should be explored. The symptom is far more significant if the pregnancy is complicated (see 'Clinical applications').

Physical examination

- Aimed at establishing the risk status of the pregnancy.
- Elevated blood pressure and proteinuria will signify pre-eclampsia complicating pregnancy.
- Symphysis–fundal height should be measured to assess fetal growth.
- Fetal movements may be palpable in the process of abdominal palpation.
- Excess amniotic fluid quantity can make maternal perception of fetal movements difficult.
- Demonstration of the fetal heart sounds is useful to reassure the parents. However, this is not clinically adequate to reassure fetal health.

Fetal assessment

Ultrasound examination for growth and liquor volume and, if needed, Doppler velocimetry should be arranged if no scan was done within the last 2 weeks.

- Ultrasound assessment is used to assess fetal growth and amniotic fluid volume.
- Doppler flow studies of the umbilical artery and the middle cerebral artery are useful indicators of uteroplacental insufficiency.
- At term and post-term a normal ultrasound assessment and fetal Doppler study do not exclude placental insufficiency. Fetal growth restriction is possible even if estimated fetal weight is within the normal range.
- Fetal biophysical profile is an assessment of current fetal status. Fetal hypoxia can be virtually excluded with a normal biophysical profile score.

Cardiotocography

Antenatal fetal heart rate monitoring is sometimes referred to as a 'non-stress test'.

- A reactive non-stress test is characterized by a normal baseline heart rate (110–160 bpm), normal baseline variability (5–25 bpm) at least 2 accelerations in a 20 min period, and absence of decelerations.
- The assessment of the fetal heart tracing is visual and subjective.
- A reactive non-stress test is a reliable sign of fetal well-being. However, it cannot predict future deterioration.
- Visual analysis of the fetal heart rate tracing is fraught with poor reproducibility.
- A computerized assessment eliminates subjective variation. It is objective, and the reproducibility is improved. Computerized CTG assessment is preferred over visual assessment using antenatal CTG.

Management

Management will depend on the underlying reason and perceived fetal risk. In a majority of cases, pregnancy assessment will be normal and reassurance is all that is needed. If the pregnancy is deemed to be at risk of fetal hypoxia, arrangements should be made for delivery. The route and timing of delivery will depend on the perceived severity of fetal compromise. Induction of labour may be advisable if it is easily possible, and fetal assessment is not grossly abnormal. Emergency caesarean section may be required if the fetus is thought to be appreciably compromised.

Limitation of fetal movements as a sign of fetal well-being

Maternal perception of fetal movements indicates fetal well-being. However during the process of fetal response to placental insufficiency, fetal movements are one of the last parameters to become abnormal prior to intrauterine death. The time-window between cessation of fetal movements and stopping of heart activity is short. Presence of normal fetal movements has no prognostic capability. In acute situations such as placental abruption or cord prolapse, fetal movements may be a useless indicator of fetal well-being. In multiple pregnancy, fetal movements of the co-twin may be continued to be perceived, even after the other has suffered intrauterine demise.

:⚙: Abnormal antenatal fetal surveillance tests

The aim of antenatal fetal surveillance is to identify fetuses which are at risk of suffering intrauterine hypoxia with resultant damage, including death. This includes each and every pregnancy, as no pregnancy is free of this risk. However, experience from screening low-risk pregnant population suggests that this approach does more harm than good when the risk of intrauterine hypoxia and the resultant sequel is low. Evidence suggests that fetal movement counting identifies fetuses at risk rather than improving outcome. Fundal height measurement has insufficient evidence of value in consistently identifying small-for-gestational-age fetuses at delivery. The primary step, therefore, is to identify those pregnancies, which are at a higher risk. Antenatal fetal surveillance is likely to be of benefit only in this group.

Biochemical tests

Historically, levels of maternal serum hormones such as oestriol and human placental lactogen were used as a test of fetal well-being. These tests are no longer used in clinical practice. A single unexplained elevated level of maternal serum alpha fetoprotein in mid trimester raises the risk of subsequent IUGR five- to tenfold. A low pregnancy-associated placental protein-A (PAPP-A) level in the first trimester increases the risk for developing pre-eclampsia and low birthweight, but the association is weak.

Fetal movements

For further details on fetal movements, please see pp. 98–100.

Ultrasound assessment

Fetal biometry

- Aimed at identifying fetal growth restriction
- Estimated fetal weight below the 10th centile is widely used as a criterion to identify small fetuses
- Many fetuses with estimated weight below 10th centile are normally grown but constitutionally small
- Serial ultrasound measurements of the fetus are more accurate than clinical examination in the identification of small babies
- Fetal abdominal circumference (AC) below the 5th centile is a sensitive indicator
- Reduced amniotic fluid volume and an advanced placental maturity are other contributory findings in growth-restricted babies.

Placental dysfunction is indicated by reduced growth velocity and increased resistance to flow in the umbilical artery. There is redistribution of blood flow so that blood is selectively shunted to important organs like the brain and the heart, with less blood flow to less important organs like extremities, GI tract, and skin. This is described as the 'head-sparing' effect or 'arterial blood flow redistribution'. In cases of placental dysfunction, the sequence of events is as follows:

Slowing of growth (small size) → Increased resistance in umbilical artery Doppler (reduced end-diastolic frequencies) → Absent/reversed end-diastolic frequencies in umbilical artery Doppler → Abnormal venous Doppler (ductus venosus Doppler) → Intrauterine death.

Box 4.1 shows a typical ultrasound report of a fetus with growth restriction due to placental insufficiency.

Fetal arterial and venous Doppler flow study

Fetal blood flow redistribution can be identified by Doppler flow studies of the umbilical arteries and fetal middle cerebral arteries (see Figs 4.1–4.3).

Box 4.1 Example of an ultrasound report of a fetus with growth restriction due to placental insufficiency

Indication:
Growth restriction.

History:
Maternal age: 27 years, blood group: A positive.
Menstrual cycle irregular. Conception Ovulation drugs.

Gestational age:
27 weeks + 4 days (by ultrasound and LMP)

Growth scan:
Fetal measurements (plotted in relation to the normal mean ± 2 SDs).

Biparietal diameter (BPD)	66.0 mm
Head circumference (HC)	219.9 m
Abdominal circumference (AC)	164.9 mm
Head/abdomen (HC/AC)	1.334
Femur length (FL)	35.0 mm
Est. fetal weight (Hadlock BPD -HC -AC -FL)	449 g

Heart: action normal. Presentation: breech. Amniotic fluid: reduced.
Placenta: Anterior high, grannum Grade 3.

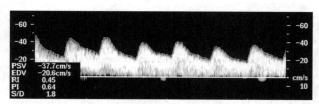

Fig. 4.1 Normal umbilical artery Doppler waveforms.

Normal umbilical artery waveforms
- The pregnancy will not develop loss of end-diastolic frequencies within a 7–10-day period, so that Doppler monitoring may be performed weekly.
- A growth-restricted fetus with normal umbilical artery waveforms will not be acidaemic, but has a 10% chance of being hypoxaemic.
- Normal umbilical artery waveforms after 36 weeks' gestation do not exclude fetal hypoxaemia and acidaemia.

Reduced/absent end-diastolic frequencies
- Loss of end-diastolic frequencies occurs only when over 75% of the placental vascular bed is obliterated. Absent end-diastolic flow is much less likely to be encountered after 36 weeks' gestation.
- Loss of end-diastolic frequencies is associated with an 85% chance that the fetus will be hypoxaemic and a 50% chance that it will also be acidaemic.
- Growth-restricted fetuses with absent end-diastolic frequencies have a fourfold increase in perinatal mortality compared to those with normal umbilical artery waveforms. The time between loss of end-diastolic frequencies and fetal death appears to differ for each fetus.
- Loss of end-diastolic frequencies precedes changes in the cardiotocograph by some days to weeks in growth-restricted fetuses.

Reversed end-diastolic frequencies
- Growth restriction with reversed end-diastolic frequencies has a tenfold increase in perinatal mortality compared to those with normal umbilical artery waveforms.
- Reversed frequencies in end-diastole are only observed in a few fetuses prior to death. This finding should be considered as a pre-terminal condition. Few, if any, fetuses will survive without delivery.

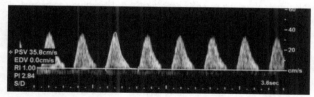

Fig. 4.2 Absent end-diastolic flow.

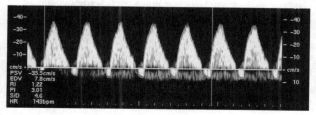

Fig. 4.3 Reversed end-diastolic flow.

A typical report showing fetal blood flow redistribution is shown as follows:

Doppler

Umbilical artery:	PI	3.01	├──┼──┤ ▸
	End-diastolic flow: reverse flow		
Middle cerebral artery:	PI	1.63	├──┼──┤
	End-diastolic flow: positive		
Ductus venosus:	PIV	0.880	├──┼──┤

Diagnosis

SGA: likely uteroplacental insufficiency.

Biophysical profile

Table 4.1 shows the criteria assessed in the biophysical profile (BPP).

Several modifications of the score are used. A score of 8 or 10 is associated with excellent perinatal outcome. Scores of 4 and 6 are borderline, whereas scores of 0 or 2 are pathological. However, there are some limitations:

- Requires access to expensive ultrasound equipment and trained operator.
- A normal BPP has limited prognostic value
- Requires at least 30 min to complete
- Lack of high-quality evidence (randomized controlled trials) to show that BPP saves lives
- The time interval between an abnormal BPP and fetal demise appears to be short.

Table 4.1 Biophysical profile score

Fetal characteristic	Score 2	Score 0
Non-stress test	At least 2 episodes of fetal heart rate accelerations over 15 bpm lasting for more than 15 sec in 30 min	Fewer than 2 episodes of fetal heart rate acceleration over 15 bpm lasting for more than 15 sec
Fetal breathing movements	At least 1 episode of fetal breathing movements lasting more than 30 sec in a 30 min period	Absent breathing movements or no episode of breathing lasting over 30 sec in 30 min
Gross body movements	At least 3 fetal movements involving the fetal spine in a 30 min period	2 or fewer movements in 30 min period
Fetal tone	At least 1 episode of active fetal limb extension with a return to flexion in 30 min period. Opening and closing of the hand is considered as normal tone	Slow extension with return to partial flexion, movements of limbs in full extension or absent limb movements.
Amniotic fluid volume	Amniotic fluid index (AFI) between 5 cm and 25 cm	AFI of below 5 cm or over 25 cm

Reprinted from *American journal of obstetrics and gynecology*, 136, Manning FA et al., 'Antepartum fetal evaluation: development of a fetal biophysical profile'. Copyright (1980) with permission from Elsevier Science and Technology.

Cardiotocography

Cardiotocography (CTG) or electronic fetal heart rate monitoring was first applied during labour. Later its use was extended to the antenatal period in order to assess the fetal well-being although it has no significant effect on perinatal outcome or interventions such as early elective delivery.

A recording of the fetal heart rate pattern for a period of 20–30 min, called the non-stress test (NST), is one of the most widely used methods of antenatal fetal surveillance. A summary of the interpretation of the NST is given in the following sections (also see Figs 4.4–4.6).

Antepartum cardiotocograph (NST)

Normal/reassuring/reactive

- At least 2 accelerations (>15 bpm for >15 sec) in 20 min, Baseline heart rate 110–160 bpm, baseline variability 5–25 bpm, absence of decelerations
- Sporadic decelerations amplitude <40 bpm are acceptable if duration <15 sec, <30 sec following an acceleration
- When there is moderate tachycardia (160–180 bpm) or bradycardia (100–110 bpm) a reactive trace without decelerations is reassuring of good health
- Interpretation/action: repeat according to clinical situation and the degree of fetal risk.

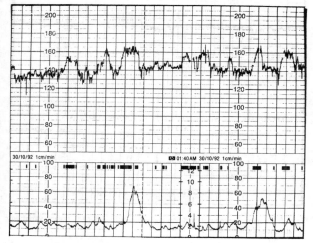

Fig. 4.4 Normal antenatal cardiotocograph.

Suspicious/equivocal
- Absence of accelerations for >40 min (non-reactive)
- Baseline heart rate 160–180 bpm or 100–110 bpm
- Reduced baseline variability (5–10 bpm for >40 min)
- Baseline variability >25 bpm in the absence of accelerations
- Sporadic decelerations of any type unless severe (see 'Pathological/ominous')
- Interpretation/action—continue or repeat CTG within 24 hours/AFI/BPP/fetal Doppler flow velocity waveform analysis.

Pathological/ominous
- Baseline heart rate <100 bpm or >180 bpm
- Silent pattern (baseline variability <5 bpm) for >40 min
- Sinusoidal pattern (oscillation frequency <2–5 cycles/min, amplitude of >10 bpm for >40 min with no accelerations and no area of normal baseline variability)
- Repeated late, prolonged (>1 min) and severe variable (>40 bpm) decelerations
- Interpretation/action—further evaluation (VAS, AFI, BPP, Doppler). Deliver if clinically appropriate.

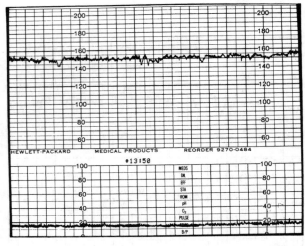

Fig. 4.5 Equivocal antenatal cardiotocograph—note reduced baseline variability and absence of accelerations.

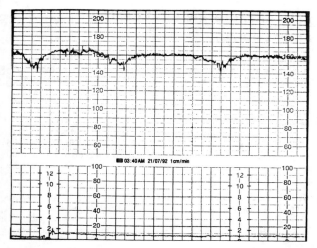

Fig. 4.6 Pathological cardiotocograph with poor variability and spontaneous decelerations.

Limitations

CTG use has the limitation of interpretation. Many studies have consistently shown sub-optimal inter- and intra-observer reliability. In order to overcome this limitation, computerized CTG is often used. The CTG information is analysed by a computer to satisfy criteria of normality. These are called 'Dawes–Redman criteria' after their developers. The algorithms for digital assessment of fetal heart rate tracing are complex, and beyond the scope of this chapter. The risk for fetal hypoxia/acidaemia is extremely low if the Dawes–Redman criteria for normality are met.

Late intrauterine fetal death and stillbirth

Definitions
Intrauterine demise of a fetus after 23^{+6} weeks of pregnancy is generally designated as a late intrauterine death (IUD). Stillbirth (SB) is defined as a baby delivered without signs of life after 23^{+6} weeks of pregnancy.

UK trends of stillbirth, perinatal death, and neonatal death
In the UK, the SB rate decreased from 5.4 per 1000 total births in 2000, to 5.2 per 1000 total births in 2009. The perinatal mortality rate showed a downward trend from 8.3 per 1000 total births in 2000 to 7.6 per 1000 total births in 2009 and the neonatal mortality rate decreased from 3.9 per 1000 live births in 2000, to 3.2 per 1000 live births in 2009.

Stillbirth: causes and associations
- Fig. 4.7 shows a break-up of causes of SB. Many SBs still remain unexplained.
- Causes of SB can be divided as associated factors and direct causes.

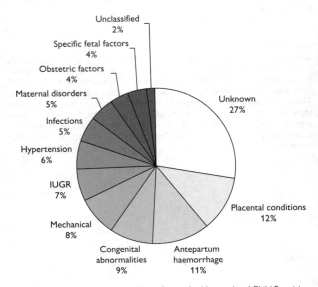

Fig. 4.7 Causes of stillbirth. Data from Centre for Maternal and Child Enquiries (CMACE). *Perinatal Mortality 2009: United Kingdom*. London: CMACE, 2011.

- As shown in Fig. 4.7, 27% of SBs were unexplained, 12% were due to placental conditions, 11% were due to APH, and 9% were due to a major congenital anomaly.[1] Several factors are identified as associated factors.
- SB is associated with several maternal conditions as shown in Table 4.2.

Table 4.2 Maternal factors associated with stillbirth

Associated risk factor	Odds ratio	95% CI
Overweight (BMI 25–30 kg/m^2)	1.23	1.09–1.38
Obesity (BMI >30 kg/m^2)	1.63	1.35–1.95
Smoking	1.36	1.27–1.46
Maternal age > 35 years	1.65	1.61–1.71
Nulliparity	1.42	1.33–1.51
Illicit drug use	1.9	1.2–3.0
Low education	1.7	1.4–2.0
Low socioeconomic status	1.2	1.0–1.4
No antenatal care	3.3	3.1–3.6
Assisted reproductive technology (singleton pregnancy)	2.7	1.6–4.7
Hypertension:	1.3	1.1–1.6
Pregnancy induced	1.6	1.1–2.2
Pre-eclampsia	2.2	1.5–3.2
Eclampsia		
Small for gestational age (weight < 10th centile)	3.9	3.0–5.1
Post-term pregnancy (>42 weeks)	1.3	1.1–1.7
Previous stillbirth	2.6	1.5–4.6
Pre-existing diabetes	2.9	2.05–4.09
Pre-existing hypertension	2.58	2.13–3.13

Data from Centre for Maternal and Child Enquiries (CMACE). *Perinatal Mortality 2009: United Kingdom*. London: CMACE, 2011.

Investigations

Tables 4.3–4.5 list mandatory investigations for the mother and cause-related tests for the mother and fetus in IUD and SB.

Table 4.3 Mandatory investigations for the mother

Test	Reason	Comment
FBC, coagulation, plasma fibrinogen	To exclude DIC	Repeat platelet count twice weekly
Blood glucose, HbA$_{1C}$	Occult diabetes	Glucose tolerance test may be normal in a few hours after IUD
Thyroid disease	Occult thyroid disorder	Thyroid stimulating hormone, free T$_3$, free T$_4$

Table 4.4 Cause-related tests for mother

Kleihauer test	To detect feto-maternal haemorrhage	Should be done as soon as possible as red cells clear quickly from circulation
Pre-eclampsia profile, bile acids	For pre-eclampsia, obstetric cholestasis	
Bacteriology-blood cultures, MSU, swabs vaginal, cervical	Suspected infections-listeria, chlamydia	Indicated in maternal fever, foul smelling liquor
Viral screen	Maternal-fetal infections	Hydrops, parvovirus, TORCH
Thrombophilia screen	Maternal thrombophilia	If IUGR, placental disease
Red cell atypical antibody screen	Immune haemolytic disease	If fetal hydrops on post-mortem
Maternal anti-Ro, anti-La antibodies	Occult maternal autoimmune disease	Evidence of hydrops, AV node calcification on post-mortem
Maternal allo-immune antiplatelet antibodies	Allo-immune thrombocytopenia	Evidence of fetal intracranial haemorrhage on post-mortem
Maternal urine	For cocaine	In drug abusers

Table 4.5 Tests for the fetus

Parental bloods for karyotype with consent	Parental balanced translocation, mosaicism	Fetal unbalanced translocation, aneuploidy e.g. 45X (Turner's syndrome)
Fetal and placental microbiology: blood, fetal swabs, placental swabs	Suspected fetal infections	With consent
Fetal, placental tissues for karyotype: fetal skin, cartilage, placenta	Aneuploidy, single-gene disorders	With consent

Legal requirements for medical certification of stillbirth and clinical governance

- SB must be medically certified by a fully registered doctor after examination of the baby.
- HM coroner should be contacted if doubt about status of birth.
- Police should be contacted if suspicion of deliberate action to cause SB.
- Standards for documentation: standard checklist use to ensure appropriate care options are offered and response to each is recorded.
- Maternity units should be aware of specific standards for IUD and SB.
- Consent for perinatal post-mortem examination should be documented using the nationally recommended form.
- All stillbirths should be reviewed in a multiprofessional setting using a standardized approach to investigate for sub-standard care and means of future prevention. Results of discussion recorded in mother's case record and discussed with parents.
- All SBs should be reported to CMACE.

Management

- Steps should be taken to expedite delivery if there is sepsis.
- Women should be tested for DIC if there is delay in induction for longer than 48 hours.
- Vaginal birth is the recommended mode of delivery. In the absence of intervention, 85% women with IUD deliver within 3 weeks of diagnosis. The risk of maternal DIC is 10% within 4 weeks from fetal death.
- Combination of mifepristone (200 mg) and vaginal misoprostol 100 mcg 6-hourly before 26 weeks, 25–50 mcg 4 hourly at 27 weeks or later.
- In women with previous LSCS, mifepristone alone can be used, induction is consultant decision.
- Women should labour in special rooms, cared for by experienced midwives.
- Women with sepsis should be treated with IV antibiotics.
- Adequate pain relief (regional anaesthesia, diamorphine) should be offered.
- Thromboprophylaxis should be given. Lactation suppression with dopamine agonists can be offered, but should not be used as routine.
- Counselling and information about support groups should be offered, bereavement services should be involved.
- Stillbirth should be certified by a fully registered doctor.
- Arrangements for burial, cremation, and spiritual guidance of all faiths should be available in the maternity unit.

Advice for future
- Women should be instructed that fertility can return quickly and ovulation can occur as early as day 18.
- Appointment is made 6–8 weeks postpartum when all reports including post-mortem are available.
- Parents should be advised about the cause of IUD and chance of recurrence depending on the cause.
- Advice about weight loss and smoking cessation should be offered where appropriate.
- Conception should be delayed until psychological issues are resolved.
- Meeting is documented with a plan outlined for future pregnancy.

Unexplained intrauterine fetal death
- Recommend birth at specialist maternity unit.
- Should have consultant-led antenatal care, screen for gestational diabetes, growth assessment.
- Vigilance for postpartum depression in women with previous stillbirths, IUD.

Reference
1. Centre for Maternal and Child Enquiries (CMACE). *Perinatal Mortality 2009: United Kingdom.* London: CMACE, 2011.

Intrapartum procedures and complications

Contributors

Eleftheria L. Chrysanthopoulou, Stergios K. Doumouchtsis, Sambit Mukhopadhyay, Kostis I. Nikolopoulos, Christiana Nygaard, Frank Schroeder, Hilary Turnbull, Dimuth Vinayagam, and Renate Wendler

Contents

Diagnosis of labour

Key learning points
- Onset of painful uterine contractions along with progressive cervical dilation is essential for the diagnosis of labour.
- Accurate diagnosis of labour is essential to avoid intervention in the latent phase.
- Labour can be diagnosed from a combination of the patient's history and physical signs on examination. Labour is diagnosed by the combination of two features:
  - regular, painful uterine activity or contractions
  - progressive cervical changes.
- Women admitted to hospital in the latent phase, and not yet in active labour, are more likely to receive medical intervention (e.g. oxytocin augmentation, electronic fetal monitoring, CS), than those admitted in active labour. Therefore, an incorrect early diagnosis of labour has significant consequences. Between 30% and 45% of women admitted to labour wards in the UK and other developed countries, are found not to be in active labour.

History
- Fundal height, lie, presentation, position, and station.
- Fetal heart auscultation using a Pinard or sonicaid or electronic fetal monitoring.

Vaginal examination
- Evidence of vaginal 'show'.
- Evidence of membrane rupture.
- Cervical changes:
  - dilatation: the increase in diameter of the cervical opening, measured in centimetres
  - effacement:
    - the progressive shortening and thinning of the cervix in labour
    - the length of the cervix is variable at the onset of labour (from a few millimetres to 3 cm), but throughout labour, the length decreases steadily to a few millimetres
  - initial cervical examination provides a baseline from which to assess progress.

Stages of labour
Labour is divided into three stages:

First stage
- Onset of labour to full dilatation of cervix with a process of cervical effacement and dilatation.
- Latent phase: the early part of the first stage of labour to 3–4 cm dilatation. It can last from a few hours to a few days.
- Active phase:
  - cervix is between 4 and 10 cm dilated
  - rate of cervical dilatation is usually 0.5–1 cm/hr
  - effacement is usually complete
  - fetal descent through birth canal is complete.

Second stage
- From full dilatation of the cervix to delivery of the baby, by a process of descent of the fetus through the birth canal.
- Early phase (non-expulsive):
  - cervix is fully dilated
  - fetal descent continues
  - no urge to push.

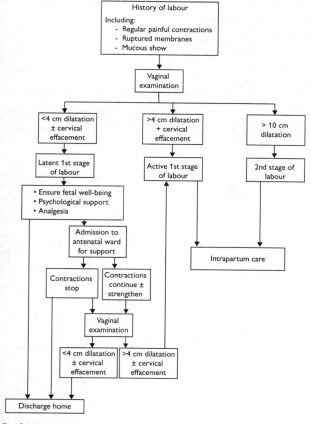

Fig. 5.1 Diagnosis of labour.

- Late phase (expulsive):
  - fetal part reaches the pelvic floor
  - urge to push
  - birth should be expected to take place by 3 hours of the start of active second stage in nulliparous and 2 hours in multiparous woman.

Third stage
- From delivery of the baby until delivery of the placenta and membranes. It usually lasts no more than 30 minutes.

Differential diagnosis
- Braxton Hicks contractions
- UTI resulting in uterine irritability
- Prolonged latent phase of labour
- Bowel symptoms.

Further reading
Cheyne H, Hundley V, Dowding D, et al. Effects of algorithm for diagnosis of active labour: cluster randomised trial. *BMJ* 2008; 337:a2396.
Holmes P, Oppenheimer LW, Wen SW. The relationship between cervical dilatation at initial presentation in labour and subsequent intervention. *BJOG* 2001; 108:1120–4.
National Institute for Health and Care Excellence. *Intrapartum Care for Healthy Women and Babies* (CG190). London: NICE, 2014.

:☠: Cord prolapse

Definition

Cord prolapse has been defined as the descent of the umbilical cord through the cervix alongside (occult) or past the presenting part (overt) in the presence of ruptured membranes.

The overall incidence ranges from 0.1% to 0.6%, whereas in the case of breech presentation, the incidence is slightly higher than 1%.

Risk factors

- Multiparity
- Low birth weight <2.5 kg
- Prematurity including preterm prelabour rupture of membranes (ROM)
- Fetal congenital abnormalities
- Polyhydramnios
- Malpresentation: transverse, oblique, and unstable lie or breech presentation
- Unengaged presenting part
- Second twin
- Low-lying placenta, other abnormal placentation
- Cord abnormalities: true knots, low content of Wharton's jelly, or a single umbilical artery.

Procedure-related risk factors

- Artificial ROM
- Vaginal manipulation of the fetus with ruptured membranes
- External cephalic version (during procedure)
- Internal podalic version
- Stabilizing induction of labour
- Placement of intrauterine catheter for pressure monitoring
- Amnioinfusion
- Induction of labour with transcervical balloon catheters.

Diagnosis

Speculum and/or digital vaginal examination:
- Should be performed when cord prolapse is suspected
- Should be performed after spontaneous ROM if risk factors are present.

Cord pulsations can be felt by the examining fingers. Should be differentiated from maternal vessel pulsations, which can occasionally be felt. In case of fetal demise, pulsations may be absent, and only the cord can be felt.

Abnormal cardiotocography

The fetal heart rate (FHR) should be auscultated after every vaginal examination in labour and after spontaneous membrane rupture.

Cord prolapse should be suspected when there is an abnormal FHR pattern, especially if such changes commence soon after membrane rupture, either spontaneous or artificial.

Management

- Cord prolapse is an acute emergency and immediate action is of crucial importance.
- A CS is the recommended mode of delivery.
- Exceptions:
  - full cervical dilatation
  - cord prolapsed of second twin after delivery of the first baby.

Immediate actions
- Call for help (preparations for immediate birth in theatre and neonatal resuscitation team).
- The presenting part should be elevated either manually or by filling the urinary bladder for prevention of cord compression.
- Minimal handling of the cord is recommended to avoid spasm of cord vessels.
- Knee–chest or Trendelenburg position may facilitate relief of cord compression.
- Tocolysis can be considered while preparing for CS if there are persistent FHR abnormalities after attempts to prevent compression mechanically and when the delivery is likely to be delayed.
- Although these measures are potentially useful during preparation for delivery, they must not result in unnecessary delay.

Cord prolapse in the community

- Women should be advised, over the telephone if necessary, to assume the knee–chest face-down position while waiting for hospital transfer.
- During emergency ambulance transfer, the knee–chest position is potentially unsafe and the left lateral position should be used.
- The woman should be transferred to the nearest consultant-led maternity unit unless a spontaneous vaginal birth is imminent.
- Minimal handling of the cord is recommended to avoid spasm of cord vessels.

Debriefing

After the incident, the patient and her partner should be offered debriefing to explain the sequence of events. They should be given an opportunity to ask questions. The developments at the time of the diagnosis are too rapid to offer adequate explanations.

☺ Abnormal fetal heart rate patterns in labour (prolonged decelerations)

Description of CTG trace features
Table 5.1 gives a description of the CTG trace features. Table 5.2 provides information about management.

Definition
Prolonged decelerations are those with duration of ≥2 minutes but <10 minutes.

Prolonged decelerations and other abnormal FHR patterns are associated with fetal risks including asphyxia, meconium aspiration, and death.

Causes
- Cord compression:
  - oligohydramnios
  - cord prolapse
  - knots.
- Uteroplacental insufficiency:
  - uterine hyperstimulation or prolonged contractions
  - placental abruption
  - uterine rupture.
- Maternal hypoxia:
  - hypotension (commonly epidural, spinal or paracervical analgesia)
  - amniotic fluid embolism
  - seizures
  - Valsalva manoeuvre.
- Fetal haemorrhage:
  - vasa praevia
  - traumatic amniocentesis.
- Fetal vagal reaction:
  - cervical examination
  - fetal scalp electrode placement
  - fetal blood sampling (FBS)
  - impending birth.
- Idiopathic.

Assessment and investigations
Consider the underlying pathophysiology and implement corrective interventions.

Examine patient:
- General observations (BP/pulse/temperature)
- Review CTG and evaluate for long-standing, gradually evolving, or subacute hypoxia
- Abdominal/vaginal examination (consider fetal response with scalp stimulation)
- FBC/G&S (clotting screen, cross-matching may be necessary).

Table 5.1 CTG trace features

Description			Features
	Baseline (bpm)	Variability (bpm)	Decelerations
Normal/ reassuring	100–160	≥ 5	None or early
Non-reassuring	161–180	< 5 for 30–90 min	Variable decelerations: dropping from baseline by ≤ 60 bpm and taking ≤ 60 sec to recover present for >90 min >50% of contractions OR Variable decelerations: dropping from baseline by >60 bpm or taking >60 sec to recover present for <30 min >50% of contractions OR Late decelerations: present for ≤30 min >50% of contractions
Abnormal	>180 <100	<5 for >90 min	Non-reassuring variable decelerations: still observed 30 min after starting conservative measures >50% of contractions OR Late decelerations: present for >30 min do not improve with conservative measures >50% of contractions OR Bradycardia or a single prolonged deceleration lasting ≥3 min

Reproduced with permission from National Institute for Health and Care Excellence (2014), from *CG190 Intrapartum care: care of healthy women and their babies during childbirth.* Manchester: NICE. Available from http://www.nice.org.uk/guidance/cg190/chapter/1-recommendations (accurate at the time of publication).

Table 5.2 Management based on interpretation of CTG traces

Category CTG is:	Definition	Interpretation	Management
Normal/ reassuring	All 3 features are normal/ reassuring	Normal CTG, healthy fetus	Continue CTG and normal care. If CTG was started because of concerns arising from intermittent auscultation, remove CTG after 20 min
Non-reassuring: need for conservative measures	1 non-reassuring feature AND 2 normal/ reassuring features	Combination of features that may be associated with increased risk of fetal acidosis. If accelerations are present, acidosis is unlikely	Think about possible underlying causes. If the baseline fetal heart rate is >160 bpm, check the woman's temperature and pulse. If either are raised, offer fluids and paracetamol. Start 1 or more conservative measures: – encourage the woman to mobilize or adopt a left-lateral position, and in particular to avoid being supine – offer oral or IV fluids. – reduce contraction frequency by stopping oxytocin if being used and/ or offering tocolysis. Inform coordinating midwife and obstetrician
Abnormal: need for conservative measures AND further testing	1 abnormal feature OR 2 non-reassuring features	Combination of features that is more likely to be associated with fetal acidosis	Think about possible underlying causes. If the baseline fetal heart rate is >180 bpm, check the woman's temperature and pulse. If either are raised, offer fluids and paracetamol. Start 1 or more conservative measures. Inform coordinating midwife and obstetrician

(Continued)

Table 5.2 (Contd.)

Category	Definition	Interpretation	Management
CTG is:			Offer to take an FBS (for lactate or pH) after implementing conservative measures, or expedite birth if an FBS cannot be obtained and no accelerations are seen as a result of scalp stimulation
			Take action in <30 min if late decelerations are accompanied by tachycardia and/or reduced baseline variability
			Inform the consultant obstetrician if any FBS result is abnormal
			Discuss with the consultant obstetrician if an FBS cannot be obtained or a third FBS is thought to be needed
Abnormal: need for urgent intervention	Bradycardia or a single prolonged deceleration with baseline <100 bpm, persisting for ≥3 min	An abnormal feature that is very likely to be associated with current fetal acidosis or imminent rapid development of fetal acidosis	Start 1 or more conservative measures
			Inform coordinating midwife
			Urgently seek obstetric help
			Make preparations for urgent birth
			Expedite birth if it persists for 9 min
			If heart rate recovers before 9 min, reassess decision to expedite birth in discussion with the woman

FBS, fetal blood sampling.

Reproduced with permission from National Institute for Health and Care Excellence (2014), from CG190. Intrapartum care: care of healthy women and their babies during childbirth. Manchester: NICE. Available from http://www.nice.org.uk/guidance/cg190/chapter/1-recommendations (accurate at the time of publication).

Management

- In cases of suspected or confirmed acute fetal compromise, delivery should be accomplished within a time appropriate for the clinical condition.
- If there is deceleration >3 minutes, medical review should be sought and preparations made to urgently expedite delivery.
- The woman should be advised to adopt the left lateral position (may improve uterine circulation).
- Oxytocin should be stopped and a full assessment of the fetal condition undertaken by an obstetrician before oxytocin is recommenced.
- In uterine hypercontractility not secondary to oxytocin infusion, tocolysis should be considered. A suggested regimen is subcutaneous terbutaline 0.25 mg.
- Administer IV fluid bolus to restore intravascular volume in case of maternal hypotension.
- Prolonged use of maternal facial oxygen therapy may be harmful to the baby and should be avoided.
- The patient should be transferred to theatre within 9 minutes.
- If the fetal heart recovers within 9 minutes the decision to deliver should be reconsidered in conjunction with the woman if reasonable.

The following timelines are a useful mnemonic

- 3 minutes: call senior obstetrician, theatre team, and anaesthetist
- 6 minutes: prepare mother for delivery
- 9 minutes: go to theatre to prepare LSSC or ventouse/forceps delivery
- 12 minutes: deliver by quickest and safest method (usually LSCS)
- 15 minutes: complete delivery.

Additional assessment

- Fetal cardiogram with continuous electronic fetal monitoring: combined assessment of the standard FHR tracing with an automated analysis of the fetal ECG.
- Digital stimulation of the fetal scalp.
- Response (acceleration in the FHR) to digital stimulation of the fetal scalp is a good predictive test.
- FBS:
  - FBS should be advised in the presence of a pathological FHR trace
  - FBS should be taken with the woman in the left lateral position.
- Contraindications to FBS include:
  - where there is clear evidence of acute fetal compromise, FBS should not be undertaken and urgent preparations to expedite birth should be made
  - maternal infection (e.g. HIV, hepatitis viruses, and herpes simplex virus)
  - fetal bleeding disorders (e.g. haemophilia)
  - prematurity (<34 weeks).

Classification of fetal blood sample results

See Table 5.3 for a classification of fetal blood sample results.

Table 5.3 Fetal blood sample results		
Lactate (mmol/L)	pH	Interpretation/action
≤4.1	≥7.25	Normal—repeat in ≤60 min if needed
4.2–4.8	7.21–7.24	Borderline—repeat in ≤30 min if needed
≥4.9	≤7.20	Abnormal—expedite delivery

Reproduced with permission from National Institute for Health and Care Excellence (2014), from *CG190 Intrapartum care: care of healthy women and their babies during childbirth.* Manchester: NICE. Available from http://www.nice.org.uk/guidance/cg190/chapter/1-recommendations (accurate at the time of publication).

Note

Management of prolonged decelerations can be extremely tenuous and is based on bedside clinical judgement, which inevitably will sometimes be imperfect given the unpredictability of these decelerations.[1]

Reference

1. Cunningham FG, Levano KJ, Bloom SL, *et al.* Intrapartum assessment. In *Williams Obstetrics* (24th ed), pp.473–503. New York: McGraw Hill, 2014.

☠ Continuous abdominal pain in labour

Intermittent pain is a normal feature of labour. Continuous pain is never considered normal and is associated with several obstetric emergencies. The common use of epidural analgesia can make diagnosis difficult and delayed.

Differential diagnosis

- Scar rupture
- Placental abruption
- Prolonged hypertonic contraction (hyperstimulation)
- Rare coincidental peritonism (e.g. splenic rupture).

Scar rupture

Usually occurs in labour.

Associations

- Previous LSCS
- Previous myomectomy
- Previous cornual ectopic/hysterotomy/perforation
- Obstructed labour (especially multiparous)
- No apparent risk factors (especially in primips—subsequent history usually reveals previous uterine instrumentation, e.g. unrevealed TOP).

Maternal risks

- Haemorrhage
- Hysterectomy
- Extension into adjacent tissues (bladder/ureters/broad ligament)
- Rarely death.

Fetal risks

- Hypoxia
- Death.

Symptoms and signs

- Change in pattern to continuous, severe pain
- Cessation of uterine contractions
- Brisk intrapartum PV bleeding
- Abnormal CTG (prolonged and profound decelerations or sudden bradycardia which is the commonest FHR change or disappearance of FHR recording and difficulty in picking up the FHR)
- Maternal tachycardia/hypotension
- Presenting part disappears out of pelvis
- Diffuse peritonism
- Can be surprisingly subtle until there is significant blood loss—have a high index of suspicion if at risk, e.g. trial of scar.

Management

- Resuscitation with IV fluids/cross-match at least 4 units of blood stat.
- Immediate laparotomy, delivery of fetus and placenta within 15 minutes (by LSCS if still in the uterus), and repair of rupture site.

- Primary closure of rupture site with haemostasis is the main aim.
- Involvement of general, vascular, and urological surgeons may be necessary if extension occurs into ureters, bladder, broad ligament, or pelvic vessels.
- Immediate neonatal resuscitation will be necessary as the neonate is often in poor condition.
- Cord gases are mandatory.
- Fully document operative findings and event timings.
- Risk management form.

Subsequent pregnancies should always be delivered by elective LSCS at 37–38 weeks.

Placental abruption in labour

Associations
- History of antepartum haemorrhage
- Pre-eclampsia, IUGR
- Polyhydramnios (usually at time of ROM)
- All other risk factors for abruption.

Maternal risks
- Haemorrhage
- DIC
- Operative delivery
- Rhesus iso-immunization.

Fetal risks
- Hypoxia
- Death
- Exsanguination.

Symptoms and signs
- Usually sudden onset of severe, continuous pain.
- Sudden intrapartum PV bleeding is common (may be massive or unrevealed).
- Abnormal CTG (*prolonged bradycardia commonest*) or decelerations associated with too frequent contractions that indicate uterine irritability.
- Maternal tachycardia/hypotension.
- Rock hard, tender uterus.

Management
- Resuscitation with IV fluids/cross-match at least 4 units of blood stat.
- Blood for FBC and clotting (abruption can trigger DIC).
- Immediate LSCS delivery of fetus and placenta within 15 minutes if fetal bradycardia, abnormal FHR changes, uterine irritability, excessive bleeding, or haemodynamic disturbance (if fully dilated then ventouse/forceps can be considered).
- Replace blood loss with whole blood (group-specific if necessary).
- Haematological advice about replacement of clotting factors and/or platelets if required.

- Needs HDU care with strict fluid balance and senior obstetric and anaesthetic input (especially if have underlying pre-eclampsia).
- Immediate neonatal resuscitation will be necessary as the neonate is often in poor condition.
- Cord gases are mandatory.
- Fully document operative findings and event timings.
- Debriefing.
- Risk management form.

:☠: **Instrumental delivery for fetal distress in the second stage of labour**

'Fetal distress' is a condition of significant impairment of oxygen transport resulting in progressive fetal hypoxia, acidosis, and asphyxia. It is the second commonest cited indication for instrumental delivery in the second stage of labour, after prolonged second stage. Fetal pH falls quicker in the second stage so delivery should be completed within 20–30 minutes of decision to deliver for 'fetal distress'.

If, in the presence of fetal distress, a difficult vaginal delivery is anticipated, then serious consideration should be given to emergency LSCS instead.

Indications for instrumental delivery for fetal distress

- Prolonged bradycardia
- Abnormal CTG
- Non-reassuring CTG with fresh meconium or abnormal FBS results
- Acute event (e.g. abruption, cord prolapse).

Choice of instrument

- The choice of the instrument depends upon individual situation where the urgency with which the baby needs to be delivered will be balanced against potential risks to the mother and the baby (Table 5.4).

Table 5.4 Advantages and disadvantages of different instruments

Instrument		Advantages		Disadvantages	
Forceps	Rotational		More effective in achieving vaginal birth	Only defensible in experienced hands, LSCS usually preferable, higher risk of CS, higher risk of maternal trauma	Higher risk of maternal trauma
	Non-rotational	Less chance of failure, safer for baby		More maternal pain and trauma	
Ventouse	Metal cup	Lower risk for maternal trauma	Less pain Less maternal trauma	Higher risk of cephalhaematoma	Likely to cause fetal trauma (scalp injury, cephalhaematoma, retinal haemorrhage)
	Soft cup	Lower risk of trauma to the baby	More chance of failure	Higher risk of failure	
	Hand-held vacuum (the Kiwi Omnicup®)	High heterogeneity of evidence		Higher risk of failure	

- *Choose the instrument that will best achieve a timely delivery*:
  - different practitioners have a preference for ventouse or forceps, according to their skills
  - forceps are particularly useful for prematurity 34–36 weeks, specific malpresentations (face, after-coming head in breech), when maternal effort is impossible or contraindicated (cardiac disease).

Contraindications

- Fetal malpresentation (brow, face mento-posterior)
- Unengaged fetal head (fetal head is above the ischial spines or more than one-fifth of the head palpable abdominally)
- Cephalopelvic disproportion
- Fetal coagulopathy or bone demineralization disorder
- Not fully dilated cervix.

Actions

- Decision to deliver (aim for 20 minutes for completion, 15 minutes for prolonged bradycardia).
- Call for help (anaesthetist/ODA/paediatrician/lead midwife).
- Obtain consent (preferably written but verbal will suffice).
- General examination of the mother (general condition, hydration, analgesia).
- In the event of an acute event (e.g. abruption), send FBC, clotting/cross-match/IV access.
- Move to theatre promptly for trial of instrumental delivery (in delivery room only if 'easy lift out').
- Reassess whole situation ('Should I be doing a LSCS?').
- Operative vaginal delivery should be abandoned where there is no evidence of progressive descent with moderate traction during each contraction or where delivery is not imminent following three contractions of a correctly applied instrument by an experienced operator.
- Forceps or CS may be considered after failed attempt to deliver by ventouse. Failure of ventouse delivery is associated with an increased risk of postpartum haemorrhage (PPH). Forceps delivery is associated with increased likelihood of third-degree perineal tears whereas CS increases the PPH rate. The neonatal morbidity is comparable regardless of whether forceps or CS is used after failed ventouse.
- Continuous fetal monitoring throughout the procedure is useful.
- Timekeeping is essential.
- If successful delivery, baby is handed straight to paediatricians.
- Cord gases are mandatory.
- Risk management form should be completed in the case of adverse outcome to the fetus or mother.
- Full, contemporaneous documentation.
- Counsel parents and explain sequence of events regardless of outcome.

Prerequisites for safe instrumental delivery

Safe instrumental vaginal delivery requires a careful assessment of the clinical situation, clear communication with the mother and healthcare personnel, and expertise in the chosen procedure (Table 5.5).

Table 5.5 Assessment and preparation checklist for instrumental delivery

Full abdominal and vaginal examination	Vertex presentation
	No more than 0–1/5ths palpable
	Pelvis is deemed adequate.
	Exclude cephalopelvic disproportion abdominally
	Full cervical dilatation and ruptured membranes
	Assessment of caput and moulding
	Fetal head below ischial spines
Preparation of mother	Aseptic technique
	Empty bladder: remove in-dwelling catheter or empty balloon
	Adequate analgesia
Preparation of staff	Anticipation of complications (e.g. shoulder dystocia, postpartum haemorrhage)
	Back-up plan in case of failure to deliver. A CS should be performed in <30 minutes

Further reading

Bhide A, Guven M, Prefumo F, *et al.* Maternal and neonatal outcome after failed ventouse delivery: comparison of forceps versus cesarean section. *J Matern Fetal Neonatal Med* 2007; 20(7):541–5.

Majoko F, Gardener G. Trial of instrumental delivery in theatre versus immediate caesarean section for anticipated difficult assisted births. *Cochrane Database Syst Rev* 2012; 10:CD005545.

O'Mahony F, Hofmeyr GJ, Menon V. Choice of instruments for assisted vaginal delivery. *Cochrane Database Syst Rev* 2010; 11:CD005455.

Royal College of Obstetricians and Gynaecologists. *Operative Vaginal Delivery* (Green-top Guideline No. 26). London: RCOG, 2011.

:☠: Shoulder dystocia

Definition
A vaginal cephalic delivery that requires the use of additional obstetric manoeuvres, following delivery of the head and failure to deliver using gentle traction. Shoulder dystocia is a bony obstruction, which occurs when the fetal shoulder impacts on the symphysis pubis (anteriorly) or, less commonly, the sacral promontory (posteriorly).

Incidence
The reported incidence of shoulder dystocia varies widely; due to the erroneous labelling of a delivery, the occurrence of shoulder dystocia can be disregarded due to poor definitions and high subjectivity. The reported incidence is between 0.57% and 0.70% of all vaginal deliveries.

Shoulder dystocia is a rare, true obstetric emergency and therefore all birth attendants should be proficient in the safe and timely management of this emergency. The management outlined in this section should be regularly rehearsed in 'skills and drills' sessions, ensuring competency for all birth attendants working in a maternity unit, especially as birth injuries caused by shoulder dystocia are an important contributor to litigation claims.

Risk factors
- Previous shoulder dystocia
- Macrosomia (>4500 g)
- Diabetes mellitus
- Raised maternal BMI
- Induction of labour
- Prolonged first stage
- Secondary arrest
- Prolonged second stage
- Oxytocin augmentation
- Operative vaginal delivery
- The single best predictor is previous shoulder dystocia
- At present there is no clinically proven predictor model that can be used
- The majority of cases occur in deliveries with no identifiable risk factors with fetal weight <4500 g.

Management
- The management of shoulder dystocia requires timely, yet controlled manoeuvres to aid delivery of the baby.
- Fetal pH drops by 0.04 per minute, hence delivery within 5 minutes is usually associated with a good outcome, provided initial pH was normal.
- Care must be taken to avoid overzealous traction being applied, as this can result in irreversible damage (e.g. brachial plexus injury).
- Good communication between birth attendant and parturient as well as other attending healthcare professionals is essential. All members of the team should be clearly informed that they are attending a shoulder dystocia emergency.

- Senior neonatal staff should be present at delivery due to the expectation of the need for neonatal resuscitation.
- Stop maternal pushing (as this can exacerbate impaction) and do not apply fundal pressure.
- Shoulder dystocia is a bony obstruction; all manoeuvres are therefore employed to create more space in the pelvis, or rotate and dislodge the shoulder to facilitate delivery.

The HELPERR algorithm for the management of shoulder dystocia
- Help— SOAPS: Senior midwife, Obstetrician, Anaesthetist, Paediatrician, & Scribe.
- Evaluate for episiotomy—increases room available for further manoeuvres.
- Legs (McRoberts manoeuvre)—hyperflexion of thighs onto abdomen increases the 'pelvic space' available.
- Pressure (directed suprapubic)—aims to rotate anterior shoulder forward off symphysis. 'CPR grip' to be used behind the fetal back.
- Enter the pelvis (Wood's screw manoeuvre)—aims to internally rotate anterior shoulder to become posterior and bring the new 'anterior' shoulder below symphysis in a 'corkscrew' fashion.
- Remove posterior arm—posterior arm flexed and swept over fetal chest to exteriorize and then perform rotation as above.
- Roll onto all fours—change in position may improve pelvic diameters and space available.

The majority of babies will be delivered using these manoeuvres. If delivery is unsuccessful, then the management algorithm should be repeated. If delivery is still not possible, the following can be performed (by the most senior obstetrician available):
- Cephalic replacement (Zavanelli procedure) and LSCS—has been successfully described.
- Symphysiotomy—not recommended unless knowledge and skill available due to maternal morbidity.
- Cleidotomy—deliberate fracture of the fetal clavicles usually only if the fetus is dead.

Post delivery
Anticipate and be prepared for postpartum haemorrhage:
- Examine perineum carefully for third-/fourth-degree tears.
- Ensure cord bloods sent.
- Fully debrief the parturient and birth partners and members of staff present.
- Provide the mother with written information (i.e. RCOG leaflet 'A difficult birth: what is shoulder dystocia?').
- Risk management documentation : *fully document* all notes in a comprehensive and legible manner, to include:
  - time of delivery of the head and time of delivery of the body
  - anterior shoulder at the time of dystocia (right or left)
  - the manoeuvres performed (timing, sequence)
  - estimated blood loss at delivery
  - cord bloods
  - vaginal/perineal examination findings.

- Return to see the mother and baby at a later stage for further debriefing.
- Arrange a 6-week postnatal consultant appointment for further counselling, if required.

Prevention

- Induction of labour *does not* prevent shoulder dystocia in non-diabetic women with suspected fetal macrosomia.
- Previous shoulder dystocia remains one of the best predictors of future shoulder dystocia.
- Elective CS should be considered in pregnancies complicated by pre-existing/gestational diabetes with an estimated fetal weight >4500 g.
- Elective CS or vaginal delivery is appropriate for future pregnancies following shoulder dystocia—this is a joint decision that should be made by the woman and her carers

Further reading

Royal College of Obstetricians and Gynaecologists. *Shoulder Dystocia* (Green-top Guideline No 42). London: RCOG, 2012.

:۞: **Acute tocolysis**

Acute tocolysis may prove to be invaluable in many intrapartum obstetric emergencies and it may help reduce maternal and fetal morbidity and mortality.

Indications
- Acute relaxation of uterus:
  - uterine hypertonus
  - fetal distress
  - Zavanelli manoeuvre
  - undiagnosed malpresentation
  - fetal entrapment during delivery, esp. for second twin (e.g. need for internal or external version)
- Acute tocolysis during CS:
  - transverse lie, especially preterm dorso-inferior, prolonged ROM, advanced labour
  - neglected shoulder presentation in advanced labour
  - preterm breech
  - second-stage CS
- Acute tocolysis for third stage of labour:
  - retained but separated placenta
  - manual replacement of uterine inversion.

Aims of acute tocolysis
- Induce uterine relaxation to allow adequate fetal perfusion and return of normal FHR.
- Possibly achieve a better fetal pH at delivery and optimize fetal condition (*in utero* fetal resuscitation).
- Ensures adequate uteroplacental circulation and reduces chances of fetal compromise.
- Increase the time available for urgent delivery without fetal asphyxia (e.g. preparation for delivery, opening of second theatre, use of regional anaesthesia vs GA).
- Allow easier access and fetal manipulation in a difficult delivery.
- Allow easier uterine manipulation.

Acute tocolytic drugs
Many agents have been used including salbutamol, terbutaline, ritodrine, ethanol, glyceryl trinitrate (GTN), nifedipine, magnesium sulfate, hexoprenaline and atosiban.

Management
- Treat underlying causes, e.g. stop or reduce oxytocin if hyperstimulation present.
- Prepare for urgent delivery if fetal bradycardia or cord prolapse (usually LSCS).
- Make appropriate plans depending upon the indications.
- *Beta adrenergics* are particularly useful in cases of hyperstimulation/ FHR changes but may even be beneficial without hyperstimulation:

- terbutaline 0.25 mg in 5 mL saline IV over 5 minutes (or 0.25 mg SC) has been shown to reduce uterine activity and improve both FHRs and subsequent cord pH, including continuing labour and achieving vaginal delivery. Its use as nebulizer, does not reduce uterine activity. Maternal side effects include palpitations, tachycardia, and hypotension. The maximal effect lasts for 20–30 minutes. If CS is performed, the neonatal outcome is expected to be better, but there is a risk of atonic PPH. Propranolol 1 mg IV may be required to reverse the effect and for oxytocin to be effective
- ritodrine 6 mg in 10 mL saline IV over 2–3 minutes has also been used. Side effects include maternal tachycardia, hypotension, and pulmonary oedema
- salbutamol inhaled via a spacing device is not effective in relaxing the uterus. Side effects include maternal tachycardia, hypotension, and pulmonary oedema. IV infusion over 1–2 minutes has been used and could be repeated after 5 minutes in sustained uterine hypertonus.
- *GTN* 5 mg in 100 mL saline (50 mcg/mL) IV—initial dose 200 mcg repeated at 1–2-minute intervals as required has also been used extensively. IV use has a more predictable uterine response during CS than the sublingual aerosol spray (400 mcg) and is preferred if available. The uterine response is rapid. Maternal side effects include flushing and hypotension. The effect is rapidly reversible with oxytocin. It can be used in a caesarean breech delivery with epidural anaesthesia, when a traumatic delivery is anticipated. Sublingual tablet for manual removal of placenta has been used with less blood loss, without any overt side effects.
- *Atosiban* has been used extensively for non-acute tocolysis, but could also be used in acute situations. Side effects include nausea, vomiting, tachycardia, hypotension, dizziness, hot flushes, and hyperglycaemia.
- Acute tocolysis for fetal distress should be considered as a temporary measure and unless the FHR returns to normal, delivery should be expedited urgently.

Contraindications

- Maternal hypotension
- Maternal haemorrhage or hypovolaemia
- Moderate/severe maternal cardiac disease.

Further reading

Abdel-Aleem H, Abdel-Aleem MA, Shaaban OM. Tocolysis for management of retained placenta. *Cochrane Database Syst Rev* 2011; 1:CD007708.

Dodd JM, Reid K. Tocolysis for assisting delivery at caesarean section. *Cochrane Database Syst Rev* 2006; 4:CD004944.

Kulier R, Hofmeyr GJ. Tocolytics for suspected intrapartum fetal distress. *Cochrane Database Syst Rev* 2000; 2:CD000035.

Royal College of Obstetricians and Gynaecologists. *External Cephalic Version and Reducing the Incidence of Breech Presentation* (Green-top Guideline No. 20a). London: RCOG, 2010.

☣ **Symphysiotomy and destructive operations**

Symphysiotomy

Symphysiotomy is the surgical division of the fibrocartilaginous symphysis pubis to open the pelvis. It is very rarely performed nowadays but still has a place in the management of certain obstetric emergencies particularly in the developing world. The procedure is increasingly hard to justify in the developed world. It should be seen as a last resort and only carried out by people experienced in the procedure or in settings where abdominal delivery carries higher risks.

Indications
- Mild–moderate obstructed labour where caesarean delivery may be inappropriate or not available.
- Severe shoulder dystocia unresponsive to all other attempts at delivery.
- Trapped after-coming head in a vaginal breech delivery.

Contraindications
- Severe cephalopelvic disproportion
- Transverse lie
- Major pelvic deformity.

Procedure
1. Only to be undertaken by an experienced practitioner.
2. Adequate anaesthesia (GA, regional, or local infiltration with opiate sedation).
3. Place in lithotomy position with two assistants holding the legs.
4. Catheterization of the bladder to identify the urethra, and empty the bladder, and retain rigid plastic or metal catheter *in situ*.
5. Identify the symphysis and make a stab incision through the skin and the symphysis cartilage just below the upper border and rotate the scalpel upwards to cut the lower fibres using the upper fibres as a fulcrum.
6. Remove the scalpel and insert it at the same point but with the blade facing upwards to extend the incision up to fully divide the symphysis (this causes less morbidity than partial division and forced abduction). With two fingers in the vagina, help to push the urethra sideways and to allow judgement on how far to incise.
7. Deal with original indication for symphysiotomy.
8. Episiotomy is recommended as the anterior vaginal wall is unsupported and tension on it can lead to avulsion and urethral damage.
9. Antibiotic prophylaxis recommended.
10. Evaluate for urethral or bladder injury.
11. Suture incision edges to achieve haemostasis.
12. Orthopaedic and physio input is vital.
13. Bladder drainage for 48 hours is recommended.
14. Physical support of the pelvis is the mainstay of treatment to aid healing.
15. Discharge is appropriate once ambulation is confident.

Risks

- Pain
- Haemorrhage
- Urethral and/or bladder injury
- Osteitis pubis and retropubic abscess
- Long-term pain and pelvic instability. May require orthopaedic intervention (plating).

Destructive operations

These are performed to remove the fetus and placenta piecemeal in the presence of fetal death or futile outcome where spontaneous vaginal delivery may not be possible and/or abdominal delivery is to be avoided. These procedures are increasingly rarely performed and should only be carried out by an experienced practitioner. In the developed world, CS is almost always preferred.

Indications

- Severe obstructed labour with fetal death (by far the commonest indication)
- Severe or lethal fetal abnormality obstructing vaginal delivery
- After severe shoulder dystocia in the event of fetal death
- After head entrapment in a breech vaginal delivery with fetal death.

Procedure

1. General anaesthesia is generally recommended.
2. Aseptic technique required.
3. Sufficient dilatation of the cervix is required, usually fully dilated, but is possible >7 cm.
4. Percutaneous drainage of any large cystic structures, e.g. cystic hygroma may facilitate delivery.
5. Craniotomy involves a cruciate incision through a suture line with either blunt forceps or sharp scissors followed by extraction of the brain tissue. The head can then be delivered by attaching Kocher forceps to the cranium and pulling down.
6. Decapitation may be used for transverse lies to facilitate vaginal removal.
7. Evisceration may also be required for the abdomen and chest where decompression is necessary to achieve delivery.
8. Cleidotomy to reduce the bi-acromial diameter may be required if there are impacted shoulders.
9. Haemorrhage should be anticipated and prevented with liberal use of oxytocics.
10. Antibiotic cover is also recommended to reduce sepsis in the puerperium.
11. Full counselling should be available for patients and staff as these procedures can be highly traumatic.

Risks

- Haemorrhage
- Infection
- Uterine perforation
- Psychological morbidity for patients and staff.

:⚙: Twin delivery

It is essential to establish chorionicity in all twin pregnancies during the antenatal period, as this will influence labour management. This requires a US scan between 10 and 13 weeks' gestation (best before 14 weeks), for assessment of viability, chorionicity, major congenital malformation, and nuchal translucency, as after this gestation US is known to be less accurate. If it is not possible to determine the chorionicity, a second opinion should be sought.

Common points of management

Survival rates for preterm twins are lower than for equivalent gestation singletons. Urgent review by an experienced neonatologist is required to assist with management in all cases of twins at high risk of preterm delivery especially in deciding whether very early gestation (24–26 weeks) should be managed expectantly rather than undergoing operative delivery such as CS.

- Steroids should be administered (two doses of betamethasone 12 mg IM 24 hours apart) where there is a significant chance of preterm delivery.
- Tocolytic agents can be used in cases of spontaneous preterm labour (cervix <4 cm) to allow maximum benefit from steroid administration.
- Hypertensive disorders (including pre-eclampsia), acute fatty liver, obstetric cholestasis, abruption, and placenta praevia more commonly complicate twin pregnancies and should always be considered even in non-specific presentations.
- A FBC at 20–24 weeks will identify women with twin pregnancies who need early supplementation with iron or folic acid, and a repeat at 28 weeks is recommended as in routine antenatal care.
- Hospitalization does not reduce the risk of preterm birth, or perinatal mortality, but may be associated with a decreased number of low-birthweight infants.
- Elective delivery of women with a twin pregnancy from 37 weeks' gestation has not been proved as better than spontaneous labour.
- Previous CS is not an absolute indication for repeat CS in an uncomplicated twin pregnancy.
- There are insufficient data on the relative benefits and risks of planned CS instead of planned vaginal birth for twin pregnancies.

Monochorionic pregnancies

- The risk of fetal loss is higher than in dichorionic, due to second-trimester loss and may have a propensity to excess neurodevelopmental morbidity.
- The role of nuchal translucency measurements in predicting TTTs is unclear. A detailed US scan which includes extended views of the fetal heart should be performed.
- Fetal US assessment should take place every 2–3 weeks in uncomplicated monochorionic pregnancies from 16 weeks and in uncomplicated cases at least nine antenatal appointments should be offered.

- Vaginal birth of monochorionic twins could be attempted unless there are accepted, specific clinical indications for CS, such as twin 1 lying breech or previous CS.
- In women with uncomplicated pregnancy, elective birth from 36 weeks 0 days, after a course of antenatal corticosteroids, should be offered.
- After the single fetal death in a monochorionic pregnancy, the risk to the surviving twin of death or neurological abnormality is high.

Monochorionic monoamniotic (MCMA) twins

- High perinatal loss rates in monoamniotic twins have been attributed mainly to umbilical cord entanglement, inter-twin transfusion syndrome, discordant fetal abnormality or fetal growth restriction, and twin reversed arterial perfusion (TRAP).
- The main differential diagnosis for monoamniotic twinning is advanced twin–twin transfusion syndrome (TTTS) in a monochorionic diamniotic twin pregnancy.
- Despite different combinations (no monitoring, CTG, and US) and frequency of monitoring, there is no discernible variation in survival rates in uncomplicated monoamniotic twin pregnancies.
- Routine use of sulindac in all monoamniotic pregnancies is not justified.
- Elective delivery at 32 weeks (after prophylactic steroids) is recommended due to the risk of sudden intrauterine death of one or both twins from a cord accident due to entanglement.
- Delivery by CS is recommended due to the risk of cord entanglement and malpresentation of second twin during delivery. At viable gestations, emergency CS should be performed in established preterm labour.

Monochorionic diamniotic (MCDA) twins

- Mode and timing of delivery remains controversial due to a paucity of data relating delivery mode and gestation to outcome. However, some obstetricians recommend caesarean delivery to avoid the risk of acute TTTS during labour or after delivery of first twin (thus compromising second twin).
- Delivery at 36 weeks is sometimes recommended to avoid the risk of worsening TTTS in the late third trimester. Pregnancies which have no evidence of TTTS, or where a laser has successfully treated TTTS, can be managed as per dichorionic diamniotic (DCDA) twins.
- The following should be considered as indication for planned caesarean delivery:
  - any evidence of TTTS during pregnancy (growth discrepancy >10%, discrepancy in amniotic fluid volume (AFV), abnormal fetal Dopplers) not successfully treated by laser ablation of communicating vessels
  - non-cephalic leading twin
  - maternal request for CS
  - any of the above in early labour (including preterm labour at a viable gestation).

Dichorionic diamniotic (DCDA) twins

- Women with uncomplicated dichorionic twin pregnancies should be offered at least eight antenatal appointments.
- Delivery by 38 weeks of gestation should be offered in women with uncomplicated pregnancies.
- Antenatal care plan should have been made in consultation with the parents resulting in a plan for delivery.
- The following should be considered as indication for planned caesarean delivery:
  - non-cephalic leading twin
  - severe growth restriction in either twin
  - either of the above in preterm labour at a viable gestation
  - maternal request
  - any of the above in early labour at term.
- On admission in labour:
  - check gestation (review US scans)
  - review US for evidence of fetal growth and well-being
  - fetal hearts simultaneously (twin cardiotocograph)
  - presentation of twin 1 (US if necessary)
  - cervical dilation
  - plans made for delivery prior to labour
  - presentation of twin 2 can be checked but is not relevant to decision regarding mode of delivery as even a cephalic twin 2 may move to a breech presentation (and vice versa).

Vaginal twin delivery

Recommendations for all women planning vaginal birth and for women with uncomplicated twins who were requesting LSCS now in advanced labour (>6 cm):

Management
- Discuss analgesia. Epidural is not mandatory but should be recommended to avoid the discomfort associated with any manipulation that may be required to assist in delivering twin 2 and to avoid the maternal risk of general anaesthetic should emergency CS be required.
- Discuss fetal monitoring and recommend continuous electronic fetal monitoring for both twins simultaneously to allow early detection of FHR abnormality. A fetal scalp electrode is used to monitor the first twin, once cervix is dilated.
- Neonatologists should be informed early of planned induction/delivery or spontaneous labour.
- Recommend IV cannulation and send blood for haemoglobin and G&S.
- Give ranitidine 150 mg PO 8-hourly during labour due to increased risk of CS or instrumental delivery.

First stage of labour managed as per a singleton fetus
Oxytocin augmentation may be used (standard dose protocols for singleton).

Second stage
- Twin 1 delivered as per singleton (spontaneous, ventouse, or forceps).
- Immediately after delivery of twin 1, check lie of twin 2 by palpation (US if required) and ensure the fetal heart is monitored effectively.
- The position of the second twin should be stabilized, keeping it cephalic.
- If lie is non-longitudinal, attempt external version to cephalic (or breech) prior to the onset of contractions.
- Await onset of contractions. If not already running, an IV oxytocin infusion can be considered if there are no contractions after 10 minutes.
- Encourage active pushing with contractions when presenting part enters pelvis.
- Do not rupture membranes until presenting part is within pelvis and contractions have re-established.
- If FHR becomes abnormal, expedite delivery as required (CS, high ventouse, breech extraction depending on clinical circumstances and experience of operator).
- If fetal heart remains normal, await descent of presenting part into the pelvis for up to 1 hour. Beyond this time, intervention to expedite delivery is required (CS, high ventouse, breech extraction depending on clinical circumstances and experience of operator).
- Ventouse may be performed with a cervix that is fully dilated or with dilatation of 8–9 cm and with the head above the ischial spines for delivery of twin 2 only. Care must be taken to ensure maternal tissues are not caught during cup application and that the cup is applied as close as possible to the flexion point on the fetal scalp.
- See comments in breech delivery regarding breech extraction.

Third stage
Recommend active management with a bolus of oxytocic given with delivery of twin 2 (IM Syntometrine® or IM/IV oxytocin 5 units) followed by oxytocin infusion 5–10 units/hr for 4–6 hours.

Caesarean delivery for twins
Twin 1 is usually delivered without difficulty as per a singleton.

Avoid rupturing the membranes of twin 2 until the head or breech is palpated in the uterine incision. Delivery can be expedited by feeling for a fetal foot through the intact membranes and gently pulling it into the uterine incision. This is often required if twin 2 is lying transverse. An IV oxytocin infusion (10 units/hr) should be used following delivery of twin 2 to reduce the risk of PPH.

Preterm twin delivery (<34 weeks)

Do not try to avoid preterm labour using bed rest at home or in hospital, IM or vaginal progesterone, cervical cerclage, oral tocolytics.

Diagnosis

- Confirm gestation, chorionicity, last presentation, and fetal growth patterns from previous US scans if available.
- Check presentation of twin 1 (US if necessary).
- Try to establish diagnosis of labour (but avoid digital vaginal examination if ruptured membranes unless mother appears to be in established labour).
- Consider sterile speculum examination to assess in possible early labour.

Further reading

Crowther CA, Han S. Hospitalisation and bed rest for multiple pregnancy. *Cochrane Database Syst Rev* 2010; 7:CD000110.

Dias T, Thilaganathan B, Bhide A. Monoamniotic twin pregnancy. *Obstetrician and Gynaecologist* 2012; 14:71–78.

Dodd JM, Crowther CA, Elective birth at 37 weeks' gestation for women with an uncomplicated twin pregnancy. *Cochrane Database Syst Rev* 2014; 2:CD003582.

Hofmeyr GJ, Barrett JF, Crowther CA, Planned caesarean section for women with a twin pregnancy. *Cochrane Database Syst Rev* 2011; 12:CD006553.

National Institute for Health and Care Excellence. *Multiple Pregnancy: The Management of Twin and Triplet Pregnancies in the Antenatal Period* (CG129). London: NICE, 2011.

Royal College of Obstetricians and Gynaecologists. *Management of Monochorionic Twin Pregnancy* (Green-top Guideline No. 51). London: RCOG, 2008.

Shub A, Walker SP. Planned early delivery versus expectant management for monoamniotic twins. *Cochrane Database Syst Rev* 2015; 4:CD008820.

⊕ Breech delivery

In breech presentation, the lie is longitudinal and the head is in the fundus. There are three types of breech presentation:
- Frank breech (65–70%): the lower extremities are flexed at the hips and extended at the knees. Presenting part is the buttocks.
- Complete breech (15%): differs in that one or both knees are flexed. Presenting part is both feet and buttocks.
- Incomplete breech (15%): one or both hips are not flexed and one or both feet or knees lie below the breech. Presenting part is one or both feet or knees.

Epidemiology

The incidence of breech presentation decreases with gestation:
- 20% at 28 weeks of gestation
- 3–4% at term.

Risk factors

- Preterm delivery
- Polyhydramnios or oligohydramnios
- Previous breech presentation (incidence of 10% for second pregnancy and 27% for third)
- Uterine abnormalities (malformations, fibroids)
- Placental locality (praevia or corneal placenta)
- Fetal abnormalities (anencephaly, hydrocephaly)
- Multiple pregnancy
- High parity
- Pelvic tumours
- Idiopathic.

Diagnosis

- Abdominal palpation (Leopold's manoeuvres)
- Vaginal examination
- US.

Fetal risks

- Hypoxia (cord prolapse especially in incomplete breech, cord compression)
- Trauma.

Planning the mode of delivery

Women should be informed that:
- Planned CS carries a reduced perinatal mortality and early neonatal morbidity and a small increase in serious immediate complications for them than planned vaginal birth.
- There is no evidence that the long-term health of babies with a breech presentation delivered at term is influenced by how the baby is born.

Indications for a caesarean delivery
- General contraindications of vaginal birth at any presentation (e.g. placenta praevia, compromised fetal condition, prolonged labour)
- Large baby (>3.8 kg)
- Suspicion of inadequacy of the pelvis
- Baby with IUGR <2 kg
- Previous CS
- Footling or kneeing breech presentation
- Hyperextended fetal neck
- If there is delay in the descent of the breech at any stage in the second stage of labour.

Vaginal breech delivery should be considered in:
- Spontaneous and normally progressing labour
- Mother and fetus healthy and well
- Any woman first diagnosed in active labour
- Any woman who admitted in advanced labour (>6 cm cervical dilation)
- Any informed and counselled woman who wishes to pursue the option of vaginal breech delivery
- Preterm labour
- Second twin breech
- Labour induction for breech presentation may be considered if individual circumstances are favourable.

Management
Vaginal breech birth should take place in a hospital with facilities for emergency CS.

During first stage
- Advise fluid-only during labour.
- Establish IV access.
- FBC and G&S (risk of emergency CS).
- Give antiemetic and antacid.
- Inform anaesthetist.
- Continuous electronic FHR monitoring.
- FBS from the buttocks during labour is **not** advised. Epidural analgesia should not be routinely advised.
- Assess progress 2–4-hourly throughout labour and expect progress 0.5–1 cm/hr.
- Labour augmentation is **not** recommended.

During second stage
- Dorsal or lithotomy position is advised.
- Commence active pushing when the buttocks are visible or 1 hour after diagnosis of full dilation.
- Pushing should **not** be commenced until the breech has reached the ischial spines.
- Considered CS if there is delay in the descent of the breech in the second stage of labour.

- Breech extraction should **not** be used routinely (causes extension of the arms and head):
  - breech extraction is the procedure where traction is applied to the groins of a frank breech or to the limbs of a complete breech to facilitate delivery. There is insufficient evidence to support or refute the policy of routinely expediting vaginal breech delivery by extraction of the baby within a single uterine contraction.
- After delivery of the buttocks, the baby is encouraged to remain back upwards, but should not otherwise be touched until the scapula is visible.
- Gentle flexion of the knees (pressure in popliteal fossa) in an extended breech to allow the legs to deliver.
- Episiotomy should be performed when indicated to facilitate delivery.
- The arms should be delivered by sweeping them across the baby's face and downwards by the index finger, or by the Lovset manoeuvre (rotation of the baby to facilitate delivery of the arms).
- If contractions become less frequent in the first stage, oxytocin infusion should be commenced, or the option of CS considered.
- Suprapubic pressure by an assistant should be used to assist flexion of the head.
- The after-coming head may be delivered with forceps, the Mauriceau–Smellie–Veit manoeuvre (pull the jaw down to flex the head) or the Burns–Marshall method (feet are grasped and with gentle traction swept in a slow arc over the maternal abdomen).
- Insertion of a weighted speculum into the vagina if there is delay in delivery of the head may allow breathing.
- Where there is head entrapment during a preterm breech delivery, lateral incisions of the cervix should be considered.
- If conservative methods fail, symphysiotomy or CS should be performed.

⑦ Abnormal lie/presentation in labour

Transverse lie in labour

The fetus is in a transverse lie when its longitudinal axis is perpendicular to the long axis of the uterus. The back may face toward or away from the cervix called dorso-inferior and dorso-superior transverse lie, respectively. It occurs in ~1/300 deliveries.

Causes
- Obstruction in pelvis:
  - fibroid in the lower segment
  - large ovarian cyst
  - placenta praevia
  - subseptate uterus
- Fetal abnormality:
  - hydrocephalus
  - neuromuscular problems (and chromosome abnormality)
- Increased uterine capacity:
  - multiparity (especially grand multiparity due to lax uterus)
  - preterm gestation
  - polyhydramnios especially with non-macrosomic baby.

Diagnosis
- On palpation—no presenting part in pelvis, fetal poles palpable laterally.
- On vaginal examination presenting part is not reached, fetal limbs or back palpable.
- Fibroid or cystic mass may be palpable (abdominal or vaginal examination).
- Concurrent antepartum haemorrhage suggests placenta praevia (vaginal examination contraindicated).
- Confirm labour—uterine contraction present and vaginal examination reveals cervical effacement and dilatation >3 cm.

Urgent issues
- ROM may result in cord prolapse (less likely if fetus is with the back down).
- If contractions are strong (advanced labour) in a multigravid woman there is a risk of uterine rupture as the labour may get obstructed. This is especially true if there is a uterine scar and immediate delivery must be undertaken.

Investigations
- Review previous US scan reports for possible cause.
- US scan on labour ward to confirm diagnosis and look for causes.
- CTG for contractions and fetal well-being.
- Take blood for G&S, FBC.

Management
- Keep nil by mouth.
- Recommend and establish IV access.
- Give antiemetic (metoclopramide 10 mg PO or slow IV) and antacid (ranitidine 150 mg PO).
- Inform anaesthetist and theatre team.
- If evidence of obstruction in pelvis delivery by immediate CS is required.
- If no evidence of obstruction and membranes are intact, attempt external version to cephalic presentation between contractions. If successful, controlled amniotomy can be considered whilst lie is maintained by a second operator. Due to the risk of cord prolapse this should be performed with facilities for immediate CS available.
- If no evidence of obstruction but membranes have ruptured, internal podalic version to breech could be considered at the limits of fetal viability (23–25 weeks' gestation) but at other gestations immediate delivery by CS is likely to be safer for the fetus.

Prior to CS remember:
- Consent for removal if ovarian cyst.
- For suspected placenta praevia, cross-match blood and request senior obstetrician to be present.
- Caesarean delivery of transverse fetus with back down can be difficult especially after membrane rupture, therefore aim to perform internal version to breech during CS before rupturing membranes. If membranes have ruptured, consider performing vertical uterine incision (De Lee) particularly for preterm gestations.
- Consider use of bolus dose of tocolytics to facilitate atraumatic delivery.

Brow presentation

A brow presentation occurs when there is poor flexion of the fetal head. This results in a much bigger presenting diameter and an average baby at term will not deliver vaginally. Smaller and preterm infants may deliver without flexion as a brow, but in larger babies vaginal delivery will only be possible if the head flexes to an occipito-anterior or occipito-posterior position or extends to become a face presentation. Good contractions are required to facilitate this flexion. However, if flexion fails to occur, the labour becomes obstructed and there is a risk of uterine rupture if the contractions are strong.

Causes
- Fetal abnormality resulting in poor fetal tone or neck hyper-extension such as neck masses or anencephaly
- Poor uterine activity
- Relative cephalopelvic disproportion (large baby or small pelvis)
- Preterm gestations
- Multiple gestation
- Prematurity
- In most cases no cause can be identified.

Diagnosis
- Diagnosis in early labour is unusual
- Abdominal palpation shows a non-engaged head
- Palpation of orbital ridges during vaginal examination.

Urgent issue

In women with a uterine scar (previous CS), immediate delivery by CS should be considered if the diagnosis of brow presentation is made in established labour at term, due to the risk of scar dehiscence if labour is obstructed.

Management
- Assess gestation and estimate fetal weight, as a low-birthweight infant is likely to deliver spontaneously even if abnormal presentation persists.
- Assess contractions:
  - good contractions are required to facilitate flexion of the fetal neck
  - commence oxytocin infusion in primigravid women with slow progress regardless of contraction pattern but only in multigravid women with slow progress and inadequate contraction pattern (<4 in 10 minutes).
- Assess and monitor progress in labour:
  - brow presentation in early labour is more likely to resolve than when diagnosis is made in advanced labour
  - remember risk of uterine rupture if contractions are strong and the head does not flex (especially in multigravid women)
  - delivery should be by CS following failure of normal cervical dilatation in the first stage of labour or failure of flexion and decent of the head on active pushing in the second stage of labour
  - assisted vaginal delivery by forceps or Ventouse is not possible, if spontaneous flexion does not occur, delivery by CS will be required.
- Give ranitidine 150 mg PO and limit oral intake due to risk of CS.
- Recommend epidural for pain relief after diagnosis (increased risk of CS).
- Monitor FHR.
- FBS is not recommended for FHR abnormality (deliver by CS).

Face presentation

A face presentation occurs when instead of flexion, the fetal head becomes fully extended. The diameter of the average fetal head is such that this presentation can deliver vaginally. However the face is a poor cervical 'dilator' and thus good contractions are required, and even then progress will often be slow. As the head delivers across the perineum by flexion in this presentation, a fetus that moves into a mento-posterior position cannot deliver vaginally as flexion will be prevented by the symphysis–pubis.

Causes
- Fetal abnormality resulting in poor fetal tone or neck hyper-extension such as neck masses or anencephaly
- Relative cephalopelvic disproportion (large baby or small pelvis)

- Grand multiparity
- Multiple gestation
- Prematurity
- In most cases no cause can be identified.

Diagnosis

- Abdominal palpation is usually unremarkable if the head is engaged.
- Smooth, rounded occiput may be palpable on the opposite side of the fetal body if the head is not engaged.
- On vaginal examination, the fetal eyes, nose bridge, and mouth can be palpated. Oedema in soft tissues may lead to the mistaken diagnosis of a breech presentation.
- Diagnosis in early labour is difficult.

Management

- Review antenatal US scan reports.
- Assess contractions (frequency and duration).
- Monitor progress in labour (examine 2–4-hourly).
- If there is delay in cervical dilatation (progress <0.5–1 cm per hour) commence IV oxytocin infusion if primigravida. In a multigravid woman, oxytocin should only be used where poor progress is thought to be due to inadequate contraction frequency (<4 in 10 minutes).
- If there is delay in the second stage, assisted vaginal delivery can be performed using long-handled traction forceps if the presenting part is mento-anterior and at the level of (or below) the ischial spines. The angle of traction is the same as for an occipito-anterior position with the head delivering once the chin is below the symphysis-pubis by flexion.

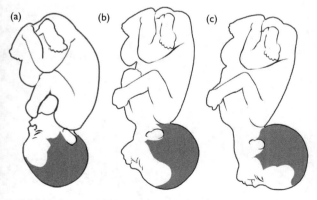

Fig. 5.2 (a) Deflexed cephalic presentation, (b) brow presentation, (c) face presentation.

- Ventouse delivery is contraindicated.
- Rotation of head—only mento-anterior position will deliver successfully vaginally. Persistent mento-posterior positions require delivery by CS.
- Head may flex during labour to become a brow (see 'Brow presentation', pp. 147–8).
- Monitor FHR.
- FBS cannot be performed for heart rate abnormality (deliver by CS).
- Skilled operators may consider the use of rotational forceps if the position is not direct mento-anterior and the head is low in the pelvis.
- CS can be difficult due to the inability to flex the head to assist with delivery.

Further reading

Cruikshank DP, White CA. Obstetric malpresentations: twenty years' experience. *Am J Obstet Gynecol* 1973; 116:1097–104.

Gemer O, Segal S. Incidence and contribution of predisposing factors to transverse lie presentation. *Int J Gynaecol Obstet* 1994; 44:219–21.

Shaffer BL, Cheng YW, Vargas JE, et al. Face presentation: predictors and delivery route. *Am J Obstet Gynecol* 2006; 194:e10–12.

☺ Anaesthetic complications on the labour ward

Anaesthetists form an integral part of the obstetric team, providing epidural analgesia or patient-controlled analgesia (PCA) with opioids for pain relief during labour. Anaesthesia is required for CS and various other operative procedures before and after delivery. In most cases neuraxial blockades are used, general anaesthesia is usually reserved for emergency operations and when regional techniques must not be performed. Whilst serious complications are rare, all anaesthetic techniques have specific risks and can lead to early and late complications.

Principles of immediate maternal resuscitation

- Call for help, place patient in left lateral position.
- Initiate life support measures (ABC approach).
- Monitor fetus and take appropriate action.
- Remember reversible causes for cardiac arrest (4H's and 4 T's).
- Consider a peri-mortem CS within 5 minutes of maternal collapse or cardiac arrest.

Complications of epidural and spinal anaesthesia

Hypotension

All neuraxial techniques cause some blockade of the sympathetic nerve system resulting in arterial and venous vasodilatation. This can lead to a decrease in maternal BP, blood flow and therefore to a significant reduction of uteroplacental perfusion.

Treatment
- Left lateral tilt
- IV fluids
- Ephedrine 5–10 mg in severe cases.

Inadvertent intravascular injection of local anaesthetics

Systemic toxicity of local anaesthetics can cause dizziness, seizures, loss of consciousness, and cardiovascular effects such as bradycardia, arrhythmia, ventricular fibrillation, and cardiac arrest. Symptoms can develop up to 1 hour after injection.

Treatment
- Stop local anaesthetic infusion.
- Left lateral tilt, ABC resuscitation.
- Administration of Intralipid® 20% at first signs of cardiotoxicity.
- 1.5 mL/kg over 1 minute followed by infusion of 0.25 mL/kg/min. Repeat bolus every 5 minutes up to 3 mL/kg or until circulation is restored (maximum dose 8 mL/kg).
- Immediate operative delivery.

Unintended dural puncture

Occurs during 0.3–2% of all epidural insertions, often unrecognized at the time of puncture, and usually (in about 85%) results in postdural puncture headache (PDPH) after 24–72 hours.

Treatment (depending on severity)
- Encourage fluid intake
- Oral pain therapy
- Epidural blood patch (sometimes a second epidural blood patch is required).

Unexpected high neuraxial block

Can be caused by the unintended placement of the epidural catheter into the subdural or subarachnoid space, by secondary catheter migration into the spinal space, or the administration of inappropriately high doses of local anaesthetics. Symptoms include hypotension, respiratory distress, and loss of consciousness.

Treatment
- Left lateral tilt, ABC resuscitation
- IV fluids
- Ephedrine or phenylephrine
- Intubation/ventilation until block resolved.

Epidural haematoma, nerve injury, or spinal abscess

Occurs more frequently in patients with undiagnosed bleeding disorders, and/or inappropriately timed anticoagulation. Infections of the puncture site can result in temporary or even permanent nerve damage.

Treatment

Prolonged nerve block or neurological symptoms in the postnatal period after epidural or spinal anaesthesia should prompt immediate examination, further investigations, and imaging (CT or MRI scan).

Urinary retention

Can occur during labour, after vaginal/operative delivery, or as a complication of neuraxial analgesia, neuraxial or general anaesthesia.

Treatment
- Temporary catheterization
- Avoid overextension of the bladder
- Parasympathomimetic drugs.

Pruritus

Frequent side effect of intrathecal, epidural, or IV opioid administration.

Treatment
- Antihistamines
- 5-HT antagonists
- Small doses of naloxone in severe cases ('titrate to effect').

Nausea and vomiting

Usually caused by hypotension associated with neuraxial anaesthesia, or as a side effect of opioids administered during/after neuraxial or general anaesthesia.

Treatment
- Check BP and treat with vasoactive drugs (e.g. phenylephrine).
- Initiate IV fluids to avoid dehydration.
- Ondansetron 4–8mg IV.
- Metoclopramide 10 mg IV or IM.

Body temperature

A small increase in maternal body temperature (usually <1.0°C and over several hours) can be seen in labouring women after the insertion of an epidural catheter. It is, however, important to exclude any other cause (e.g. infection) for a rise in maternal temperature.

Complications of systemic opioid administration

The systemic administration of opioids requires careful monitoring of the mother to avoid sedation, respiratory depression, and hypoxaemia. Regardless of whether opioids are administered intrathecally, epidurally, intravenously, intramuscularly, or by PCA, all opioids can cause respiratory depression, nausea, vomiting, as well as pruritus (and should be treated as outlined earlier in this section).

All conventional opioids used in clinical practice will cross the placenta and can lead to fetal bradycardia and neonatal respiratory depression. Remifentanil, which has an ultra-short length of action, is rapidly redistributed and metabolized in the mother and in the fetus. However, it still can lead to short periods of bradycardia and respiratory depression.

Complications of general anaesthesia

With advances in anaesthetic techniques, better airway management and modern anaesthetic drugs, general anaesthesia has a very low risk for serious complications.

Aspiration of gastric content/acid

This is a serious complication and will frequently require intensive care therapy and ventilatory support. The risk of aspiration in pregnant women is increased due to a decreased lower oesophageal sphincter tone, decreased gastric motility, and increased secretion of gastric acid, especially during the second half of pregnancy.

Treatment
- Intubation/ventilation
- CXR
- Intensive care treatment (± bronchoscopy?).

Hypoxaemia

More frequent at induction of anaesthesia due to a decreased functional residual capacity (FRC) in the pregnant woman.

Treatment
- Sufficient pre-oxygenation
- Difficult airway protocol in obstetric anaesthesia (limited number of intubation attempts).

Fetal depression due to transplacental transfer of anaesthetic agents

Treatment
- Avoid administration of opioids/sedatives before the neonate is delivered.
- Neonatal resuscitation.
- Inform paediatrician in advance of delivery.

Post-delivery procedures and complications

Contributors

Maya Basu, Stergios K. Doumouchtsis, George Iancu, Christiana Nygaard, Justin Richards, and Dimuth Vinayagam

Contents

☼ Retained placenta

Definition
A placenta is considered retained if not delivered (partly or completely) within 30 minutes after birth despite adequate attempts to deliver it in cases of active management of the third stage of labour in the third trimester (98% are expelled by then). In cases of expectant management (physiological management of third stage), a placenta is considered retained if not delivered after 60 minutes. In the second trimester, the risk of retained placenta is usually higher.

Epidemiology
The incidence of retained placenta varies greatly worldwide, ranging from 0.01% to 6.3% of vaginal deliveries, depending on the population studied and definition used. It is a considerable cause of maternal morbidity and mortality, especially in the developing world.

Pathophysiology
In some cases, the placenta is simply trapped behind a partially closed cervix; in other cases, it is superficially adherent to the uterine wall or invading the myometrium or adjacent organs (morbidly adherent placenta).

Risk factors
- Gestational age is one of the most important factors (<26 weeks)
- Previously retained placenta (commonest) (risk 2–4-fold higher)
- Maternal haemoglobin level <8.5 g/dL at onset of labour
- BMI >35 kg/m²
- Pre-eclampsia
- Induction of labour, prolonged first, second, or third stage of labour, precipitate labour
- Grand multiparity (≥4)
- Maternal age (≥35 years)
- Known placental abnormality e.g. succenturiate lobe/double placenta
- Uterine abnormalities(congenital müllerian fusion defects)
- Placenta praevia
- Previous CS/uterine trauma, e.g. multiple curretage and placenta praevia associated with previous uterine surgery (predisposes to morbid adherence—placenta accreta/increta/percreta).
- Stillbirth, IUGR (abnormal placentation).

Complications
- Postpartum haemorrhage (PPH): the need for intervention is supported by observations that the risk of haemorrhage increases with the length of time the placenta is retained
- Intrauterine infection and sepsis
- Uterine inversion (if over-zealous traction applied)
- Hysterectomy
- Maternal death.

Prevention
Active management of the third stage (oxytocin/ergometrine, cord clamping, controlled cord traction) significantly reduces the risk of PPH, but possibly increases the risk of retained placenta compared to physiological management.

Retained placenta
If partial closure of the cervix and/or a contracted lower uterine segment is inhibiting delivery of the placenta, glyceryl trinitrate (nitroglycerine) can be administered to relax the uterus and facilitate delivery (reduces the need of manual removal and blood loss).

Management
(See Fig. 6.1.) IV infusion of oxytocin should not be used to assist the delivery of the placenta.

For women with a retained placenta, oxytocin injection into the umbilical vein with 20 IU of oxytocin in 20 mL of saline is recommended, followed by proximal clamping of the cord.

Assess degree of bleeding and haemodynamic status
- If actively bleeding or haemodynamically compromised *act quickly*—immediate treatment for PPH should include:
  - calling for appropriate help
  - uterine massage
  - IV fluids
  - uterotonics.
- IV oxytocin infusion (40 IU in 500 mL normal saline).
- Repeat bolus of oxytocin (IV), ergometrine (IM, or cautiously IV), IM oxytocin with ergometrine (Syntometrine®), misoprostol, carboprost (IM).
- Blood for FBC and G&S (crossmatch 2–4 units if Hb <10 g/dL or active bleeding).
- Catheterize the bladder.
- Judicious attempt at controlled cord traction, with a hand on the abdomen to secure uterine fundus.
- Avoid excessive traction.
- If undelivered after 30 minutes, manual removal under anaesthesia and antibiotic prophylaxis is recommended.
- Anticipate PPH at all stages.

Manual removal of placenta (MROP)
(See Fig. 6.2.)
- Perform in theatre.
- Adequate anaesthesia (usually epidural/spinal).
- The bladder should be emptied.
- Sterile technique (operator to use gauntlet gloves).
- Prophylactic broad-spectrum antibiotic cover (e.g. ampicillin or first-generation cephalosporin).
- Use hand to progressively dilate cervix.
- Tocolysis is rarely required unless access to the cavity is manually impossible.

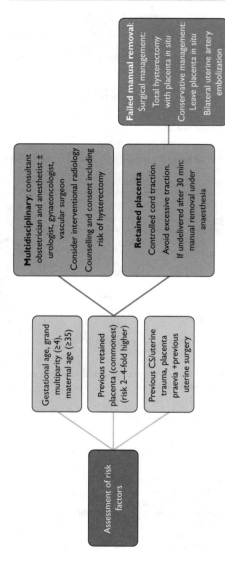

Fig. 6.1 Algorithm for the management of abnormal adherent placenta.

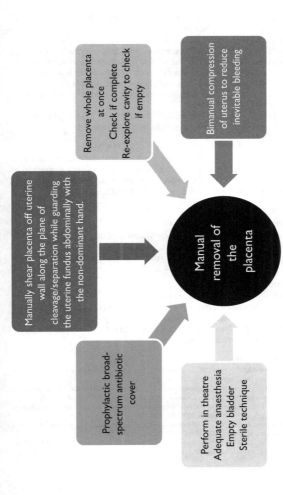

Fig. 6.2 Algorithm for manual removal of the placenta.

- Manually shear placenta off uterine wall along the plane of cleavage/separation while guarding the uterine fundus abdominally with the non-dominant hand.
- Remove placenta wholemeal if possible and check whether it is complete.
- Re-explore cavity to check if empty.
- Bimanual compression of uterus to reduce inevitable bleeding.
- Repair any perineal or vaginal tears as appropriate.
- Although high-quality randomized trials show that the use of oxytocin has little or no effect, administration of oxytocin into the umbilical vein (at least 20 units) is used to reduce the incidence of need for MROP. This may be a measure to consider in low-resource settings where safe MROP may not be easily accessible.
- If manual removal fails, instrument extraction using ring forceps or other large-headed forceps.
- If extracted placenta is incomplete and excessive bleeding ensues, curettage with a large, blunt curette might be needed.

In the event of non-delivery of the placenta

When the placenta is morbidly adherent (placenta accreta/increta/percreta) and does not separate at manual removal or is very difficult, then no further attempts should be made to deliver it as there is an increased risk of heavy bleeding and the need for hysterectomy.

Options

If bleeding is minimal and does not continue
- Leave the placenta undisturbed (antibiotic and oxytocic cover)
- Placenta tends to autolyse and separate and get extruded
- Methotrexate is of questionable use (no reduction in rates of PPH).

If active bleeding
- Balloon tamponade
- Emergency arterial embolization
- Surgical haemostasis: oversewing of the placental bed, compression sutures, pelvic devascularization, hysterectomy—preferable if the family is complete and no desire for future fertility or the bleeding is causing haemodynamic disturbance.

Further reading

Abdel-Aleem H, Abdel-Aleem MA, Shaaban OM. Tocolysis for management of retained placenta. *Cochrane Database Syst Rev* 2011; 1:CD007708.

Chongsomchai C, Lumbiganon P, Laopaiboon M. Prophylactic antibiotics for manual removal of retained placenta in vaginal birth. *Cochrane Database Syst Rev* 2014; 10:CD004904 .

Doumouchtsis S.K, Arulkumaran S. The morbidly adherent placenta: an overview of management options, *Acta Obstet Gynecol* 2010; 89:1126–33.

Nardin JM, Weeks A, Carroli G. Umbilical vein injection for management of retained placenta. *Cochrane Database Syst Rev* 2011; 5:CD001337.

NICE. *Intrapartum Care for Healthy Women and Babies* (CG190). London: NICE, 2014. http://www.nice.org.uk/guidance/cg190

☺ Postpartum haemorrhage

PPH is defined as a blood loss in excess of 500 mL following vaginal delivery (1000 mL following CS). It is not only the absolute value of blood loss that is important; other clinical parameters must also be taken into consideration. The mother with the low BMI or severe anaemia will have less ability to compensate following blood loss, and if she becomes haemodynamically unstable, then this too constitutes a PPH. Complications of PPH include haemorrhagic shock, DIC, adult respiratory distress syndrome, and end-organ damage (e.g. renal failure).

PPH is divided into primary or secondary PPH:
- Primary PPH: blood loss in excess of 500 mL from the time of delivery for 24 hours.
- Secondary PPH: blood loss in excess of 500 mL from 24 hours post delivery up until 6 weeks postpartum.

There are ~500,000 maternal deaths worldwide every year. Up to 50% of these can be attributed to obstetric haemorrhage. The Confidential Enquiries into Maternal Deaths and Morbidity 2009–2012 report, published in 2014, showed a slight increase in overall mortality rate compared to the 2006–2008 report but this does not represent a significant increase in mortality (a rate of 0.49/100,000 maternities in 2009–2012 cf. 0.39/100,000 in 2006 to 2008). However, it means that obstetric haemorrhage is the third leading cause of direct maternal death.

Risk factors
- Previous PPH
- Antepartum haemorrhage
- Prolonged labour
- Augmented labour
- Multiple pregnancy
- Polyhydramnios
- Maternal obesity.

Causes
- Tone: uterine atony is the most prevalent cause of PPH.
- Trauma: this may be genital tract injury (cervical, vaginal tears, or episiotomy), uterine rupture, or traumatic bleeding encountered at CS (e.g. from angular extensions).
- Tissue: retained placenta/placental membranes.
- Coagulation failure: failure of appropriate clotting is a rarer cause of PPH than the above-mentioned causes, often the coagulation failure (i.e. DIC) can occur following massive bleeding from placental abruption, sepsis, or pre-eclampsia. Hereditary coagulopathies must also be taken into account.
- Infection: this is the commonest cause of secondary PPH. Retained products of conception can be the focus of infection and should be excluded.

Prevention

- The list of risk factors given earlier is by no means complete. Risk factors (both antenatal and intrapartum) need to be identified and taken into consideration when formulating care plans (place of birth, IV access, G&S, etc.).
- Active management of the third stage of labour reduces maternal blood loss and therefore reduces the risk of PPH.
- Prophylactic oxytocics reduce the risk of PPH by 60% and should be offered routinely for management of the third stage.

Management and resuscitation

- Management involves early recognition and prompt diagnosis, maternal resuscitation to correct haemodynamic instability, and identification and treatment of the underlying cause.
- In massive obstetric haemorrhage (>1500 mL), a multidisciplinary approach is essential, including a senior obstetrician, anaesthetist, and haematologist.
- Effective management requires the presence of auxiliary staff such as porters, healthcare assistants, receptionists, and theatre staff.
- An initial assessment of the degree of blood loss and haemodynamically instability is vital, and efforts should be made to ensure that blood loss is not underestimated.
- Resuscitation involves the ABC approach.

Pharmacological management

- Oxytocin 5–10 IU IM bolus (if not given at delivery).
- Oxytocin infusion 40 IU in 500 mL N/saline at a rate of 125 mL/hour (10 IU/hour).
- Ergometrine 0.5mg IM or IV (contraindicated in hypertension).
- Misoprostol PR 800–1000 mcg can be administered rectally: 4 or 5 tablets.
- Carboprost 250 mcg IM can be given every 15 minutes up to a maximum of 8 doses (2 mg). Contraindicated in asthma.

If bleeding is persisting, approaching 1000–1500 mL, or not settling with initial uterotonics, then transfer to theatre is the most appropriate course of action. The most senior obstetrician available should be present.

Surgical management

- Examination under anaesthesia (EUA): this should take place to assess the genital tract for tears (vagina and cervix). The uterine cavity should also be explored to exclude retained tissue.
- Direct uterine massage: this is an extension of bimanual compression which enables direct myometrial compression.
- Uterine packing/tamponade: an effective method to control haemorrhage, using a Sengstaken or Bakri balloon. The balloon is instilled with up to 500 mL of warm saline to act as an intrauterine tamponade, which may arrest bleeding. If bleeding persists, then laparotomy would be the next step.

- Compression sutures: the B-lynch technique envelopes and compresses the uterus to arrest bleeding. If manual compression is of value, then compression sutures should be performed.
- Pelvic devascularization: ligation of blood vessels that supply the uterus. This would commence with ligation of the uterine arteries followed by tubal branches of both ovarian arteries. Internal iliac ligation would be the next step, although this would have to be performed by a senior surgeon.
- Uterine artery catheterization: this requires input from interventional radiologists. The need for specialized equipment and the availability of radiologists able to perform this preclude its widespread use.
- Hysterectomy: this should be the last resort, as a life-saving procedure, only performed when all other conservative measures have failed.

Fluids and blood products

- Replacing lost fluid and blood is an essential part of resuscitation. Replacement of blood and clotting factors is important to restore the oxygen capacity and prevent further haemorrhage by loss of coagulation factors (i.e. DIC).
- Crystalloid: up to 2 L of Hartmann's.
- Colloid: up to 1–2 L of colloid until blood is available.
- Blood: this should ideally be cross-matched. If cross-matched blood is not available, give unmatched group-specific blood or O Rh-negative blood.
- Fresh frozen plasma: 4 units with every 6 units of red cells or if the prothrombin time/activated partial thromboplastin time is >1.5 × normal value.
- Platelet concentrate: if platelet count is <50 × 10^9/L.
- Cryoprecipitate: if fibrinogen is <1 g/L.
- Patients require HDU level care following PPH (especially >1500 mL):
  - senior input from obstetrics/anaesthetics/haematology
  - observe for ongoing bleeding/heavy lochia, abdominal wounds, drains
  - 15-minute observations
  - accurate fluid balance charts, hourly urine output measurement
  - CVP monitoring
  - arterial line.
- Patients and staff involved must be fully debriefed by the most senior obstetrician attending, at the earliest available opportunity.
- Documentation should include the following:
  - staff attending and timing of arrival
  - timings and sequence of administration of the pharmacological agents used
  - timings of surgical intervention where relevant
  - maternal condition and observations throughout
  - timing of fluid and blood products given.

- The mnemonic HAEMOSTASIS can be used as a stepwise algorithm for the management of atonic PPH:
  - H: Ask for Help and Hands on the uterus (uterine massage)
  - A: Assess and resuscitate (vital signs, IV fluids, blood and blood products to restore the oxygen-carrying capacity)
  - E: Establish aetiology, ensure the availability of uterotonics, empty the bladder (catheterize)
  - M: Massage uterus
  - O: Oxytocics—oxytocin infusion/prostaglandins—IV/IM/PR/ intramyometrial
  - S: Shift to theatre—bimanual compression, aortic pressure or anti-shock garment
  - T: Tamponade balloon/uterine packing—after exclusion/ management of tissue/trauma
  - A: Apply compression sutures—modified B-Lynch compression sutures
  - S: Systemic pelvic devascularization—uterine/ovarian/internal iliac vessels
  - I: Interventional radiology. If appropriate, uterine artery embolization can be performed
  - S: Subtotal/total hysterectomy.

Further reading

Chandraharan E, Arulkumaran S. Surgical aspects of postpartum haemorrhage. *Best Pract Res Clin Obstet Gynaecol* 2008; 22(6):1089–102.

Doumouchtsis S, Papageorghiou A, Arulkumaran S. Systematic review of conservative management of postpartum haemorrhage: what to do if medical treatment fails. *Obstet Gynecol Surv* 2007; 62(8):540–7.

Knight M, Kenyon S, Brocklehurst P, et al. Saving Lives, Improving Mothers' Care – Lessons Learned to Inform Future Maternity Care from the UK and Ireland Confidential Enquiries into Maternal Deaths and Morbidity 2009–12. Oxford: National Perinatal Epidemiology Unit, University of Oxford; 2014.

Mishra N, Chandraharan E. Best practice in labour and delivery. In Warren R, Arulkumaran S (eds) *Postpartum Haemorrhage*, pp.160–70. Cambridge: Cambridge University Press, 2009.

Moore J, Chandraharan E. Management of massive postpartum haemorrhage and coagulopathy. *Obs Gynaecol Reprod Med* 2010; 20(6):174–80.

Royal College of Obstetricians and Gynaecologists. *Prevention and Management of Postpartum Haemorrhage*. Green-top Guideline No. 52. London: RCOG, 2009.

:O: Vaginal and perineal lacerations

More than 85% of women sustain perineal trauma after vaginal delivery and up to two-thirds of these women will require suturing. Perineal trauma may occur either spontaneously during vaginal birth or a surgical incision (episiotomy) is intentionally made to enlarge the diameter of the vaginal outlet. It is also possible to have a spontaneous tear in addition to an episiotomy. The episiotomy incision begins at the posterior fourchette and may be mediolateral (incision directed laterally to avoid the anal sphincter) or midline (directed vertically towards but not including the anus). Although the midline episiotomy is associated with less bleeding, less pain, and better healing, it is more likely to extend and involve the anal sphincter. Midline episiotomies are preferred in North America and mediolateral episiotomies are preferred in Europe.

Perineal lacerations are classified as follows:[1,2]

- First degree: laceration of the vaginal epithelium or perineal skin only.
- Second degree: involvement of the perineal muscles but not the anal sphincter.
- Third degree: disruption of the anal sphincter muscles which should be further subdivided into:
  - 3a: <50% thickness of external sphincter torn
  - 3b: >50% thickness of external sphincter torn
  - 3c: internal sphincter also torn.
- Fourth degree: a third-degree tear with disruption of the anal epithelium.

It is also possible to get an isolated laceration of the rectal mucosa (buttonhole) without involvement of the anal sphincter.

Aetiology

- Normal vaginal delivery
- Instrumental delivery
- Shoulder dystocia
- Malpresentation and malposition
- Big baby.

Diagnosis

Symptoms
- Bleeding
- Pain.

Signs
- Anaemia or shock may occur with severe PPH or haematoma.
- Perineal tears may be associated with involvement of the anal sphincter (third- or fourth-degree tears).
- Fever may develop if infection develops.

Management

- Manage shock.
- Perform rectal examination to exclude anal sphincter involvement.
- Vaginal examination to establish extent of tear.
- Ensure adequate analgesia (top-up epidural or inject local anaesthetic).
- First-degree tears may not need suturing unless associated with bleeding.
- It is recommended that all second-degree tears should be sutured unless it is the explicit wish of the woman to the contrary.
- If multiple lacerations are present, each laceration should be repaired individually ensuring anatomical and cosmetic restoration.
- Repair of a second-degree tear (including episiotomy) is performed in layers approximating the vaginal epithelium and perineal muscles using a continuous, non-locking method and subcuticular suturing of skin. Vicryl Rapide™ is associated with less perineal pain and need for suture removal.[1,3] Rectal examination should be performed after repair to check for inadvertent insertion of sutures through the anal epithelium.
- All third- and fourth-degree tears must be repaired in the operating theatre under regional or general anaesthesia.[2-4] If torn, the anal epithelium is repaired with interrupted 3-0 Vicryl™ sutures with the knots tied in the anal canal. The internal anal sphincter is approximated using mattress sutures with 3-0 PDS® sutures. The external sphincter can be repaired by the end-to-end or overlap technique using 3-0 PDS® sutures. The perineal body should be reconstructed in the same manner as described for second-degree tears.
- All women with third- and fourth-degree tears should be prescribed antibiotics as a single IV dose intraoperatively, followed by 7 days of oral antibiotics. Laxatives should be prescribed for 7–14 days. Hospital follow-up is essential in order to screen for bladder, bowel, and vaginal symptoms, as well as debrief the patient and provide advice for subsequent pregnancies.

Prevention

- Restrictive rather than liberal use of episiotomy
- Mediolateral rather than midline episiotomy
- Vacuum extraction is preferable to forceps
- Antenatal perineal massage can be beneficial.

References

1. Royal College of Obstetricians and Gynaecologists. *Methods and Materials Used in Perineal Repair*. Green-top Guideline No. 23. London: RCOG Press, 2004.
2. Royal College of Obstetricians and Gynaecologists. *The Management of Third- and Fourth-Degree Perineal Tears*. Green-top Guideline No. 29. London: RCOG Press, 2015.
3. Fernando R, Sultan A, Kettle C, et al. Method of repair for obstetric anal sphincter injuries. *Cochrane Database Syst Rev* 2006; 3:CD002866.
4. Thakar R, Sultan AH. Management of obstetric anal sphincter injuries. *Obstetrician and Gynaecologist* 2003; 5:31–9.

☠ Uterine inversion

Uterine inversion is a complication of the third stage of labour, whereby after delivery of the fetus, the uterus is partially (the fundus, though inverted, does not herniate through the cervix) or completely inverted and protrudes through the cervix, in or outside the vagina.

Uterine inversion can be classified by severity in four degrees:

- First-degree (incomplete) inversion involves extension of the inverted fundus to the cervical ring.
- In second-degree (incomplete) inversion, the fundus protrudes through the cervical ring but the inverted uterus remains within the vagina.
- In third-degree (complete) inversion, the inverted fundus extends to the introitus.
- Fourth-degree inversion is a total inversion where the vagina is also inverted.

Puerperal uterine inversion can occur after a vaginal delivery or CS. It can be acute (<24 hours postpartum), subacute (>24 hours postpartum), or chronic (> 1 month postpartum). Chronic, non-puerperal uterine inversions may rarely occur and are usually associated with uterine tumours.

The incidence of uterine inversion varies widely from 1:2000 to 1:50,000 deliveries depending upon the management of the third stage of labour. It is more likely to occur in primiparous patients and when there is a fundal placenta, morbidly adherent placenta, uterine abnormalities, and/or short cord.

Aetiology

- Most commonly it occurs due to mismanagement of the third stage involving fundal pressure and/or excessive cord traction performed before placental separation. Downward traction on the fundus, usually in combination with uterine atony, may result in partial or complete uterine inversion.
- Too rapid withdrawal of the placenta during manual removal or at CS.
- It may also occur without mismanagement of the third stage when there is a sudden rise in intra-abdominal pressure when the uterus is relaxed, e.g. coughing or vomiting.
- A short umbilical cord, fundal implantation of the placenta, morbidly adherent placenta, and uterine anomalies are contributing factors.

Diagnosis

Symptoms

- Severe lower abdominal pain
- Bleeding per vagina.

Signs

- Placenta may or may not be *in situ*
- Shock out of proportion to blood loss due to increased vagal tone
- Haemorrhage, present in 94% of cases
- Uterine fundus not palpable per abdomen (in incomplete cases there may be a dimple in the fundal area)
- Pelvic examination showing a mass in the vagina or outside the introitus.

Management

- *Help*: assistance, including an experienced obstetrician, an anaesthetist, and a senior midwife is summoned immediately. The blood bank should be notified urgently and blood and blood products requested.
- *Manage shock*: early recognition, rapid, systematic assessment, and simultaneous initiation of resuscitation with aggressive fluid and blood replacement are essential. The level of consciousness should be ascertained and airway maintained. Continuous monitoring of blood pressure, pulse, respiratory rate, oxygen saturation, and urine output is mandatory. Oxygen administration should be commenced. Two wide-bore IV cannulae are inserted to enable fluid resuscitation and blood transfusion. Blood samples are sent for urgent FBC, crossmatch of 4–6 units, and clotting screen. IV crystalloid infusion is commenced. If the patient is in shock with bradycardia, IV atropine is administered. Oxytocin infusion should be stopped until the uterus is replaced. At the same time, appropriate analgesia is administered and preparations are made for transfer to theatre.
- *Attempt to reposition the uterus*: the earlier the repositioning the more likely the success.[1] Delay in replacement of the uterus is associated with formation of a cervical ring and increasing oedema and congestion of the uterus. Do not attempt to remove the placenta if still attached to the uterus. Immediate non-surgical techniques are successful in most cases. The uterine fundus can be replaced manually or by hydrostatic pressure.

Techniques to replace the uterus

Manual replacement (the Johnson manoeuvre)

Manual replacement of the uterus is preferable under general anaesthesia as it requires the uterus to be relaxed. Tocolytic drugs (e.g. magnesium sulfate, ritodrine, terbutaline) may be used to relax the cervical ring to facilitate replacement.[2]

The technique for replacement of the uterus is to cup the fundus in the palm of the hand, with the fingertips at the junction of the cervix and the corpus, and lift the entire uterus out of the pelvis towards the umbilicus. This position is maintained for a few minutes until firm contraction of the uterus occurs. If the placenta is not delivered it is removed manually at this stage.

Hydrostatic repositioning (O'Sullivan technique)

- Ensure that there are no tears in the vagina, cervix, or uterus. Infuse warm saline into the vagina (via a rubber tube held 1–2m above the patient) while the vagina is blocked by the assistant.[3] As the vaginal vault is distended with fluid, the fornices are ballooned and stretched, pulling on the constricting cervical ring and facilitating spontaneous reduction of the uterus. Alternatively an IV giving set can be attached to a silicone Ventouse cup inserted in the vagina, which can produce a better seal.[3]
- Surgical management: this is attempted if conservative treatment fails. It involves performing a laparotomy and the uterus is repositioned by the following techniques:

- *Huntington's technique:* Allis forceps are placed within the dimple of the inverted uterus. Gentle traction is applied on the clamps with further placement of forceps on the advancing fundus
- *Haultain's technique:* this involves incising the cervical ring posteriorly with a longitudinal incision. This facilitates enlargement of the constricted cervical ring and replacement of the uterus. The incision is sutured. After repositioning the uterus, oxytocics should be administered to prevent recurrence.

Prevention

Avoid mismanagement of third stage. Cord traction should not be applied until signs of placental separation appear, i.e. trickle of blood at introitus, lengthening of the cord, and globular, hard contracted uterus on palpation.

References

1. Watson P, Besch N, Bowes WA. Management of acute and subacute puerperal inversion of the uterus. *Obstet Gynecol* 1980; 55:12–16.
2. Johnston R, Cox C. Uterine inversion. In Johanson R, Cox C, Grady K, *et al.* (eds) *Managing Obstetric Emergencies and Trauma: The MOET Course Manual*, pp.183–4. London: RCOG Press, 2002.
3. O'Sullivan J. Acute inversion of the uterus. *BMJ* 1945; 2:282–3.

Further reading

Baskett TF. Acute uterine inversion: a review of 40 cases. *J Obstet Gynaecol Can* 2002; 24(12):953–6.

Bhalla R, Wuntakal R, Odejinmi F, *et al.* Acute inversion of the uterus. *Obstetrician and Gynaecologist* 2009; 11:13–18.

Brar HS, Greenspoon JS, Platt LD, *et al.* Acute puerperal uterine inversion. New approaches to management. *J Reprod Med* 1989; 34(2):173–7.

Calder AA. Emergencies in operative obstetrics. *Baillieres Best Pract Res Clin Obstet Gynaecol* 2000; 14(1):43–55.

Livingston SL, Booker C, Kramer P, *et al.* Chronic uterine inversion at 14 weeks postpartum. *Obstet Gynecol* 2007; 109(2 Pt2):555–7.

Paterson-Brown S. Obstetric emergencies. In Edmonds DK (ed) *Dewhurst's Textbook of Obstetrics and Gynaecology*, pp.145–58. Oxford: Blackwell Publishing, Inc., 2007.

Shamsudin F, Morton K. Novel correction technique of chronic puerperal inversion of the uterus. *J Obstet Gynaecol* 2007; 27(2):197–8.

Thomson AJ, Greer IA. Non-haemorrhagic obstetric shock. *Baillieres Best Pract Res Clin Obstet Gynaecol* 2000; 14(1):19–41.

Vijayaraghavan R, Sujatha Y. Acute postpartum uterine inversion with haemorrhagic shock: laparoscopic reduction: a new method of management? *BJOG* 2006; 113(9):1100–2.

☼ Vulval/perineal haematoma

A haematoma may occur in the vulval/perineal and vaginal area either immediately following delivery or in the postpartum period. They occur infrequently, with an incidence of between 1:500 and 1:900 pregnancies.

Aetiology
- Frequently related to episiotomy.
- Risks factors include nulliparity, macrosomia, prolonged second stage, vulval varicosities, clotting disorders, and pre-eclampsia.
- Can occur despite delivery with intact perineum (~20%).

Diagnosis
Symptoms
- Pain in the perineal area.
- Swelling of the perineal area.
- Occasionally may present with shock in spite of no obvious swelling. This can occur when there is a paravaginal haematoma. The classical presentation is pain, restlessness, urinary retention, and rectal tenesmus a few hours after delivery.

Signs
- Tender swelling of the perineal area. Overlying skin may appear purple and glistening.
- Signs of shock depending on the amount and rate of blood loss.

Management
- Management of shock if present.
- Surgical evacuation by incision and drainage if the haematoma is large and expanding. Incision should preferably be made in the vagina to avoid scar formation. Achieve haemostasis. Often no obvious bleeding points are seen. A large vulval haematoma may require a drain or pack *in situ*.
- Angiographic embolization can be considered when primary surgical management has failed.
- If small (i.e. <5 cm) and not expanding use ice-packs and pressure dressings.
- Appropriate analgesia.

Prevention
- The perineum should be carefully examined after delivery and in the immediate postpartum period.
- Episiotomy should be restrictive.

Further reading
Carroli G, Mignini L. Episiotomy for vaginal birth. *Cochrane Database Syst Rev* 2009; 1:CD000081.
Mirza FG, Gaddipati S. Obstetric emergencies. *Semin Perinatol* 2009; 33(2):97–103.

:☼: Resuscitation of the newborn

Only 1–2% of newborns will require active resuscitation at delivery. The need for resuscitation is often unpredictable thus it is essential that all personnel who attend deliveries are able to methodically assess the baby, and provide initial neonatal resuscitation.[1–3]

Preparation

Examples of deliveries where babies may require resuscitation include:
- Emergency CS
- Instrumental deliveries
- Meconium-stained liquor
- Fetal distress
- Cord prolapse
- Breech deliveries
- Multiple births
- Preterm deliveries <37 weeks' gestation
- Infants of diabetic mothers
- Congenital abnormalities (antenatal diagnosis).

Equipment
Ideally prepare and check prior to the delivery:
- Resuscitaire with air/oxygen mix: turned on
- Heater: turned on
- Suction: checked with selection of catheter sizes
- Clock: set to zero
- Stethoscope
- Laryngoscope: two sizes, good light source
- Face masks: size 00, 0/1
- Pressure delivery system, usually T-piece set to 25–30 cm H_2O
- Resuscitation/Ambu bag: 500 mL
- Umbilical venous catheter and cord ties
- Drugs: see p. 175.

Assessment and action

Before assessment it is important to dry and cover the baby to prevent heat loss.

The ABC(D) of resuscitation are:
- **A**irway
- **B**reathing
- **C**irculation
- **D**rugs/volume.

Each step should take ~30 seconds.

Progression to next step is dependent on completion of previous step. See the newborn life support algorithm for a summary (Fig. 6.3).

1. At delivery:
- If concerned **CALL FOR HELP**.
- Start clock.
- Dry and wrap baby on resuscitaire.

Newborn Life Support

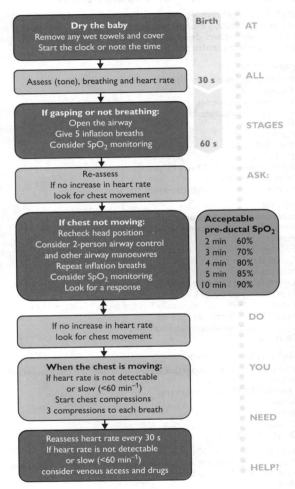

Fig. 6.3 Newborn life support. Reproduced with the kind permission of the Resuscitation Council (UK).

- Assess:
  - breathing—quality and quantity
  - heart rate—assess at apex with stethoscope or palpate at base of cord; assess as slow <60, adequate >100. If a pulse oximeter is readily available this is the most reliable way to assess heart rate and oxygen saturation following delivery[4]
  - colour—centrally pink, pale or cyanosed; peripheral cyanosis is common and unimportant if baby otherwise well
  - tone—active, reduced or floppy.
2. Obviously healthy: good respiratory effort and good heart rate, pink and active → dry and give to mother.
3. Poor respiratory effort or apnoea, good heart rate →
   - open airway by positioning head in neutral position (see Fig. 6.4a)
   - stimulate, by rubbing with towel

If no response proceed as below.
4. Poor respiratory effort or apnoea, slow heart rate, cyanosis, floppy → **CALL FOR HELP** if not already done so.

Airway

Before the baby can breathe the airway must be open:
- Open airway by positioning head in neutral position (see Fig. 6.4a).
- Most newborns have a prominent occiput causing head to flex—consider raising shoulders with shoulder support if on flat surface.
- If floppy may need a chin lift, jaw thrust (Fig. 6.4b), or Guedel airway.

Breathing

If the baby is not breathing
- Use face mask and T-piece or Ambu bag to administer **5 inflation breaths** at 30 cm H_2O for **2–3 seconds** using air.[5-7]
- Re-assess.
- Effective inflation indicated by an **increase in heart rate**.
- If no increase in heart rate **did the chest move** with inflation breaths?

If no increase in heart rate and no chest movement consider:
- Is head in neutral position (see Fig. 6.4a)?
- Jaw thrust—open airway by positioning fingers behind angle of jaw and push jaw forward (see Fig. 6.4b).
- Two-person jaw thrust with one operator holding face mask with two hands whilst second operator provides intermittent positive pressure ventilation.
- Guedel airway.
- Do you need a longer inflation time and/or higher inflation pressure?
- Is airway blocked? Observe under direct vision and, if indicated, suction under direct vision at 8–12 kPa (60–100 mmHg) negative pressure.

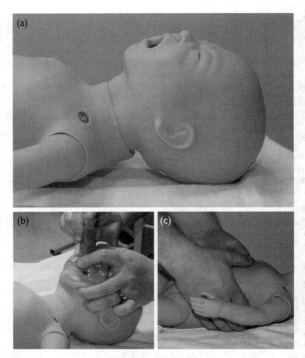

Fig. 6.4 (a) Neutral position. Newborn babies have a prominent occiput and thus adopt a flexed head posture when prone. (b) Ventilation breaths with single person jaw thrust and face mask in place. (c) Position of hands for cardiac compressions.

If inflation breaths are effective, but no spontaneous respiration
- Continue with 1-second ventilation breaths at 30–60/minute; use appropriate pressure to give effective chest movement, this is usually lower than inflation breaths, e.g. 20–25 cm H_2O for term baby.
- Proceed to endotracheal intubation only if you are experienced. Most babies can be ventilated for the initial resuscitation with facemask intermittent positive-pressure ventilation (IPPV) as long as the chest movement is good.

Reassess after 30 sec of effective ventilation breaths.

Circulation

Do not proceed to cardiac compressions until effective ventilation with adequate chest movement is achieved.

The commonest cause of slow heart rate is ineffective lung inflation. If heart rate remains slow despite adequate ventilation:
- Provide chest compressions by:
  - encircling chest with both hands, placing thumbs over lower third of sternum and fingers around back of chest (see Fig. 6.4c), or
  - two-finger technique—place index and middle finger over lower third of sternum.
- Depress lower third of sternum by depth of 1/3 or 2–3 cm for term baby.
- Provide three compressions to one effective ventilation at ratio of 3:1 or 30 cycles/minute (120 events/minute).

Reassess after 30 seconds.

Drugs

If heart rate remains slow, <60 bpm, despite effective lung inflations and cardiac compressions, gain IV access via catheterization of umbilical vein or peripheral venous access. Administer:

Adrenaline (epinephrine)
- 0.1 mL/kg 1:10,000 IV stat followed by 2–3 mL saline flush.
- Continue CPR.
- Repeat adrenaline every 3 minutes.
- Try 0.3 mL/kg if third dose necessary.
- If no IV access, first dose can be given via endotracheal tube but higher doses of 0.5–1.0 mL/kg 1:10,000 should be given.

Sodium bicarbonate
Administer 2–4 mL/kg 4.2% $NaHCO_3$ followed by 2–3 mL saline flush.

Glucose
2–3 mL/kg 10% glucose followed by 2–3 mL saline flush.

Volume
If evidence of hypovolaemia, especially acute blood loss, give 10–20 mL/kg of 0.9% saline, or O Rh-negative blood.

When to stop resuscitation

In a newborn baby with no cardiac activity, and with cardiac activity that remains undetectable after 10 minutes, it is appropriate to consider stopping resuscitation.[2] Ideally a senior paediatrician should be involved in this decision.

Post resuscitation

- Cord gas: arterial cord pH and base deficit should be measured and documented in all cases where there has been fetal distress or neonatal resuscitation.
- Documentation: needs to be full, logical, and clear with a legible signature.

Special considerations

1. Temperature
- Overheating is linked to adverse outcome and should be avoided.[8]
- Preterm babies: hypothermia increases adverse outcomes[9] and exacerbates acidosis, hypoxia, and RDS. There is good evidence that placing babies in an occlusive wrap or clear polythene bag prevents heat loss in babies <28 weeks,[10] and many units are doing this for babies <30 weeks.

2. Premature babies ≤35 weeks
If possible, anticipate delivery, allowing time for senior staff to be present and to communicate with parents outlining the prognosis and discussing the parents' wishes.

ABC assessment and action should proceed as for term babies with the following precautions:
- Temperature—see point 1, 'Temperature'.
- Lower pressure is usually required for inflation breaths, e.g. 20–25 cmH$_2$O; once functional residual capacity and effective chest movement is established, the pressure should be reduced to maintain adequate, not overenthusiastic chest movement—try 15–20 cmH$_2$O.
- Babies with severe RDS may need higher pressure for inflation breaths e.g. 30 cmH$_2$O.
- Babies requiring intubation <30 weeks should receive surfactant as soon as possible by a skilled operator. This is often administered in the labour ward.
- Do not give adrenaline under 27 weeks.
- Continuous positive airway pressure (CPAP): many premature babies, including some extremely preterm babies may not need intubation in the labour ward. There is evidence that CPAP commenced at birth, is safe and effective.[11]

3. Extremely premature babies 23–24 weeks—at the margins of viability
- <23 weeks:
  - standard practice should be not to resuscitate.[12]
- 23^{+0}–23^{+6} weeks:
  - anticipate delivery to allow senior staff to attend and appropriate communication
  - if baby has spontaneous respiration and HR >60 resuscitation with endotracheal intubation may be initiated; if the baby does not improve and the HR remains absent or very low at 10 minutes then further resuscitation should be withheld. Do not give adrenaline
  - if the baby is in poor condition with poor/absent respiration, low/absent HR, often with extensive bruising, it may be kinder not to attempt resuscitation and to give the baby to the mother
- 24–26 weeks:
  - these babies should be resuscitated but the same principles apply
  - commence ABC resuscitation as described earlier
  - stop resuscitation if poor response at 10 minutes
  - do not give adrenaline.

4. Meconium-stained liquor

Perineal suction and routine tracheal intubation for suction have been shown to be of no benefit.[9,10]

Assessment and action:
- Good respiratory effort and pink:
  - dry and give to mother
  - observe as inpatient for 24 hours.
- Poor respiratory effort:
  - **CALL FOR HELP**
  - assess airway under direct vision; if meconium present then suction under direct vision with a large-bore catheter (e.g. size 10 or above) at 8–12 kPa (60–100 mmHg) until airway patent. Withdraw catheter as suction applied
  - repeat if meconium still in airway
  - once meconium removed, if respiration ineffective then further appropriate ABC management should be initiated
  - trainees are sometimes incorrectly concerned with how long they should suction for before commencing facial IPPV; once airway patency has been established with suction under direct vision, then inflation breaths should be given with further ABC resuscitation as necessary
  - babies requiring extensive resuscitation need admission to NICU
  - babies who are well after resuscitation should stay with their mother but must be reviewed at 1 hour of age and at regular intervals for 24 hours. Any concerns, particularly tachypnoea with respiratory rate >60 bpm, should be reported to a paediatrician immediately.

5. Air versus O_2 for resuscitation

Recent evidence has demonstrated increased adverse outcome in babies resuscitated with 100% O_2 compared to those resuscitated with air alone.[11] The safest O_2 concentration to use for resuscitation has not been established and it is certainly possible to achieve successful resuscitation with air alone. Current UK resuscitation guidance is to commence resuscitation with room air, and only add O_2 if the baby is failing to respond despite good chest movement.

Poor response to resuscitation

Consider DOPE:
- **D**isplaced tube (e.g. in oesophagus or right main bronchus)
- **O**bstructed tube
- **P**neumothorax—transilluminate or observe for hyperinflation of affected side
- **E**quipment failure:
  - are air or O_2 supplies depleted or disconnected?
  - is pressure setting on T-piece too low or malfunctioning?

other causes:
- maternal opiates
- congenital diaphragmatic hernia—scaphoid abdomen
- severe asphyxia—review history
- severe anaemia—review history and check haematocrit or packed cell volume (beware: values may be high if recent haemorrhage).

References

1. Wyllie J, Richmond S. *The Resuscitation Guidelines 2010*, Chapter 11. 2010. [Online] <http://www.resus.org.uk/pages/nls.pdf>
2. Perlman JM, Wyllie J, Kattwinkel J, *et al.* Part 11: Neonatal Resuscitation: 2010 International Consensus on Cardiopulmonary Resuscitation and Emergency Cardiovascular Care Science With Treatment Recommendations. *Circulation* 2010; 122:S516–S538.
3. Richmond S, Wyllie J. European Resuscitation Council Guidelines for Resuscitation 2010, Section 7. Resuscitation of babies at birth. *Resuscitation* 2010; 81:1389–99.
4. Kamlin COF, Dawson JA, O'Donnell CP, *et al.* Accuracy of pulse oximetry measurement of heart rate of newborn infants in the delivery room. *J Pediatr* 2008; 152:756–60.
5. Davis PG, Tan A, O'Donnell CPF, *et al.* Resuscitation of newborn infants with 100% oxygen or air: a systematic review and meta-analysis. *Lancet* 2004; 364:1329–33.
6. Rabi Y, Rabi D, Yee W. Room air resuscitation of the depressed newborn: a systematic review and meta-analysis. *Resuscitation* 2007; 72:353–63.
7. Saugstad OD, Ramji S, Vento M. Resuscitation of depressed newborn infants with ambient air or pure oxygen: a meta-analysis. *Biol Neonate* 2005; 87:27–34.
8. Petrova A, Demissie K, Rhoads GG, *et al.* Association of maternal fever during labor with neonatal and infant morbidity and mortality. *Obstet Gynecol* 2001; 98:20–7.
9. Acolet D, Elbourne D, McIntosh N, *et al.* Project 27/28: inquiry into quality of neonatal care and its effect on the survival of infants who were born at 27 and 28 weeks in England, Wales, and Northern Ireland. *Pediatrics* 2005; 116:1457–65.
10. Vohra S, Roberts RS, Zhang B, *et al.* Heat Loss Prevention (HeLP) in the delivery room: a randomized controlled trial of polyethylene occlusive skin wrapping in very preterm infants. *J Pediatr* 2004; 145:750–3.
11. Morley CJ, Davis PG, Doyle LW, *et al.* Nasal CPAP or intubation at birth for very preterm infants. *N Engl J Med* 2008; 358:700–8.
12. Wilkinson AR, Ahluwalia J, Cole A, *et al.* Management of babies born extremely preterm at less than 26 weeks of gestation: a framework for clinical practice at the time of birth. *Arch Dis Child Fetal Neonatal Ed* 2009; 94:2–5.

Further reading

Resuscitation Council (UK). *Resuscitation at Birth: Newborn Life Support Course Manual*. London: Resuscitation Council (UK), 2010.

Sepsis in pregnancy

Contributors
Stergios K. Doumouchtsis and Austin Ugwumadu

Contents

Maternal sepsis

The onset of maternal sepsis may be insidious. Obstetric patients who are young, fit, and healthy compensate well, but may deteriorate rapidly. The signs and symptoms may be non-specific. Early diagnosis and treatment is essential in order to prevent septic shock and severe maternal morbidity and mortality.

Causes
- Chorioamnionitis
- Postpartum endometritis
- Pyelonephritis
- Wound infection
- Others including peritonitis, pneumonia, cellulitis, and pancreatitis.

Organisms frequently identified in women with maternal sepsis
- Group A streptococci
- Group B streptococci
- *Ureaplasma urealyticum*
- *Mycoplasma hominis*
- *Staphylococcus aureus*
- *Escherichia coli*
- Proteus species
- Klebsiella species
- Bacteroides species
- *Gardnerella vaginalis*
- *Neisseria gonorrhoeae*
- *Chlamydia trachomatis*.

Risk factors
Delivery conditions
- Prolonged rupture of membranes
- Postpartum haemorrhage
- Multiple vaginal examinations
- Caesarean delivery
- Prolonged labour.

Maternal conditions
- Nulliparity
- Anaemia (due to poor nutrition, sickle cell, thalassemia)
- Obesity
- Impaired glucose metabolism and diabetes mellitus
- Impaired immunity
- Invasive procedures
- Infections:
  - HIV/AIDS
  - pelvic infections.

Symptoms

- Uterine tenderness:
  - before delivery: chorioamnionitis
  - after delivery: endometritis
- Constant severe abdominal pain
- Vaginal discharge
- Nausea vomiting diarrhoea
- Generalized rash:—suspect toxic shock syndrome
- Conjunctival suffusion: suspect toxic shock syndrome.

Signs

- Hypothermia (<35.0°C)
- Pyrexia (>38.0°C once, or 37.5°C on two occasions 2 hours apart):
  - normal temperature does not exclude sepsis
  - swinging pyrexia—may indicate a persistent focus of infection and warrants investigation
- Hypoxia (< 90% saturation on room air)
- Hypotension (systolic BP < 90 mmHg)
- Oliguria (<0.5 cc/kg/hr)
- Tachycardia (> 100 bpm; >90 bpm in puerperium): differential diagnosis includes VTE, or an underlying cardiac condition
- Tachypnoea (respiratory rate > 20/min): exclude other pathologies including VTE, amniotic fluid embolism, pulmonary oedema, and pneumonia
- Impaired consciousness
- Leucocytosis (white blood cell (WBC) counts < 2.0 × 10^9/L; > 12.0 × 10^9/L or < 2000/mm^3; > 12 000/mm^3):
  - leucopenia (often an indicator of worsening sepsis)
- DIC/abnormal clotting
- Failure to respond to treatment
- Fetal: fetal heart beat abnormality or intrauterine death.

Investigations

- Blood cultures
- FBC (leucocytosis or low WBC counts are concerning, but during pregnancy the WBC count may reach 15,000 and up to 20,000 during labour)
- Biochemistry:
  - U&Es (raised blood sugar in the absence of diabetes also points to sepsis)
  - LFTs
  - Inflammatory markers—CRP
  - Serum lactate:
    - check within 6 hours of suspicion of sepsis
    - >4 mmol/L indicates tissue hypoxia
  - lactate dehydrogenase (LDH)
  - Amylase

- Radiology:
  - Pelvic US (for pelvic collection or retained products of conception)
  - Chest X-rays
  - US or CT scan abdomen
- Urine cultures
- Stool cultures
- Swabs:
  - vagina
  - throat
  - wound
  - other
- For women who develop signs or symptoms of infection during labour or delivery:
  - swabs from placenta, baby, and vagina
  - placenta histology and microbiology
  - lumbar puncture (if appropriate).

Management

- Fluid resuscitation
- IV broad-spectrum antibiotics
- Electronic fetal monitoring
- Avoidance of epidural and NSAIDs
- Modified Early Warning Score (MEWS)
- Consider central monitoring
- Expedite delivery if intrauterine infection is suspected
- Consider steroids to enhance fetal lung maturity if preterm and delivery is imminent:
  - women with severe sepsis or septic shock warrant broad-spectrum therapy until the causative organism and its antibiotic sensitivities have been defined
  - duration of therapy should be typically 7–10 days; longer courses may be appropriate depending on clinical response
  - advice should be sought from a consultant microbiologist as soon as possible
  - the following broad-spectrum IV antibiotic regimens are common options for genital tract sepsis:
    - co-amoxiclav 1.2 g 8-hourly plus metronidazole 500 mg 8-hourly or
    - cefuroxime 1.5 g 8-hourly plus metronidazole 500 mg 8-hourly or
    - cefotaxime 1–2 g 6- to 12-hourly plus metronidazole 500 mg 8-hourly
    - In cases of allergy, clarithromycin (500 mg twice daily) or clindamycin (600 mg to 1.2 g by IV infusion three or four times daily) plus gentamicin for Gram-negative bacteria are alternatives.

:O: Postpartum infections

Background

Puerperal sepsis is a polymicrobial condition, which occurs in a small minority of women, suggesting that the pathogenesis involves more than just a source of potentially pathogenic bacteria. As pregnancy progresses, there is a 10-fold increase in the population of protective *Lactobacillus* species and a progressive decline in the number of potentially pathogenic anaerobes including *Prevotella bivia*, *Bacteroides* species, peptococci, peptostreptococci, and *Escherichia coli*, a possible adaptation of the genital tract flora designed to protect the fetus from exposure to harmful bacteria at the time of birth. By the third postpartum day, and regardless of the mode of delivery, the numbers of anaerobic organisms rise again to levels higher than in the antenatal period. This latter rise is believed to be due to a combination of withdrawal of trophic hormone support from the genital tract and the presence of lochia and necrotic decidua all of which conspire to set the scene for postpartum infections.

Endometritis

Endometritis is the commonest puerperal infection and usually presents within 5 days of delivery.

Risk factors

- CS (27% vs 1.2% in women who had vaginal delivery)
- Multiple vaginal examinations during labour
- Prolonged rupture of membranes
- Use and duration of internal monitoring devices
- Prolonged labour
- Group B streptococcal colonization
- Anaemia, diabetes mellitus, obesity.

Diagnosis

Criteria for diagnosis include fever, chills and rigors, uterine tenderness, abdominal pain, purulent or foul smelling lochia, leucocytosis, and exclusion of another focus of infection. There may be tachycardia. Localizing signs may be absent if the infection is due to group A or B streptococci.
   Obtain cervical and vaginal samples for culture.

Treatment

If febrile and unwell—IV broad-spectrum antibiotics with anaerobic cover, e.g. cephalosporin or clindamycin and gentamicin. Once the woman becomes afebrile for 24 hours the antibiotic therapy should be discontinued. There is no need for additional oral treatment.

Septic pelvic thrombophlebitis

This is thought to be due to bacterial injury to the pelvic (ovarian) venous endothelium. The diagnosis should be considered in any patient with a persistent temperature despite appropriate antibiotic therapy and prior soft tissue pelvic infection.

Clinical features
- Persistent fevers may be the only presenting sign.
- Progressively worsening abdominal pain usually right > left.
- Nausea, vomiting, or abdominal distension may be present.
- Bowel sounds may be normoactive or absent.
- Tachycardia.
- Tachypnoea and respiratory distress if pulmonary embolus has occurred.
- The thrombosed ovarian vein (usually right) may be palpable as an abdominal or adnexal mass.

Investigations
- US scan
- CT scan.

Treatment
- Broad-spectrum antibiotic therapy.
- Anticoagulation with heparin was a traditional adjunct to therapy but this is no longer recommended.
- Surgical ligation/excision of the affected vein is reserved for patients with acute abdomen or not responding to medical therapy.

Urinary tract infection

This is a common cause of postpartum pyrexia and is usually caused by *E. coli* although enterococci, group B streptococci, and other Gram-negative aerobic bacilli may be responsible occasionally. Symptoms include dysuria, frequency, nocturia, fever, and backache. Physical examination may reveal tenderness in the renal angles. A clean-catch midstream specimen of urine for culture is helpful in diagnosis. Sterile pyuria may reflect bladder inflammation from trauma during labour and delivery.

Risk factors
- Physiologic hydroureter of pregnancy
- Asymptomatic bacteriuria
- Intra-partum catheterization.

Treatment
Parenteral cephalosporin and gentamicin initially until urine cultures and antibiotic sensitivities become available.

Mastitis and breast abscess

Staphylococcus aureus is the main causative agent of sporadic, epidemic, and endemic mastitis. Fever, malaise, and breast pain and tenderness are the usual presenting features. Breast abscess may develop in untreated cases. Beware that breast engorgement may produce signs and symptoms which are identical to infective mastitis.

Treatment
A penicillinase-resistant penicillin such as flucloxacillin or erythromycin should be administered. Other measures include breast support, ice packs, and analgesics. Breastfeeding should continue unless abscess develops.

Wound and episiotomy infections

Around 5–15% of CS wounds become infected depending on the definition of wound infection used. The presence of erythema, induration, pain, and fluid exudate are suggestive signs. If the wound breaks down, debridement and secondary closure is now recommended instead of the traditional approach of debridement and dressing, and allowing healing by secondary intention. Clinicians should maintain a high index of suspicion in order to recognize life-threatening wound complications such as necrotizing fasciitis, clostridial myonecrosis (gas gangrene), and nonclostridial bacterial synergistic gangrene (Meleney's gangrene).

A simple episiotomy infection usually presents with localized erythema, oedema, and exudate, which are limited to the surrounding skin and subcutaneous tissue. If the findings are more extensive, a deeper infection may be present. The wound should be opened, explored, drained, and debrided, and appropriate antibiotics administered. Most of these will heal by granulation but if perineal muscles or anal sphincter is involved, the wound should be re-sutured once the infection settles down, say in about 5–10 days. The patient should avoid sexual intercourse and have sitz baths three to four times daily.

Complications associated with complex psychosocial needs

Contributors

Joanna Bécares Doumouchtsi, Jonathan Dominguez-Hernandez, and Astrid Osbourne

Contents

Substance misuse in pregnancy

Introduction

Substance misuse involves the regular use of recreational drugs, over-the-counter medications, prescription medications, alcohol, or volatile substances (such as solvents or inhalants) to an extent where physical dependence or harm is a risk (to the woman and/or her unborn baby).[1]

Substance misuse, among other complex social factors, has been associated with an increased risk of maternal death and/or infant death in the perinatal period. Fifty-three (11%) of all the women whose deaths were assessed between 2006 and 2008, including coincidental and late causes, had problems relating to substance misuse.[2] Of these, 31 were known drug addicts, 16 were occasional users, and six women were solely alcohol dependent. Ten women were both drug and alcohol dependent. In England and Wales, there are 250,000–350,000 children affected by parental substance misuse.[3]

Commonly used drugs

- Cannabis ('hash' and marijuana)
- Stimulants (such as amphetamine, cocaine, and ecstasy)
- Hallucinogens (e.g. LSD and 'magic mushrooms')
- Opioids (e.g. heroin, methadone, dihydrocodeine, and buprenorphine)
- Benzodiazepines (e.g. diazepam and temazepam)
- Volatile substances (e.g. 'gas' and 'glue')
- Crystal methamphetamine
- Alcohol
- Tobacco
- Other drugs (such as cyclizine, ketamine, gamma hydroxybutyrate or 'GHB', 'poppers', steroids, and antidepressants).

Complications associated with substance misuse in pregnancy

- Blood-borne viruses
- Deep vein thrombosis
- Pulmonary embolism
- Bacterial endocarditis
- Venous leg ulcers
- Asthma
- Malnutrition and general poor health
- Chaotic lifestyle and indulging in risky behaviour
- Mental illness
- Domestic abuse
- Child protection issues.

Management

Principles of care
- Women-centred care should be provided.
- The woman should be treated as a healthy pregnant woman having a safe delivery of a healthy baby, only complicated by the

pharmacological effects of the substance misused on mother and baby and its implications on the woman's lifestyle and capacity to parent.
- The aim should be to improve maternal and neonatal outcome, minimizing the impact of substance abuse.
- Treatment and care should take into account women's individual needs and preferences.
- Management must be pragmatic, multidisciplinary, and confidential.
- The multidisciplinary team dedicated to care for pregnant women that misuse substances should include professionals with knowledge and skills needed for the optimal delivery of care.

Treatment options
- Ideally abstinence; however in pregnancy this may not be realistic.
- Stabilize on methadone (preferred option in the UK).
- Detoxification: usually in the second trimester, however could be at any gestation. Detoxification can be carried out at any stage during pregnancy provided that drug withdrawal is gradual and drug dosage whether prescribed or illicit does not fluctuate.
- Pregnant women should have priority into in-patient/community treatment at drug services, but only after assessment by a drug key worker.
- Should a woman request a reduction/detoxification of her drug treatment the specialist midwife and drug service must be contacted. In-patient treatment within the maternity services is not usually appropriate.
- Admission to maternity/gynaecology services may be indicated based on obstetric/gynaecological grounds and advice sought for the drug dependency from Drug Services at the earliest opportunity.
- After discussion with the prescribing agency, the agreed drugs should be prescribed on the prescription chart.
- Never initiate emergency treatment of drug misuse problems without obtaining specialist advice.

Antenatal care
Initial assessment
- Medical, obstetric, and psychosocial history
- Drugs: past and present
- Forensic history
- Blood tests and immunization.

The assessment of drug misuse should include:
- Smoking
- Alcohol
- Illicit drug use including 'over-the-counter' and prescribed medication
- Method of administration
- Partner's involvement and possible drug use
- Any contact with other services.

If parenting skills are to be assessed, this should be carried out by the appropriate agency by competent professionals, looking at what is needed rather than what should be done.

Suggested additional booking investigations
- Hepatitis C virus (HCV) antibodies
- HCV RNA
- CMV
- Toxoplasmosis
- Liver function test (LFT)
- Gamma glutamine transferase (G-GT)
- Urine toxicology with consent.

Suggested antenatal investigations
- 28 weeks: FBC, LFT, GTT, HCV RNA (if hepatitis C positive)
- 34 weeks: FBC, LFT, GTT, HCV RNA
- 37 weeks: HCV RNA (HIV if still engaging in at-risk activities)
- Fetal growth scans at 28 and 32 weeks.

Multidisciplinary team referrals/ liaison
- Specialist midwife, e.g. substance misuse/perinatal mental health/ child safeguarding
- Consultant paediatrician/neonatologist
- Family services and social work team
- Perinatal mental health team if there is any psychological or psychiatric history or concerns.

For referrals, consent should be gained. If there is an immediate risk of harm to a child, consent is *not* required for referral to family services and the social work team.

Recreational or occasional use
It is important to ascertain the difference between recreational use/ social use and drug dependence. A drugs worker or the specialist midwife in substance misuse is the most appropriate professional to carry out this assessment in the first instance.

Labour and delivery
On admission
- Established labour should be confirmed
- Urine specimen for drug toxicology screening
- The notes should be reviewed for details of:
  - substance abuse
  - alcohol use
  - evidence of IUGR
  - child protection issues (as outlined in the 'Social Alert' report).

The midwife in charge of the woman's care is responsible for informing the various agencies/departments of admission. These should include:
- Consultant obstetrician
- Midwife in charge of delivery suite
- Specialist midwives
- Allocated social worker (or duty social worker if out of normal working hours)
- Neonatal unit (NNU).

Care in labour
- The care in labour should be as normal.
- Analgesics should be given as required.
- There is no contraindication to an epidural. Poor venous access may be a complication. The woman may need a central line in the case of an emergency.
- Cyclizine should not be used as it can act as a stimulant.
- Invasive procedures; fetal blood sampling and a fetal scalp electrode, should be avoided if the woman is hepatitis C positive.
- The paediatrician should be present for delivery if there are any concerns with the baby (e.g. IUGR, meconium, history of illicit drug usage around the perinatal period).
- Naloxone should not be given to the baby for respiratory depression, because it causes rapid withdrawal symptoms in the baby.
- Before prescribing methadone, the prescriber must be familiar with the local policy.

Postnatal care
- Bonding between the mother and baby must be encouraged at delivery if appropriate.
- The baby may be admitted to the NNU for observations for withdrawal from opiates if necessary. However, the baby should not be taken immediately to the NNU unless medically indicated.
- On transfer to the postnatal ward, the relevant professionals should be informed (e.g. social worker and health visitor).
- The midwives on the postnatal ward and nurses on the NNU should promote, observe, and document bonding with the baby. The decision as to whether this baby goes home with his/her mother will be based on these observations.
- The prescribing agency should be made aware of admission and confirm the dosage prescribed.
- Midwives or NNU staff may be requested to attend a discharge-planning meeting prior to discharge.

Breastfeeding
Women who are well stabilized on reasonably low doses of prescribed drugs may breastfeed their babies, as the potential benefits far outweigh the risks. Drug use is not an absolute contraindication to breastfeeding. Breastfeeding provides natural immunity to babies and also reduces the severity of neonatal withdrawal and may be appropriate in some women.

Contraindications to breastfeeding include an HIV-positive mother and a mother who is taking sedative drugs, e.g. benzodiazepines.

Neonatal
Neonatal abstinence syndrome (NAS) should be discussed in the antenatal period with involvement of a neonatologist. The onset and severity of neonatal withdrawal symptoms is variable and difficult to predict. Onset usually occurs within 24–72 hours of birth, but it can be delayed by up to 7–10 days. Methadone tends to produce withdrawal symptoms with a later onset, longer duration, and greater severity.

Withdrawal symptoms
- High-pitch crying
- Irritability and restlessness
- Tremor/shakiness (fits indicate medical complications)
- Feeding difficulties
- Sleeping difficulties (not settling after feeds)
- Vomiting/and or diarrhoea
- Fever
- Nappy rash (usually due to frequent loose stools).

Specific drug problems

Cannabis use in pregnancy

Cannabis is the most common drug used in pregnancy. The consequences are similar to use of nicotine. Regular use is associated with low birth weight and prematurity.[4]
- Cannabis does not produce physical dependence.
- The hazards of cannabis use include:
  - acute effects: intoxication, lethargy, and lung damage
  - long-term effects: may precipitate or exacerbate psychosis
  - indirect harm: financial costs.

Alcohol use in pregnancy

Alcohol, like tobacco, is socially acceptable and differs from other drugs especially illicit drugs taken in pregnancy. There are no established safe limits of alcohol that can be taken in pregnancy. Heavy alcohol consumption during pregnancy increases the risks of low birthweight, preterm birth, and SGA, whereas light to moderate alcohol consumption shows no effect. Preventive measures during antenatal consultations should be initiated.

Adverse effects of alcohol misuse during pregnancy

Fetal alcohol syndrome:
- Growth retardation
- Learning disability
- Hypotonia
- Microcephaly
- Hyperactivity
- Poor coordination
- Liver damage
- Neurological
- Cardiac
- Lungs and stomach
- Reproductive
- Small intestines and pancreas, joints and muscles.

Recommended investigations

The normal booking bloods plus:
- LFT
- GGT
- HCV antibodies
- HCV RNA

- Additional tests to be repeated at 28 weeks, 34 weeks, and 37 weeks of gestation
- Fetal growth scans should be arranged at 28 and 32 weeks.

Women **must not** be told to stop drinking, as sudden cessation of dependent/heavy drinking is dangerous to the mother (risk of seizures). Women need to be referred to an alcohol service so that an adequate assessment of the level of drinking, tolerance, and dependence can be made before a reduction in alcohol consumption can start. Alcohol detoxification needs careful supervision by obstetricians and alcohol specialist.

References

1. National Institute for Health and Care Excellence. *Pregnancy and Complex Social Factors: A Model for Service Provision for Pregnant Women with Complex Social Factors* (Clinical Guidance 110). London. NICE, 2010. Available at: https://www.nice.org.uk/guidance/cg110.
2. Centre for Maternal and Child Enquiries (CMACE). Saving Mothers' Lives: reviewing maternal deaths to make motherhood safer: 2006–08. The Eighth Report on Confidential Enquiries into Maternal Deaths in the United Kingdom. *BJOG* 2011; 118(Suppl. 1):1–203.
3. Advisory Council on the Misuse of Drugs. *AMCD Inquiry: 'Hidden Harm' Report on Children of Drug Users.* London: ACMD Inquiry, 2011.
4. National Children's Bureau. *Drug Use in Pregnancy.* [Online] Available at: http://www.ncb.org.uk/media/424056/adultdrugprobs_pres3.pdf

Further reading

National Institute for Health and Care Excellence. *Antenatal and Postnatal Mental Health: Clinical Management and Service Guidance* (Clinical Guidance 192). London: NICE, 2014. Available at www.nice.org.uk/guidance/cg192.
Patra J, Bakker R, Irving H, *et al.* Dose–response relationship between alcohol consumption before and during pregnancy and the risks of low birthweight, preterm birth and small for gestational age (SGA)—a systematic review and meta-analyses. *BJOG* 2011; 118(12):1411–21.
Royal College of Obstetricians and Gynaecologists. *Alcohol Consumption and the Outcome of Pregnancy* (RCOG Statement No. 5). London: RCOG, 2006.

Violence against women and children: safeguarding children and infants

Violence against the weakest in society is a phenomenon that exists throughout all cultures, in all countries, and has transcended all periods of human history. Healthcare professionals have a duty to respond appropriately when violence against anyone in their care occurs; however, violence against women and children is more common than any other and carries the most severe consequences for family units, including future development of children.

Violence exists against men and within same-sex relationships; a violent culture within a relationship is destructive. While this chapter will acknowledge all perpetrators and survivors of violence, the focus for action by health carers, will be upon violence against women within domestic relationships. That is, within families and includes close family connections; this is by far the most common form of violence. The effect on children, the safety of children, and the action required by health carers to protect children will also be discussed.

One in four women in England and Wales experience some form of domestic violence in their life. Of these, one in eight will have violence initiated during pregnancy.

Definitions

Crown Prosecution Service UK

'Any form of physical, sexual or emotional abuse which takes place within the context of a close relationship. In most cases the relationship will be between partners (married, cohabiting or otherwise) or ex-partners.'

Women's Aid

Domestic violence is usually defined as 'physical, emotional, sexual and other abuse by someone (usually but not always a man) of a person (usually but not always a woman) with whom they have or have had some form of intimate relationship such as marriage, in order to maintain power and control over that person'.

The absence of a standardized definition of violence and abuse and the lack of a standard measurement means that it is difficult to establish precisely how many women really are experiencing some form of violence or abuse.

Detection of violence by health professionals

Doctors, nurses, midwives, and a broader range of professional health providers are well placed to detect violence against women and children. Most particularly in the UK, women are invited to interface with healthcare by health screening, such as cervical smear testing, breast screening, contraceptive care, and antenatal care in pregnancy. Babies and children are regularly monitored through the national health process of examination, immunization, and school health services. These opportunities should be used productively to identify possible problems and initiate higher surveillance and action where indicated.

Health professionals may see the following when women come forward for routine care, particularly in pregnancy:

- Women with low self-esteem—not making eye contact
- Male (or female) chaperone speaking for her and not leaving her alone
- Regular interface with medical services for mild or non-existent problems, e.g. backache during pregnancy
- Unexplained injuries or inadequately explained injuries
- Eating disorders
- Nervousness and depression
- Repeated unplanned pregnancies
- Repeated miscarriage
- Injury to the pregnant abdomen and genitalia
- Multiple bruises of differing ages
- Vaginal bleeding during pregnancy
- Premature labour
- Low-birth-weight baby
- Physical injuries to the baby evident at birth
- Non-attendance for planned routine care
- After birth: removal of perineal sutures
- Cessation of breastfeeding, usually sudden and unexpected
- Early sexual activity after childbirth
- Abused girls: early teen pregnancy and a history of multiple termination of pregnancy
- Self-harming.

Healthcare professionals need to know what is locally available to them when they wish to refer on suspected safeguarding issues for both women who are subject to violence and children. Violence is unlawful and should/can involve law enforcement.

It is necessary to reassure the victim of violence, particularly women, that they are to be supported and that their children are a key concern. This does not automatically mean the breakup of the family.

For women who are subject to domestic violence, the healthcare professional must:

- Listen, understand, and never blame the woman, she may have never confided in anyone before.
- Never offer a personal opinion.
- Respect the decisions she makes.
- Always tell the woman if you are making a referral to other agencies, particularly to social services.
- Outline what is available to support the woman—Women's Aid telephone number and website.
- Offer to arrange for photographs of her injuries and keep them in a safe place, she may want to use them later. General practitioners are ideally placed for this.
- Explain safety strategies for the woman. When violence is irrupting, steer it toward the lounge or bedroom, where soft furnishings will help protect. Try to exit bathrooms and kitchens.
- Keep copies of documents like passports, rent books, and birth certificates, and house keys.

- Try to keep a little money hidden away for a taxi in the event of a hasty exit.
- If possible, confide in a trusted neighbour so that you can signal when the police should be called.

Domestic and family violence may not entirely disappear, but health workers can provide surveillance, understanding, support, safety, and zero tolerance towards it.

Further reading

Cawson P, Wattam C, Brooker S, et al. *Child Maltreatment in the United Kingdom: A Study of the Prevalence of Child Abuse and Neglect.* London: NSPCC, 2000.

Coleman K, Reed E. *Homicides, Firearms Offences and Intimate Violence 2005/2006: Supplementary Volume 1 to Crime in England and Wales 2005/2006.* London: Home Office, 2007.

Department of Health Taskforce. *Violence Against Women and Girls.* London: Department of Health, 2010.

D'Gregorio P. Obstetric violence: a new legal term introduced in Venezuela. *Int J Gynecol Obstet* 2010; 111:201–2.

Dobash RE, Dobash RP. *Women, Violence and Social Change.* London: Routledge, 1992.

Hunt SC. *Poverty Pregnancy and the Healthcare Professional.* London: Books for Midwives, 2004.

McIntosh T, Ashwin C. From public to private: the history of domestic abuse in Britain. *Pract Midwife* 2012; 15(2):20–1.

Moore M. Reproductive health and intimate partner violence. *Fam Plann Perspect* 1999; 31(6):302–6.

National Commission of Inquiry into the Prevention of Child Abuse. *Childhood Matters: Report of the National Commission of Inquiry into the Prevention of Child Abuse: Volume 2 Background Papers.* London: The Stationery Office, 1996.

O'Donnell A, Fitzpatrick M, McKenna P. Abuse in pregnancy – the experience of women. *Irish Medical Journal* 2000; 93(8):229–30.

Sperlich M, Seng JS. *Survivor Moms: Women's Narratives of Birthing, Mothering, and Healing after Sexual Abuse.* Eugene, OR: Motherbaby Press, 2008.

Walaby S, Allen J. *Domestic Violence, Sexual Assault and Stalking. Findings from the British Crime Survey 2004.* London: Home Office, 2004.

Women's Aid website: http://www.womensaid.org.uk/.

Miscellaneous topics in obstetrics

Contributors

Olujimi Jibodu, Sambit Mukhopadhyay, Leonie Penna, Paul Simpson, and Vladimir Rivicky

Contents

☼ Emergency cerclage

Emergency cerclage is the insertion of a suture in the cervix in response to shortening or dilatation in the second trimester, to reduce the risk of threatened preterm birth. It may delay delivery by up to 5 weeks. It may be indicated after 24 weeks but the need has to be weighed against the significant prospect of fetal viability from 24 weeks. Where neonatal facilities are inadequate, emergency cerclage after 24 weeks may be appropriate to delay for *in utero* transfer or further fetal maturity.

Indications

- Mid-trimester cervical dilatation visualized on speculum examination for vaginal bleeding or discharge. Fetal membranes may be found exposed in the vagina. This procedure is known as rescue cerclage.
- US finding of shortening of the cervix to 25 mm or less before 24 weeks, along with dilatation of the internal os (funnelling). The US scanning is usually for previous history of one or more mid-trimester cervical dilatation leading to pregnancy loss or extreme premature live birth.

Contraindications

- Painful uterine contractions with progressive cervical effacement and dilatation. This combination of signs suggests established preterm labour.
- Rupture of fetal membranes.
- Lethal fetal abnormality, structural or chromosomal.
- Fetal death.
- Clinical features of sepsis/chorioamnionitis.
- Chorioamnionitis confirmed by amniocentesis.
- Heavy vaginal bleeding.

Improved outcome with:

- Cervical dilatation <4 cm
- Fetal membranes not protruding beyond external cervical os
- Gestation above 20 weeks when cerclage needed.

Preparation and procedure

- The usual procedure is a McDonald suture, inserted vaginally, as close as possible to the level of the cervico-vaginal junction. Abdominal cerclage may also be performed as a rescue procedure but may not offer any advantage and has the major drawback of needing delivery by LSCS or a repeat abdominal procedure to remove it.
- Informed written consent should be obtained. Preoperative discussion should include risks of ROM during the cerclage procedure. The procedure should not be continued if membranes inadvertently rupture.
- FBC and CRP are useful only when they support a clinical suspicion of chorioamnionitis. Amniocentesis may be performed to confirm infection.

- Confirmed vaginal infection should be treated but antibiotic prophylaxis is not of proven benefit.
- Exclude lethal fetal abnormality or fetal death by US scan.
- Tocolysis (e.g. with indometacin), prolonged nursing in Trendelenburg position, or percutaneous amnioreduction have all been used with variable effect in reducing membranes bulging beyond the external os.
- Anaesthesia may be general or regional on agreement of the woman, obstetrician, and anaesthetist.
- Lithotomy position is needed on the operating table. Two assistants may be necessary to achieve optimal vaginal retraction.
- Maintain aseptic technique.
- Protruding fetal membranes may be reduced by gentle pressure with a wet swab or a Foley catheter balloon with 30–50 mL saline. A Trendelenburg tilt of the operating table is useful.
- Grasp anterior and posterior lips of the cervix, each with sponge holders (e.g. Rampley's).
- Use appropriate suture (e.g. Mersilene tape), inserted as a purse-string, starting at 12 o'clock, out and back in at 9, 6, and 3 o'clock, and finally back out at 12 o'clock. The suture is then knotted at 12 o'clock, after pulling the ends gently until the cervical os is closed. A secondary loop may be placed to allow grasping and traction for removal.

Complications

- Cervical laceration. A soft, effaced cervix can be easily torn while trying to place a suture in it.
- Fetal membranes may be inadvertently ruptured while a cervical cerclage is being performed. The procedure should be discontinued.
- Cerclage may not achieve the desired effect. The suture needs to be removed if labour becomes established.
- Vaginal discharge and light bleeding may persist while the suture is in place. The patient should be reassured and no treatment is necessary.

Removal

- The suture should be removed electively from 36 weeks' gestation or as soon as possible if membranes rupture or labour becomes established.
- If delivery is by LSCS, the suture may be left in place until LSCS is performed.
- To remove the suture, grasp the suture or knot (at 12 o'clock) and cut the main loop proximal to the knot.
- Examine the removed suture for completeness.
- Await spontaneous or induced labour if vaginal birth is intended.

Further reading

Norwitz ER. *Transvaginal Cervical Cerclage*. UpToDate®, 2015. http://www.uptodate.com/contents/transvaginal-cervical-cerclage
Royal College of Obstetricians and Gynaecologists. *Cervical Cerclage* (Green-top Guideline No. 60). London: RCOG, 2011, reviewed 2014.

⚙ Trauma in pregnancy

Trauma is common in pregnancy, the majority (>90%) are minor. Adverse pregnancy outcome occurs in up to 4% of minor injuries and fetal loss is in the range of 40% in critical maternal injury.

Causes

These include road traffic accidents (RTAs), falls, domestic accidental and non-accidental injury, assault, and penetrating trauma. Some of these result in fatality (coincidental maternal mortality). Awareness of domestic violence is important as it often starts, or when pre-existing, worsens, in pregnancy.

Anatomical and physiological effects of pregnancy

- Blood volume increases by up to 50% in pregnancy.
- Up to 30% of blood volume may be lost before pulse and blood pressure change.
- Uterine perfusion may be compromised while maternal pulse and blood pressure are still maintained.
- Reduced venous return in supine position, due to inferior vena cava (IVC) compression by the enlarged uterus.
- Blood loss into uterus/abdomen may be concealed.
- Uterine size and position in late pregnancy render it more prone to trauma.
- Fetus may be more immediately affected than mother.
- Delayed gastric emptying increases risk of vomiting and aspiration.

Approach to management

Unless contraindicated, the pregnant woman should always be nursed and transported with a 15–30° left tilt, using a wedge or rolled-up clothing or in left lateral position. For major trauma, the paramedic/trauma team often carries out immediate resuscitation. The woman is then transferred to an appropriate secondary or tertiary centre, depending on nature, extent, and severity of injuries. The emergency department is a more appropriate place than the labour ward for the pregnant woman with non-obstetric trauma.

In the UK and many Western countries, women carry a copy of their maternity records, which provides a synopsis of the antenatal care and test results.

Initial assessment is as for any trauma patient, maternal resuscitation is the first priority. Advanced Trauma and Life Support® (ATLS®) principles of resuscitation allow uniform and consistent care. Fetal assessment only follows stabilization of maternal condition. Multi-disciplinary working and early involvement of obstetricians by trauma team and vice versa is crucial.

Primary survey

This reveals immediately life-threatening problems.

A = airway control using chin lift, suction, or oropharyngeal airway as appropriate. Note increased risk of aspiration in pregnant women.

Avoid moving neck/tilting head if possibility of neck injury. Establish cervical spine control/apply cervical collar/sandbags. Call anaesthetist early for airway problems.

B = breathing/ventilation: give O_2 once airway control is achieved. Pulse oximetry valuable in monitoring, ensuring ≥ 95% O_2 saturation.

C = circulation: CPR if cardiac arrest; control of haemostasis/IV lines using large-bore cannulae (two 14–16 G) and aggressive infusions. Warm infusions when large volumes used. Blood group usually known or recorded in hand-held notes so cross-match is rapid. When matched blood is not available and the woman is not known to have any red cell antibodies, O-negative or group-specific blood may be used. Central venous access may be crucial when peripheral veins are inaccessible, e.g. in severe shock or extensive burns (although siting a central line is more hazardous). US is useful in identifying peripheral veins that are difficult to locate. Interosseous needles have recently come into use and should become more widely available and valuable.

Once neck injury is excluded, left lateral position or 15–30° left tilt will relieve IVC pressure and improve venous return.

D = disability (neurological) assessment: with orientation and responsiveness, pupillary reaction, motor response, and Glasgow coma scale. Levels are alert, voice responsive, pain responsive, unconscious (note that unresponsiveness may be due to hypovolaemia).

E = exposure: (to allow full/physical examination).

Primary survey—resuscitation phase
Problems that need immediate attention are dealt with as they are identified.

Fetal viability and well-being are assessed after maternal primary survey/resuscitation. Depending on maternal and fetal status, delivery may be indicated. Determine gestation (refer to hand-held notes or clinical estimation if history is not available) and listen for fetal heart. US assessment may be done when patient is stabilized. Electronic FHR monitoring may be used if appropriate.

Secondary survey
Secondary survey identifies and deals with problems that are not immediately life-threatening. It is performed when the maternal condition is stable and involves more detailed assessment and investigations. Maternal health remains the overriding priority and X-rays, CT, and MRI scans are safe in pregnancy and when needed should not be delayed or withheld because of pregnancy. Reference ranges that apply to pregnancy should be used in interpreting test results, e.g. Hb of 10–11 g/dL is not unusual in pregnancy. This is due to plasma volume expansion exceeding red cell mass expansion, resulting in a physiological anaemia. Relative leucocytosis is normal. Some ECG changes may be normal for pregnancy.

Adequate exposure should be done without compromising warmth, to allow complete physical evaluation. Up to 50% of the mortality in severe trauma patients is due to head injuries so an early neurological assessment is essential. All neck injuries should be considered life-threatening and receive prompt and adequate attention.

When a chest tube is indicated, it should be placed 1–2 intercostal spaces higher than would otherwise have been indicated to allow for the elevation of the diaphragm that occurs in pregnancy.

▶ Return to ABC if any deterioration in status.

▶▶ Unless trauma is primarily obstetric, obstetric evaluation is part of the secondary survey. Unstable neck or spine injuries and femoral fractures contraindicate pelvic examination as the positioning will worsen these conditions.

Definitive care phase
This is dictated by the type and severity of injury.

General measures
Urinary catheter allows examination of urine for haematuria as a sign of pelvic trauma and urine output as an indicator of renal perfusion. Urine output of 30 mL/hour or more indicates good renal perfusion.

Kleihauer test is useful in determining feto-maternal haemorrhage (FMH) and dose of Rh globulin for Rh-negative women. To avoid undue delay, 250 U IM up to 20 weeks' gestation and 500 U after 20 weeks can be given while awaiting test result.

Check tetanus immunization status if indicated by nature of injuries.

Additional treatment options
Emergency (perimortem) LSCS may be necessary if mother has cardiopulmonary arrest and CPR is unsuccessful for 4 minutes, despite left lateral tilt. ▶▶ Basic skin preparation is sufficient, anaesthesia is not immediately needed and haemostasis is not an issue.

▶ Maternal resuscitation should continue through the LSCS. The fetus is relatively resilient to maternal hypoxia for short periods but the *primary* aim of the perimortem LSCS is to facilitate maternal resuscitation.

Other indications for LSCS in pregnant trauma patients are:
• Inadequate exposure during laparotomy for other abdominal trauma
• Unstable pelvic or lumbosacral fracture with patient in labour
• Uterine rupture.
• Placental abruption.

Laparotomy may be necessary for abdominal injury. Peritoneal/pelvic haemorrhage may be diagnosed by US showing large volume of free fluid.

DVT risk increases in pregnancy. Hypovolaemia and immobilization increase the risk. Thromboprophylaxis with LMWH should be considered but only after risk of haemorrhage is controlled.

▶ Consider the possibility of drug or alcohol intoxication depending on the nature or circumstances of trauma.

Persistent shock in trauma patients
Life-threatening problems in the chest
• Airway obstruction
• Tension pneumothorax
• Open pneumothorax
• Massive haemothorax
• Flail chest
• Cardiac tamponade.

Other systemic problems
- Neurogenic shock
- Uncorrected hypothermia
- Hypoxia
- Acid–base/electrolyte imbalances.

Pregnancy-specific traumas
- Placental abruption
- Uterine rupture
- Eclampsia and its complications
- Amniotic fluid embolism (AFE).

Seat belts

Maternal serious injury or death is more likely if the unrestrained woman is ejected from the moving vehicle. Seat belts are protective at all stages of pregnancy. Unrestrained passengers are likely to have impact injuries with the interior of the vehicle or be ejected, with potentially severe injuries to head, face, chest, abdomen, and pelvis. Maternal mortality risk when the passenger is ejected from a moving vehicle is about 30% compared with 5% when restrained.

The three-point lap and shoulder restraint is best, reducing the likelihood of moderate to critical injury by 50% and fatal injury by 45%. It should be worn correctly, with the shoulder belt passing between the breasts and over the top of the fundus and the lap belt passing below the uterus. Injuries sustained with this belt in place include sternum, clavicle, and rib fractures. Hollow viscus and lumbar spine injuries may occur with lap-only belts and clavicle, cervical spine, rib, and liver injuries with shoulder-only belts. Airbags may cause abrasions to face and chest.

Blunt trauma

This is the commonest type of trauma in pregnancy, the main cause being from RTAs. Most injuries are relatively minor and even major injuries are more likely to be non-obstetric. Obstetric complications include preterm labour, FMH, placental abruption, and uterine rupture.

Blunt trauma also results from falls and physical assault. Recurrent presentation with minor blunt trauma should raise the suspicion of domestic violence as this is known to either start or worsen in pregnancy.

Major peritoneal haemorrhage is more likely in advanced pregnancy because of the large blood supply to the uterus. Haemorrhage may develop slowly and repeated assessment is necessary to detect any deterioration in physical condition.

Placental abruption is the commonest cause of fetal death when the mother has sustained blunt injury. There may not be obvious abdominal injury to raise the suspicion of fetal trauma. Signs include vaginal bleeding, tense and tender uterus, FHR abnormalities, and maternal haemodynamic parameters are worse than would be explained by the apparent injuries or blood loss. Placental abruption may not be clinically obvious for several days after blunt trauma to the gravid uterus.

In addition to the priority management of the mother's trauma, obstetric management will depend on the duration of gestation, maternal condition, and the degree of fetal compromise if any. A particular complication to exclude and monitor is coagulopathy.

▶ Corticosteroids should be given to improve fetal lung maturity when gestation is under 34 weeks and delivery can be delayed, even by just a few hours.

▶ Vaginal delivery is not excluded in the presence of placental abruption. LSCS should be avoided if maternal condition is stable and there is coagulopathy or a dead fetus.

Preterm labour

It may be difficult to determine if uterine activity after blunt trauma is due to labour or placental abruption. If preterm and placental abruption is considered unlikely, tocolysis may be used, especially if the mother is being transferred between units or circumstances dictate that it is of benefit to improve fetal lung maturity with corticosteroids. Atosiban is now commonly used as a tocolytic but some of the older tocolytic agents, e.g. β-mimetics and nifedipine have side effects, e.g. tachycardia, similar to signs of blood loss.

Uterine rupture

This is uncommon as uterine muscle elasticity reduces the risk of rupture. Increased risk of rupture with maternal pelvic fracture and scarred uterus from previous LSCS. Fetal mortality risk is close to 100% with traumatic uterine rupture. Absence of fetal heart sounds, easily palpable fetal parts, and shock disproportionate with injury are leading signs. Management includes obstetric and surgical laparotomy at which other visceral injury should be excluded or appropriately managed if found.

Feto-maternal haemorrhage (FMH)

Risk of FMH is up to 30%, vs 8% in pregnancies with no reported trauma. Nature and severity of maternal trauma do not correlate well with FMH. Sequelae include Rhesus isoimmunization in Rh-negative women carrying Rh-positive fetuses, fetal anaemia, and fetal demise. Kleihauer testing is used to quantify the volume of FMH and dose of Rh globulin that needs to be given to the Rh-negative mother.

Penetrating injury

This is uncommon and may be due to stab or gunshot. In early pregnancy, the uterus is pelvic and the pattern of injury is similar to that in non-pregnant women. In late pregnancy, the uterus is large and central in the abdomen. The viscera are displaced superiorly and laterally. Fetal injury is more likely and visceral injury less likely. The high associated perinatal mortality rates may be due directly to the injury or the complications of resultant premature delivery. When bowel is affected by penetrating injury, multiple wounds are more likely, due to the compression of more bowel in a smaller area. Laparotomy should be undertaken by joint obstetric and surgical team but if uterus is not involved, delivery may not be necessary.

Burns

Burns may be due to contact with a hot surface, flame, scalds, chemical, or electrical burns. Most are minor, resulting from domestic accidents. More severe burns may occur from house fires and accidents with hot or flammable liquids or gases. Severity and extent are described in terms of depth (full or partial thickness) and the % total body surface area affected. The 'rule of nines' used to estimate area of burns is easy to remember and use but underestimates the increased surface area of the abdomen in pregnant women.

Classification
- Minor: partial thickness <10% of surface area
- Major: partial or full thickness burns >10%
- Moderate: 10–19%
- Severe: 20–39%
- Critical 40% or more.

Obstetric complications of major burns include premature labour and delivery and fetal death. Early delivery may be considered to optimize maternal management. Corticosteroids should be considered if gestation is <34 weeks and the maternal condition permits the necessary delay, even if this is for a few hours. LSCS, if necessary can be performed through burnt skin without additional morbidity.

Maternal mortality risk
- <40% burns: <3% mortality
- 40–59% burns: 50% mortality
- 60% burns: 90–100% mortality.

Fetal mortality risk
- 20% maternal burns: fetal mortality unlikely
- 20–39% maternal burns: 10–27% fetal mortality
- 40–59% maternal burns: 45–53% fetal mortality
- 60% burns: up to 100% fetal mortality.

▶ If the fetus is of viable age, delivery is indicated if maternal burns are 50% or greater. With major burns, fetal loss tends to be within 5 days of burns.

Management
Women with minor burns need analgesia and appropriate wound dressing. Initial management of women with major burns is similar to all trauma victims. Subsequent care should involve burns team. Factors to be considered include surface area involved, depth of burns, body parts affected (facial burns imply higher risk of inhalation injury), inhalation, and associated injuries.

Inhalation injury from burns
Concurrent inhalation injuries may affect the prognosis. Immediate or delayed airway obstruction may occur so secure and maintain airway early, including by endotracheal intubation if necessary.

Suspect inhalational injury when:
- Fire in enclosed space
- Voice alteration
- Facial burns or singed facial and nasal hair
- Coughing up sooty/dark sputum
- Respiratory distress.

If inhalational injury suspected, check ABGs for carbon monoxide (CO). CO crosses the placenta and achieves higher concentrations (10–15× maternal levels) in the fetus. The fetus also needs a longer time than the mother to eliminate CO.

Fibreoptic bronchoscopy may be undertaken to assess the respiratory tract, if the situation indicates and facilities permit.

Signs of CO poisoning
- 10–20% CO: palpitations, headaches, nausea
- 20–40% CO: dizziness, confusion, agitation, incoordination, memory loss
- >40% CO: dyspnoea, coma, and death

Management
- 10–20% CO blood levels: treat with 100% O_2 by facemask. Time to restore fetal levels to normal may be 5× that of mother, so extended therapy is needed.
- 20% CO or more/neurological features irrespective of CO level: treat with hyperbaric O_2.
- Most pulse oximeters are unable to distinguish carboxyhaemoglobin from oxyhaemoglobin so their use may be unreliable in CO poisoning.

Electrocution

Electrocution is very rare and is predominantly from domestic accidents. Cardiac arrest is the commonest cause of maternal death from electrical injury. Cardiac arrhythmias may be delayed so continuous cardiac monitoring is prudent.

Injuries are varied, including those due to falls from the shock. Early consultation and joint management with a trauma team with appropriate experience is advisable.

The fetus is very vulnerable to electrocution and mortality risk is high if it is in the path of the current (e.g. hand–foot path). Fetal outcome therefore does not correlate well with the degree of maternal injury. When the fetus survives the initial shock, continuous monitoring is indicated. If at term, delivery should be considered, as the fetal effects of electrocution are difficult to assess. If delivery is not indicated, regular fetal monitoring including growth scans is advised.

Further reading

Knight M, Kenyon S, Brocklehurst P, et al. Saving Lives, Improving Mothers' Care – Lessons Learned to Inform Future Maternity Care from the UK and Ireland Confidential Enquiries into Maternal Deaths and Morbidity 2009–12. Oxford: National Perinatal Epidemiology Unit, University of Oxford; 2014.
Woollard M, Hinshaw K, Simpson H, et al. (eds) Pre-Hospital Obstetric Emergency Training: The Practical Approach. Oxford: Wiley-Blackwell, 2010.

⑦ Transfer and transport of pregnant women

It is sometimes necessary to transfer pregnant women for:
- Failure to progress during labour at home
- Failure to progress during labour at peripheral or midwifery unit
- Transfer to specialist unit for investigation or treatment of maternal medical illness
- *In utero* transfer of fetus for neonatal intensive care. This is the commonest indication for maternal transfer between hospitals.

A systematic approach to transfer includes *A*ssessment, *C*ontrol, *C*ommunication, *E*valuation, *P*reparation, and *T*ransport (*ACCEPT*).

Assessment for transfer

Transfer of any ill patient from one location to another is often necessary for better care than available at the starting point. The risks of staying must outweigh the risks of transfer so it is important that the right patient is transferred at the right time, by the right personnel to the right place using the right mode of transport, with the right care in transit. For ill or potentially ill babies, neonatal outcome is improved by birth in the unit where the neonatal intensive care or surgery will take place.

Transfer may be initiated by clinicians already caring for the patient or paramedics if from home or the site of an accident. Appropriate briefing at every point of the handover of care helps to optimize care in transit and on delivery to destination. The NHS Institute for Innovation and Improvement recommends the use of the *S*ituation, *B*ackground, *A*ssessment, *R*ecommendation (SBAR) aide-memoire for communicating in situations of handover of care.

Some maternal conditions are not suitable for transfer, e.g.:
- Fulminating pre-eclampsia
- Ongoing haemorrhage
- Imminent delivery.

In these circumstances, delivery and/or stabilization may have to be undertaken in the referring unit and the baby transferred for neonatal intensive care or the mother transferred as indicated. It is important to avoid separating mother and baby so obstetric and neonatal units need to liaise to ensure appropriate arrangements are made for both.

Controlling the transfer

Many regions now have integrated transfer teams (e.g. Embrace in Yorkshire and Humberside region of UK) who coordinate many aspects of *in utero* and neonatal transfer. Many regions also have a 'neonatal network' and pathways for transfers. The transfer team should have clear lines of duty set out, if not already existing. This should include leadership, tasks to be performed during the transfer, and who performs them. A named person (e.g. the transferring consultant) will have overall responsibility for the transfer.

Communication

Decisions and responsibility for transfers must be taken at consultant level, even when regional transfer teams are used. The clinicians initiating a transfer should agree with the receiving unit that a transfer is appropriate and the facilities to undertake the appropriate care are available. These include:

- Antenatal bed (liaise with obstetric team)
- Appropriate intrapartum facilities (liaise with obstetric team)
- Appropriate expertise (liaise with obstetric and paediatric surgery teams)
- Neonatal intensive care cot (liaise with neonatology team).

The need to transfer should then be discussed with the patient and/or relatives.

► It is vital that full and accurate information be provided. A copy of medical records or summary should be provided for the transfer. This will be handed to the receiving unit.

Evaluation

This determines the necessity and clinical urgency of the transfer, based on severity of the patient's illness. It also determines the mode of transport and the accompanying personnel. Transfer categories are:

- Intensive
- Time critical
- Ill and unstable
- Ill and stable
- Unwell
- Well.

Preparation for transfer

The maternal and fetal conditions must be stable before transfer so that the additional stress of travel can be withstood. Inadequate resuscitation before transfer is likely to cause deterioration in maternal or fetal condition in transit. Appropriate personnel, IV fluids, drugs, oxygen, and equipment, including neonatal respiratory support must be available in the ambulance.

The mother should be secured to the trolley, which is in turn secured to the ambulance. Wedging is important to prevent aortocaval compression. All lines, drains, monitoring, and drug administration equipment also need to be secured. Accompanying persons should be securely seated and restrained. It may, however, become necessary during a transfer for procedures to be carried out (e.g. delivery of a baby). It may be necessary for the ambulance to remain stationary for this and resume the trip afterwards.

Arrangements for the return trip for the accompanying staff and relatives must be confirmed before setting out on the trip. The ambulance is not obliged to return them to their base.

Apart from the ambulance crew, the patient may be accompanied by a midwife. Other accompanying personnel will depend on the indication for transfer and potential problems anticipated. If there is a risk of delivery, especially if preterm, it may be more appropriate for that to be undertaken at the referring unit and the neonate transferred (*ex utero*) instead.

Tocolysis is usually used to reduce the risk of delivery in transit. Corticosteroids are administered concurrently to promote fetal lung maturity if the fetus is <34 weeks.

Transportation

Appropriate ambulance transportation is arranged either by the referring unit or the regional transfer team. The mode and type of transportation is determined by:

- Nature and severity of maternal or fetal illness
- Urgency of transfer
- Needs and potential problems in transit
- Geographical factors, e.g. accessibility by road
- Distance to travel
- Traffic conditions on the route
- Weather conditions

Most transfers are over relatively short distances and road ambulances are most appropriate. Air ambulances are more expensive but more appropriate if the distance is long or road access is restricted or unfavourable.

Seek expert advice if long-distance air ambulance is considered necessary. Effects of the plane's microclimate need to be considered and air flight may be contraindicated.

If the patient is a trauma victim, continuous assessment and maintenance of resuscitation principles (ABC) is necessary.

Handover

At the destination, the patient should be directly handed over to a senior member of the receiving unit. The NHS Institute of Innovation and Improvement *SBAR* guide is useful. Medical records and details of monitoring or events during the transfer should be passed on.

Further reading

Driscoll P (ed). *Safe Transfer and Retrieval: The Practical Approach* (2nd ed). Oxford: BMJ Books/ Blackwell Publishing, 2006.

Obstetric collapse

Causes

Obstetric collapse may occur at any time during pregnancy. Sudden loss of maternal consciousness is potentially the most serious emergency occurring during pregnancy. The differential diagnosis will depend on whether the woman is antenatal, intrapartum, or postnatal:

- Non-serious 'collapse' vaso-vagal episode
- Haemorrhagic shock:
  - Obstetric:
    - APH
    - PPH
  - Non-obstetric:
    - aortic dissection
    - hepatic rupture
    - rupture of splenic artery aneurysm
    - rare causes (AV malformations, other aneurysms).
- Uterine inversion
- Cardiogenic shock:
  - myocardial infarction
  - cardiomyopathy
  - cardiac disease
- Adrenal crisis
- Pulmonary embolism
- Septic shock
- Anaphylactic shock
- AFE
- Cerebrovascular accident
- Hypoglycaemia
- Drug toxicity.

The Resuscitation Council (UK) has proposed an 'aide-memoire' for the common reversible causes of collapse in any woman known as the '4H's (hypovolaemia, hypoxia, hypo/hyperkalaemia and other electrolyte disturbances and hypothermia) and the '4T's (thromboembolism, toxicity, tension pneumothorax, tamponade (cardiac)) with the addition of eclampsia and intracranial haemorrhage for the pregnant woman.

Management

- Assessment and initial management must occur simultaneously.
- Call for help (cardiac arrest team may be required).
- Commence basic life support.
- If breathing spontaneously give high-flow oxygen via face mask with reservoir bag in all cases.
- If antenatal and >24 weeks' gestation use wedge for left lateral tilt.
- Insert two large bore (16 G minimum) IV cannulae.
- Commence monitoring (automated BP/pulse), pulse oximeter, cardiac rhythm monitor).
- Insert urinary catheter.

Investigations
- FBC, U&Es, LFTs coagulation screen on all
- G&S
- Serum lactate
- CRP and blood cultures (suspected septic shock)
- Fibrinogen and fibrinogen degradation products (possible DIC)
- Blood gases
- 12-lead ECG
- Request portable CXR
- Abdominal US.

Making a diagnosis
- Rapid review of antenatal notes for risk factors.
- Obtain history of events immediately prior to collapse.
- Some diagnoses such as obstetric haemorrhage are obvious; others will require investigation.
- Examine woman to assess cardiac and respiratory status (JVP, heart auscultation and full respiratory assessment).
- Examine woman for specific signs (abdominal tenderness, neurology).

Diagnosis-specific management

Perimortem caesarean delivery

Management principles
- Request CS set immediately in all cases of antenatal cardiopulmonary arrest (>24 weeks' gestation).
- If advanced life support with effective tilt is unsuccessful after 5 minutes, commence to assist in maternal resuscitation.
- Crash call senior paediatrician to assess baby (delivery is to assist resuscitation not to save baby).
- Request sterile gloves, scalpel, and blade.
- Shaving, swabbing, and draping the abdomen is unnecessary in this circumstance.
- Vertical or horizontal (Cohen's) abdominal incision are acceptable, whichever the operator feels will be quickest.
- Vertical uterine incision saves time by avoiding need to reflect bladder.

Amniotic fluid embolism

Consider diagnosis in any woman collapsing intrapartum or immediately after delivery. AFE may occur in women delivered by CS. Recent rupture of membranes is not essential for diagnosis. Initial presentation is of massive right-sided heart failure. Severe left-sided heart failure and DIC may follow in women who survive the initial presentation.

Management principles
- Ventilation with 100% O_2.
- Maintenance of cardiac output with crystalloid and inotropes.
- Admission to intensive care unit for invasive monitoring.
- Aggressive treatment of coagulopathy (platelets, fresh frozen plasma, and cryoprecipitate).

- Requires urgent delivery if antenatal and successful resuscitation (assisted vaginal delivery if possible or CS).
- Anticipate possible massive PPH and manage promptly.

Septic shock

Consider the possibility in any woman with previous diagnosis of infection, prolonged rupture of membranes, immunocompromise, or post CS.

Consider possibility of appendicitis.

Management principles

- Administer crystalloid and inotropes.
- Culture for source of infection prior to commencing broad-spectrum IV antibiotics in appropriate doses.
- If antenatal and resuscitation successful, deliver only if signs of fetal compromise.

Adrenal crisis

Consider in any woman taking high-dose steroids.

Management principles

- Crystalloid fluid replacement.
- Fluids to replace electrolyte imbalance (hyponatraemia, hyperkalaemia occur with Addisonian crisis).
- 50% glucose if hypoglycaemia (glucocorticoid deficiency).
- Give hydrocortisone 100 mg IV.
- If antenatal and resuscitation successful, deliver only if there are signs of fetal compromise.

Anaphylaxis

Consider possibility of latex allergy or if new drug was recently administered.

Management principles

- Give 0.5 mL of adrenaline 1 in 10,000 (may require repeat and infusion 0.1 mg/min if BP remains low).
- Crystalloid volume expansion.
- Antihistamines (chlorphenamine 10–20 mg IV) infusion.
- Maintain BP and adequate renal perfusion judged by urinary output—dopamine 2–10 mcg/kg/min is useful.
- Hydrocortisone 200 mg IV.
- Inhaled salbutamol if bronchospasm (or IV 250 mcg).
- If antenatal and resuscitation successful, deliver only if there are signs of fetal compromise.
- Full allergy testing on recovery and avoid stimulus in future.

Magnesium toxicity

Magnesium sulfate toxicity is very rare with standard doses but consider possibility of drug error or in women with impaired renal function.

Management principles
- Stop magnesium infusion and withhold until levels available.
- Give 10 mL of 10% calcium gluconate IV over 2 minutes.
- Send blood for magnesium levels.
- If antenatal, consider expediting delivery (CS or assisted vaginal delivery) as pre-eclampsia is now further complicated.

Further reading

Resuscitation Council (UK). *Resuscitation Guidelines 2010*. [Online] https://www.resus.org.uk/resuscitation-guidelines/

Royal College of Obstetricians and Gynaecologists. *Maternal Collapse in Pregnancy and the Puerperium* (Green-top Guideline No 56). London: RCOG, 2011.

⑦ **Pharmacotherapeutics in obstetrics**

Analgesics

Simple analgesics like paracetamol or a combination of paracetamol and codeine phosphate are often used in pregnancy for non-specific abdominal pain, UTI, headache, and any musculoskeletal pain, after ruling out serious pathology. Opiates are commonly used for pain relief in labour and postoperatively.

Paracetamol (acetaminophen)

Side effects and dosage are not different from non-pregnant patients. Pharmacokinetics also do not differ significantly. Simple analgesia is more effective if taken regularly. It should be used with caution in patients with hepatic and renal impairment.

Entonox®

A 50:50 mixture of nitrous oxide and oxygen, which provides transient analgesia whilst maintaining consciousness. It is most often self-administered through a demand valve.

Pethidine (meperidine)

Pharmacology

This is a synthetic opioid analgesic, predominantly a μ-receptor agonist. Its main action is on the CNS and the neural elements in the bowel.

Use

Moderate to severe pain, obstetric analgesia, and perioperative analgesia.

Dose

- 1 mg/kg (max. 150 mg), typically 50–150 mg by SC or IM route
- Can be repeated 1–3 hours later if necessary
- Maximum dose 400 mg in 24 hours
- Better avoided within 3 hours of delivery (neonatal respiratory depression).

Pharmacokinetics

Onset of analgesic effect is within 10 minutes after SC or IM injection. Though it is absorbed by all routes of administration, rate of absorption after IM injection may be erratic. Peak plasma concentration occurs at about 45 minutes. It is metabolized chiefly in the liver, with a half-life of 3 hours. It crosses the placenta and can cause neonatal respiratory depression.

Side effects

- Nausea, vomiting, constipation
- Drowsiness
- Larger dose can cause respiratory depression and hypotension
- Ureteric and biliary spasm
- Bradycardia, tachycardia, palpitations
- Hallucination, mood change

- Pruritus
- Convulsion
- Dependence.

Drug interactions
- Monoamine oxidase (MAO) inhibitors cause CNS excitation or depression (up to 2 weeks after discontinuation).
- Chlorpromazine and tricyclic antidepressants increase the CNS depressant effects.
- Selegiline can cause hyperpyrexia and CNS toxicity
- Cimetidine inhibits metabolism of pethidine
- Ritonavir (antiviral) increases the plasma concentration.

Contraindications
- Acute respiratory depression
- Acute alcoholism
- Raised intracranial pressure
- Head injury
- Phaeochromocytoma (risk of pressure response to release of histamine)
- Severe renal impairment.

Morphine
Pharmacology
It is an opioid analgesic (μ-receptor agonist) more commonly used in an acute pain and postoperative setting.

Dose
- 2.5–20 mg 2–4-hourly dependent on need, SC or IM or IV
- Oral morphine solution: 10–20 mg 2–4-hourly is a particularly useful postoperative analgesia
- Antiemetic prophylaxis is often required when the IM or IV route is used.

Pharmacokinetics
The plasma half-life is 3–4 hours. It is conjugated by the liver to morphine-6-glucuronide, a more active analgesic. This is then excreted by the kidneys and so the dose must be adjusted in renal failure. Neonates are poor conjugators and so morphine should be avoided in labour and the neonatal period.

Side effects
- Nausea, vomiting, constipation
- Drowsiness
- Larger dose can cause respiratory depression and hypotension
- Ureteric and biliary spasm
- Bradycardia, tachycardia, palpitations
- Hallucination, mood change
- Pruritus
- Convulsion
- Dependence.

Antiemetics

Nausea and vomiting in pregnancy is a common experience affecting 50–90% of all pregnant women. Hyperemesis gravidarum is the most severe manifestation of the spectrum of nausea and vomiting of pregnancy. It requires hospitalization for IV fluid therapy and antiemetics. A variety of antiemetics are used in pregnancy.

None of them are licenced for use in pregnancy but fortunately teratogenic effects on human fetuses have not been reported with any of the commonly used antiemetics.

The previously used Food and Drug Administration (FDA) A–X classification of such drugs has been replaced. For further information about the new FDA classification of drugs used in nausea and vomiting in pregnancy and for up-to-date safety information please see http://dailymed.nlm.nih.gov/dailymed.

The antiemetics commonly used in pregnancy are as follows.

First line

Phenothiazines

- Prochlorperazine: severe: 12.5 mg IM 8-hourly or 5 mg PR three times a day; mild: 5mg PO three times a day.
- It is a dopamine antagonist and acts centrally by blocking the chemoreceptor trigger zone.
- Side effects: extrapyramidal symptoms (tremor, dystonia and tardive dyskinesia), drowsiness and antimuscarinic symptoms (dry mouth, constipation, difficulty with micturition and blurred vision).

Metoclopramide

- Metoclopramide 10 mg three times a day, PO, IM, or IV.
- This has a promotility action. It has both central as well as peripheral antidopaminergic effects.
- Side effects: extrapyramidal symptoms, hyperprolactinaemia, and drowsiness.

Second line

Antihistamines

- Cyclizine 50 mg three times a day, PO, IM, or IV.
- It is a sedating antihistamine, which acts centrally on the chemoreceptor trigger zone.
- Side effects: drowsiness, headache, psychomotor impairment and antimuscarinic symptoms.

Third line

Ondansetron

- Ondansetron 4–8 mg twice a day, PO, IM, or IV.
- A 5-HT$_3$ antagonist, acting in both the GI tract and the CNS. It is particularly useful in patients receiving cytotoxics and in postoperative nausea.
- Side effects: constipation, headache, flushing, and less commonly arrhythmias and seizures. IV administration can lead to dizziness and transient visual disturbance.

Antibiotics

The following antibiotics are considered safe in pregnancy:
- Penicillins
- Co-amoxiclav (except in the third trimester due to the risk of necrotizing enterocolitis in the neonate)
- Cephalosporins
- Erythromycin
- Clindamycin.

Antibiotics are used in obstetrics for various infections e.g. UTI, respiratory tract infection, and also for prophylaxis, e.g. ruptured membranes, cardiac valve abnormality (during labour), prevention of group B streptococcal (GBS) infection in baby during labour, etc.

Prevention of GBS infection in the baby is an important indication for antibiotic treatment. GBS infection can cause fatal neonatal septicaemia. Penicillins are commonly used as prophylaxis in labour.

For women in labour, the recommended doses of penicillin G are 3 g (or 5 mega units) IV initially and then 1.5 g (or 2.5 mega units) at 4-hourly intervals until delivery. For women who are allergic to penicillin, clindamycin should be prescribed; the recommended dose is 900 mg IV every 8 hours until delivery.

To optimize the efficacy of antibiotic prophylaxis, the first dose should be given at least 2 hours prior to delivery.

Elective caesarean sections

Women undergoing planned CS in the absence of labour or membrane rupture do not require GBS antibiotic prophylaxis, irrespective of their GBS status, since the risk of neonatal GBS disease is extremely low.

Current NICE guidance recommends antibiotic prophylaxis (usually a single dose cephalosporin) prior to the start of surgery.

Other situations

- Antibiotic prophylaxis for GBS is unnecessary for women with preterm rupture of the membranes—unless they are in established labour.
- If chorioamnionitis is suspected, broad-spectrum antibiotic therapy, including an agent active against GBS should replace GBS-specific antibiotic prophylaxis.
- Pharmacokinetics of some common antibiotics is discussed in the 'Antibiotics' section above.

Anticoagulants

Anticoagulants are used in pregnancy for prophylactic as well as therapeutic reasons. Prophylactic use is during prolonged bed rest or the postoperative period in high-risk cases. Therapeutic use is during PE or DVT. They are also used throughout pregnancy if there is higher risk of DVT or PE due to personal or family history.

Antenatal risk factors for VTE as classified by NICE:
- Reduced mobility for ≥3 days
- Active cancer
- Age >35 years
- Critical care admission
- Dehydration

- Excess blood loss or blood transfusion
- Known thrombophilias
- Obesity (BMI >30 kg/m^2)
- Medical co-morbidity (heart disease, metabolic, endocrine, or respiratory pathologies, infectious or inflammatory conditions)
- Personal history or first-degree relative with history of VTE
- Pregnancy-related risk factors (OHSS, hyperemesis gravidarum, multiple pregnancy, pre-eclampsia)
- Varicose veins with phlebitis.

Low-molecular-weight heparins (dalteparin, enoxaparin, tinzaparin)

Pharmacology
- LMWHs are as effective as the unfractionated heparin. They have a longer duration of action and are given once or twice daily by the SC route. Doses are calculated based on early pregnancy weights.
- The standard prophylactic regimen does not need monitoring.

Dosage
See Table 9.1.
Therapeutic dalteparin (based on early pregnancy weight)
- 100 units/kg twice daily antenatally
- 200 units/kg once daily postnatally.

Therapeutic enoxaparin
- 1 mg/kg twice daily antenatally
- 1.5 mg/kg once daily postnatally.

Therapeutic tinzaparin
- 175 units/kg once a day.

Side effects
- Haemorrhage
- Thrombocytopenia: rare unless previously exposed to unfractionated heparin
- Hyperkalaemia
- Hypersensitivity.

Table 9.1 Prophylaxis of venous thromboembolism (VTE) daily doses

	Dalteparin	Enoxaparin	Tinzaparin
<50 kg	2500 units	20 mg	3500 units
50–90 kg	5000 units	40 mg	4500 units
91–130 kg[a]	7500 units	60 mg	7000 units
131–170 kg[a]	10000 units	80 mg	9000 units

[a] Give as two divided doses.

Drug interactions
Cautious use with NSAIDs and aspirin.

Contraindications
- Haemophilia and other haemorrhagic disorders
- Thrombocytopenia
- Peptic ulcer, recent cerebral haemorrhage
- Severe hypertension
- Known hypersensitivity
- Cautious use during spinal or epidural anaesthesia due to risk of spinal haematoma.

Anticonvulsants

Magnesium sulfate

Pharmacology
Magnesium sulfate has been shown to be very effective in the management of eclampsia, a life-threatening obstetric emergency. It prevents recurrent seizures. The exact mechanism of action of magnesium sulfate is not known.

Dosage
Regimens for management of eclampsia and for seizure prophylaxis in severe pre-eclampsia are the same:
- Loading dose: 4 g IV (over 5–10 minutes)
- Maintenance infusion rate of 1 g/hr for 24 hours after last seizure
- Additional IV bolus of 2 g can be given in cases of seizure recurrence.

Monitoring
Monitoring of pre-eclampsia and for clinical signs for overdose is essential:
- BP (every 15–60 minutes depending on severity)
- Urine output (minimum of 100 mL in last 4 hours)
- Respiratory rate (should be >16 breaths/min)
- Patellar reflexes (lost in overdose).

Calcium gluconate (10%–10 mL) can be used for management of magnesium toxicity.

Side effects
It can cause nausea, vomiting, thirst, and skin flushing but the more serious side effects are due to toxicity. These are arrhythmia, drowsiness, confusion, loss of tendon reflex, and respiratory paralysis.

Drug interaction
Profound hypotension has been seen with nifedipine and IV magnesium sulfate in pre-eclampsia. Parenteral magnesium enhances the effect of non-depolarizing muscle relaxants.

Diazepam
This is a benzodiazepine, which enhances GABA-mediated synaptic inhibition. Regular use is avoided in pregnancy due to risk of neonatal withdrawal symptoms, but it can be used for seizure control (e.g. status epilepticus). It was used in the past to treat eclamptic convulsions but magnesium sulfate has now been proven to be more effective.

Antihypertensives

The aim of treating hypertension in acute obstetric emergencies like severe pre-eclampsia and eclampsia is primarily to prevent serious maternal complications.

Hydralazine or labetalol infusion is preferred. Sometimes nifedipine is used sublingually to achieve a quick control of severe hypertension. Methyldopa, takes longer to control BP; hence it is not the drug of choice in cases of emergency.

Hydralazine
Pharmacology

This is a vasodilator and acts by direct relaxation of arteriolar smooth muscles. The decrease in BP is associated with a selective decrease in vascular resistance in coronary, cerebral, renal, and placental circulations.

Dosage
- The usual dose is administered as a slow IV 5–10 mg (diluted with 10 mL normal saline). This may be repeated after 20–30 minutes.
- Infusion 200–300 mcg/min, with a maintenance dose of 50–150 mcg/min is used in most units.

Side effects
- Flushing, palpitation, tachycardia, headache, fetal heart rate abnormalities due to reduction *in utero* placental circulation
- Fluid retention
- Arthralgia and myalgia
- Abnormal liver function, jaundice
- Pyridoxine responsive polyneuropathy.

Drug interactions
- Anaesthetics, analgesics, antidepressants, alcohol, anxiolytics, beta blockers, muscle relaxants, and nitrates all increase the hypotensive effect.
- Corticosteroids decrease the hypotensive effect.

Labetalol
Pharmacology

This is a combined α1 and β receptor antagonist. It lowers BP by reducing vascular resistance. Cardiac output at rest is not reduced.

Dosage
- Oral: 100 mg twice daily, can be increased to 800 mg twice daily. If dose is higher, should be divided into 3–4 doses. Maximum dose 2.4 g daily.
- IV injection: 50 mg over 1 minutes, repeated after 5 minutes. Maximum dose 200 mg.
- IV infusion: 2 mg/min until a satisfactory response is seen.
- In acute hypertensive crisis in pregnancy a dose of 20 mg/hr, doubled every 30 minutes, may be required (maximum dose of 160 mg/hr).

Side effects
- Postural hypotension
- Headache, tiredness
- Rashes
- Liver damage.

Contraindications
- History of obstructive airways disease
- AV block
- Severe peripheral arterial disease
- Phaeochromocytoma.

Nifedipine
This is a calcium channel blocker and relaxes vascular smooth muscle and dilates coronary and peripheral arteries.

Dosage
Different preparations have different dosages, but usual initial dose is 10 mg, twice daily, orally.

Side effects
- Headache, palpitation
- Tachycardia
- Gravitational oedema, rash.

Contraindications
- Cardiogenic shock, congestive cardiac failure
- Advanced aortic stenosis
- Porphyria.

Methyldopa
Pharmacology
This is a centrally acting antihypertensive which acts via an active metabolite. It is not used in cases of emergencies, but for long-term control of BP. It should be changed to another agent postnatally due to the association with postnatal depression.

Dosage
Oral—250 mg three times a day gradually increased to a maximum dose of 3 g daily.

Side effects
- GI disturbances, dry mouth
- Sedation, headache, dizziness, depression
- Hepatotoxicity is an uncommon but serious toxic effect
- Haemolytic anaemia, bone marrow depression.

Contraindications
- Depression
- Active hepatitis
- Phaeochromocytoma
- Porphyria.

Corticosteroids

The RCOG guidance states 'Antenatal steroids are associated with a significant reduction in rates of neonatal death, RDS and intraventricular haemorrhage and are safe for mothers'. These are given when preterm birth is expected at gestations between $24^{+0}/40$ and $34^{+6}/40$.

Glucocorticoids

Dosage
- Betamethasone 12 mg IM once daily (two doses)
- Dexamethasone 6 mg IM twice daily (four doses) or 12 mg IM twice daily (two doses).

Side effects
- Headache, malaise, and nausea
- Petechiae
- Facial erythema
- Urticaria
- Leucocytosis
- Hyperglycaemia
- Hypersensitivity reactions.

Contraindications
- Overt systemic infection is the major contraindication.
- Caution should be taken with diabetic patients as the administration of steroids can destabilize glycaemic control and often necessitates cover with IV insulin as a sliding scale.
- The mineralocorticoid side effects of hypertension and water retention are negligible with high-potency glucocorticoids but care must be taken in patients with cardiomyopathy or poor cardiac reserve.

Tocolytics

These are used in cases of preterm labour. Different drugs are used in different hospitals. The following are commonly used drugs.

Atosiban

This is an oxytocin receptor antagonist, which is licensed for the inhibition of uncomplicated preterm labour between 24 and 34 weeks' gestation.

Dosage
Initially 6.75 mg over 1 min by IV injection, then 18 mg/hr for 3 hr, followed by 6 mg/hr for up to 45 hours by infusion. Maximum duration of treatment is 48 hours.

Side effects
Nausea, vomiting, tachycardia, hypotension, headache, dizziness, hot flushes, hyperglycaemia.

Contraindications
- Eclampsia or severe pre-eclampsia
- Intrauterine infection
- Intrauterine fetal death
- Placenta praevia, abruption
- Abnormal fetal heart rate.

Nifedipine

This is a dihydropyridine calcium-channel blocker which is not licensed in the UK as a tocolytic and therefore the responsibility for its use lies with the prescribing doctor. It has comparable effectiveness to atosiban in delaying birth and is associated with better neonatal outcomes when compared to beta-2 agonist drugs.

Dosage

- Initial dose is 10 mg sublingually or PO every 15 minutes for the first hour.
- Maintenance dose is 20 mg PO three times a day.
- Dose can be increased to 160 mg/day depending on uterine activity but doses of >60 mg/day are associated with more adverse events.

Side effects

- Hypotension
- Headache and dizziness
- Palpitations
- GI upset.

Contraindications

- Cardiogenic shock
- Aortic stenosis
- Acute porphyria.

Terbutaline

This is a beta-2 agonist that is used for short-term tocolysis in situations of uterine hyperstimulation. A dose of 250 mcg SC is given, which can be repeated 15 minutes later if needed.

Induction agents

Various techniques are available for the induction of labour. A membrane sweep at term increases the chance of spontaneous labour (1 in 8 chance) and facilitates any subsequent induction of labour.

Dinoprostone

This is a prostaglandin E_2 analogue. It is recommended by NICE as the preferred method of induction of labour.

Dosage

- 3 mg PV: two separate doses 6 hours apart.
- Can be repeated 24 hours later if not in labour.

Risks

- Informed consent is required before use.
- There is a risk of uterine hyperstimulation and possible fetal compromise secondary to hypoxia.
- There is also a risk of uterine rupture leading to maternal haemorrhage and risk of amniotic fluid embolus.

Side effects

- Nausea and vomiting
- Diarrhoea
- Flushing, shivering, headache, dizziness and hypotension

- Hypertension
- Convulsions
- Pyrexia and raised white cell count.

Uterine stimulants

These are used to stimulate or increase uterine contractions. The main uses are induction of labour, augmentation of labour, prevention or treatment of PPH, management of retained placenta.

Oxytocin

This is an octapeptide produced in the hypothalamus and released from the neurohypophysis. The plasma half-life is only a few minutes. It stimulates both the frequency and the amplitude of uterine contractions. These effects are dependent on oestrogen and the immature uterus is resistant to these effects. It is similar in structure to vasopressin and so also has an antidiuretic hormone effect.

Use

Induction and augmentation of labour, as well as prophylaxis and treatment of PPH.

Dosage

30 IU of oxytocin in 500 mL of normal saline will give 1 milliunit (mU) per minute if run at 1 mL/hr. Maximum recommended dose is 20 mU/min. Infusion is commenced at 2 mU/min and escalated at 2 mU/min every 30 minutes until contractions lasting 40 seconds recur 4–5 times in every 10 minutes. The dosage schedule is indicated in Box 9.1.

In severe PPH an IV infusion of up to 40 IU in 500 mL of fluid is given at a rate sufficient to control uterine atony.

Side effects

- Uterine hyperstimulation leading to fetal distress
- Water intoxication and hyponatraemia if given in high doses with electrolyte free solutions: muscle cramps, confusion, and coma
- Nausea, vomiting
- Arrhythmia
- Headache.

Drug interactions

- Inhalational anaesthetics reduce oxytocic effect
- Prostaglandins have uterotonic effect.

Box 9.1 Concentration of oxytocin

- 2–16 mU/min is physiological range
- 5–10 mU/min initiates uterine activity comparable to early labour
- 10–15 mU/min generates uterine activity similar to late first stage of labour
- 20–25 mU/min produces activity similar to second stage of labour.

Contraindications
- Mechanical obstruction to delivery
- Fetal distress
- Severe cardiovascular disease
- Severe pre-eclampsia.

Ergometrine
Pharmacology

This is an ergot alkaloid and has a very powerful uterotonic action. It produced a forceful and prolonged uterine contraction so that resting tone is increased and a sustained myometrial contracture is maintained. This is very effective in controlling atonic uterine bleeding.

Use

Postpartum bleeding, bleeding after miscarriage.

Dosage

500 mcg IM injection.

Side effects
- Nausea, vomiting, headache, dizziness, tinnitus
- Transient hypertension
- Vasoconstriction
- Abdominal pain, chest pain.

Drug interactions

Risk of ergotism with erythromycin.

Contraindications
- Severe hypertension, eclampsia
- Induction of labour, first, and second stage of labour
- Vascular disease
- Severe hepatic and renal impairment
- Severe cardiac disease
- Impaired pulmonary function.

Carboprost
Pharmacology

Prostaglandin F2α is produced in the uterus and is a luteolytic hormone in some subprimate species. Its main use is to control bleeding in atonic PPH where the uterus has failed to respond to ergometrine and oxytocin.

Dosage

250 mcg deep IM injection, to be repeated if necessary after 15 minutes. Maximum dose is 2 mg (8 doses).

Side effects
- Nausea vomiting, diarrhoea
- Hyperthermia and flushing
- Less frequently raised BP and dyspnoea and pulmonary oedema.

Contraindications

Cardiac, renal, pulmonary, and hepatic disease.

Further reading

Joint Formulary Committee. *British National Formulary* (70th ed). London: BMJ Group and Pharmaceutical Press, 2015.

National Institute for Health and Care Excellence. *Caesarean Section* (CG 132). London: NICE, 2011, reviewed 2014.

National Institute for Health and Care Excellence. *Inducing Labour* (CG70). London: NICE, 2008, reviewed 2014.

Royal College of Obstetricians and Gynaecologists. *Antenatal Corticosteroids to Prevent Respiratory Distress Syndrome* (Green-top Guideline No 7). London: RCOG, 2004, reviewed 2014.

Royal College of Obstetricians and Gynaecologists. *Reducing the Risk of Thrombosis and Embolism During Pregnancy and Puerperium* (Green-top Guideline No. 37a). London: RCOG, 2015.

Royal College of Obstetricians and Gynaecologists. *Tocolysis for Women in Preterm Labour* (Green-top Guideline No. 1b). London: RCOG, 2011.

Schaefer C, Peters PWJ, Miller RK (eds). *Drugs During Pregnancy and Lactation: Treatment Options and Risk Assessment* (3rd ed). London: Academic Press Inc, 2014.

Sweetman SC (ed). *Martindale: The Complete Drug Reference* (38th ed). London: Pharmaceutical Press, 2014.

Part 2

Gynaecology

Abnormal menses and bleeding

Contributor
Tahir Mahmood

Contents

Abnormal uterine bleeding

Physiological basis of menstrual bleeding

Progesterone withdrawal is thought to trigger menstrual bleeding by initiating the local production of large amounts of prostaglandin (PG)-$F_{2\alpha}$ and endothelin 1. Some arterial bleeding may be augmented by the presence of vasodilating PGE_2 and PGI_2 in the first 2 days of menses. Further contribution is made by the endometrial stroma which also produces PGE_2 and PGI_2 with platelet inhibiting and vasodilating activity.

There is also increased production of cytokines, especially interleukin 1 and tumour necrosis factor alpha by local mast cells and endometrial vascular endothelial growth factor expression also increases with the onset of hypoxia.

Plasminogen activator inhibitors are also decreased around menstruation.

Normal cycle length ranges between 22 and 35 days in the mid-reproductive years. The range of normal duration varies between 3 and 8 days.

Causes of abnormal uterine bleeding

- Endocervical polyps
- Adenomyosis
- Submucous leiomyoma
- Endometrial hyperplasia and malignancy
- Disorders of systematic haemostasis (von Willebrand disease has been noted in up to 13% of cases in one series)
- Ovulatory dysfunction (failure of consistent and predictable ovulation results in absent or inconsistent release of progesterone from the ovary manifesting as oligo/anovulation; isolated or chronic anovulation as seen in polycystic ovaries (PCO)
- Around the menarche, the relative immunity of the hypothalamic–pituitary–ovarian axis frequently results in a transient oligoanovulatory environment
- Untreated hypothyroidism
- Iatrogenic causes:
  - anticoagulants (LMWH and warfarin)
  - drugs affecting ovulation (tricyclic antidepressants and phenothiazines act through dopamine metabolism causing ovulatory dysfunction)
  - systematically administered agents such as steroids (oestrogens, progestins, and androgens)
  - intrauterine systems, i.e. inert devices such as copper-loaded IUCD or the levonorgestrel-releasing intrauterine system (LNG-IUS)
- Endometrial causes, i.e.:
  - local disturbances of endometrial molecular mechanisms within ovulatory cycles
  - increased local levels of PGI_2—leads to reduction in the ability of endometrium to attain effective haemostasis
  - enhanced fibrinolysis through increased endometrial levels of tissue plasminogen activator

- Post-traumatic arteriovenous malformations in the uterus (following uterine curettage for retained placental tissue)
- Chronic endometrial infection and/or inflammation.

A structured management strategy

The purpose of history taking is to establish:
- The patient's normal menstrual pattern
- The features of the abnormal bleeding including timing, volume, and associated symptoms such as dysmenorrhoea
- Mid-cycle unilateral pelvic pain is suggestive of ovulation
- To assess the impact of heavy menstrual bleeding (HMB) or abnormal uterine bleeding on quality of life
- Identify risk factors for a systematic disorder of haemostasis. This includes enquiring about the following:
  - history of HMB since menarche
  - history of epistaxis once to twice a month, frequent gum bleeding; easy bruising and family history of bleeding disorders
  - family history of hereditary non-polyposis, colorectal cancer syndrome (this group of women are at increased risk of developing uterine cancer)
  - past history of PPH, surgical-related bleeding, bleeding associated with dental work
- Physical examination:
  - to determine that the bleeding is not arising from obvious lesions of the perineum, perianal area, the lower genital tract, or extra-genital region and is definitely uterine in origin
  - look for signs suggestive of PCO (note: women with high BMI would have increased risk of anovulation and unpredictable bleeding)
- Investigations:
  - consider checking haemoglobin, haematocrit, thyroid function test if underactive thyroid is suspected, and PCO screening if history and signs are suggestive of it.

Abdominal and pelvic examination

Pelvic examination should help to find out if uterine enlargement is symmetrical or asymmetrical and to rule out any concomitant pelvic masses. It should also help to differentiate between *non-genital tract causes of bleeding*, which are as follows:
- Lacerations
- Tumours
- Anal fissures
- Urethral caruncle.

Speculum examination

Should rule out vaginal traumatic lacerations and tumours.
  Cervix:
- Ectropion
- Cervicitis
- Polyps
- Sometimes, you may find a lost tampon higher up in the vaginal canal, just behind the cervix. It should be removed
- Cervical suspicious lesions.

If ectropion or cervicitis is noted, screening should be considered for *Chlamydia trachomatis* infection.

Indications for uterine evaluation

Endometrial biopsy is a blind procedure and quite ineffective at diagnosing intrauterine focal lesions and polyps are quite often missed. In an ideal situation, endometrial sampling should be done along with diagnostic hysteroscopy.

Histology assessment should be considered in the following groups:
- High-risk age group (age >40)
- Obesity (weight >90 kg)
- History of chronic anovulation, infertility, or diabetes
- Family history of endometrial cancer
- Prolonged exposure to unopposed oestrogens or tamoxifen
- Where trial of treatment with medical treatments has failed.

Transvaginal ultrasound scanning (TVS): to measure double thickness of endometrium, also called endometrial echocomplex (EEC). A homogenous, thin EEC <5 mm without any adjacent leiomyoma is reassuring.

Ultrasound is generally useful for evaluation of myomas in the myometrium. TVS is as sensitive as MRI for the diagnosis of diffuse adenomyosis.

Colour flow Doppler ultrasound is useful in detecting blood flow and for the detection of arteriovenous malformations. It has also a place in distinguishing focal adenomyosis from leiomyoma.

Management plan
- Management of anaemia
- Antifibrinolytics
- Non-steroidal anti-inflammatory drugs
- LNG-IUS
- Combined oral contraceptive
- Oral progestogens
- Injected progestogens
- Danazol
- Gonadotrophin-releasing hormone analogues
- Esmya® (ulipristal acetate) for uterine fibroids
- Endometrial ablation
- Uterine artery embolization
- Myomectomy
- Hysterectomy.

Pre-menarcheal bleeding
- Utero-vaginal bleeding that occurs prior to menarche must always be considered abnormal.
- The most common causes of such bleeding are inflammation and infections of the vulva and perineum.
- Sexual abuse has to be considered.

Causes

Hormonal

- Hormonal (precocious puberty, sex steroid-producing tumours such as granulose, theca, embryonal, others)
- Combination contraceptives
- Vaginal/cervical neoplasm such as adenocarcinoma and rhabdomyosarcoma.

Inflammatory

- Sexually transmitted infection (chlamydia, gonorrhoea, condyloma)
- Parasites (amoebiasis, fungal, *Enterobius vermicularis* (pinworm))
- Bacterial (*Staphylococcus aureus*, beta-haemolytic *Streptococcus*)
- Chemical (soap, cosmetics)
- Dermatological (lichen sclerosis).

Trauma

- Sexual abuse
- Instrumentation
- Physical activity related (accidental causes such as bicycle riding, falling on sharp object)
- Social (poor hygiene, foreign body)
- Urological (haematuria)
- Idiopathic.

Management

- History should be taken from the patient's parents separately to ascertain the nature of symptoms, duration, and the associated history.

Examination

- It is useful to spend time explaining why examination is needed and how it will be performed in a very relaxed environment, especially for younger children. The room should be nicely decorated with plenty of toys for their attention diversion.
- Examination of younger children may be successful while they are sitting in their parent's or guardian's lap (positioning for vulval examination can be done with the child lying supine with legs in a 'frog leg' or 'butterfly' position).
- For visualization of the vagina, the 'knee chest' position may be best.
- If adequate examination is not feasible in the clinic then examination under anaesthesia may be required.
- General examination. Assess Tanner staging of both breasts and pubic hair as early menarche is a relatively common cause of physiological pre-menarcheal bleeding.
- Look for any evidence of bruising.
- Observation of child's interaction with parents or guardians is important.

Vulva/hymen
- May be facilitated by using a colposcope, especially in the case of abuse.
- Should also consider potential non-genital tract source of bleeding in the peri-urethral or perianal region.
- In case of abuse, always look for non-specific findings which include labial adhesions, vaginal discharge, vulval/introital or anal erythema, anal fissures and anal dilatation, hymenal tags—acute laceration or ecchymosis.
- Foul smelling discharge could be associated with a foreign body in the vagina, e.g. toilet paper, small toys, coins, etc.

Acute uterine bleeding
Reasons are not always clear but may be associated with the following:
- Localized lesions such as submucosal leiomyoma.
- Acute bleeding may occur from a structurally normal endometrial cavity or an unsuspected cervical tumour.
- Most often occurs among women with disorders of ovulation as there is a lack of progesterone-dependent endometrial haemostatic factor.
- Frequently seen in peri-menarcheal girls.
- Medical disorders such as PCO, hyperprolactinaemia, hypothyroidism and drugs which affect dopamine metabolism.
- Other factors such as psychological stress, rapid changes in weight, and excessive exercise.

Initial evaluation
- Ensure that patient is haemodynamically stable; if not, set up an IV line.
- Check haemoglobin levels and cross match if required.
- β-hCG estimation to rule out pregnancy and an ectopic pregnancy.
- Ascertain by examination that bleeding is indeed uterine in origin.
- Consider investigations for an inherited disorder of haemostasis if history is suggestive.
- Endometrial biopsy may be suboptimal due to the influence of intrauterine blood clots.

Management
- High-dose oestrogen plus progestin combined monophasic pill administered 3–4 times a day with gradual reduction once bleeding has stopped
- Progestin such as medroxyprogesterone acetate 60–120 mg on day 1 and then continuing 20 mg per day for the next 10 days. The other option is to start with high-dose norethisterone, such as 10 mg twice a day till bleeding has stopped and then gradually reduce it to complete a course of 3 weeks.
- Surgical: consider intrauterine tamponade using Foley's catheter balloon.
- Hysteroscopy and uterine curettage.
- Thermal balloon ablation.
- Uterine artery occlusion.
- In rare circumstances, hysterectomy may be considered.

Heavy menstrual bleeding

Normal cycle length ranges between 22 and 35 days in the mid-reproductive years. The range of normal duration varies between 3 and 8 days. The proportion of menstrual fluid that is red cells is about 25% with the remaining fluid volume likely derived from the serous, endometrial transudates. In women with HMB, the mean whole blood component is increased to around 50%.

HMB has been defined as excessive menstrual blood loss, which interferes with a woman's physical, emotional, social, and sexual quality of life and which can occur alone or in combination with other symptoms. Whether HMB is a problem, it should be determined not by measuring blood loss but by the woman herself. In the UK, 5% of women present with this problem in acute hospitals and the incidence increases with age (>30 years) and parity.

Causes

In the majority of women there are no pathological features other than an imbalance of hormonal production or imbalance in prostaglandin production. HMB may be the result of either ovulatory or anovulatory cycles.

Aetiology

- *Disorders* of endometrial function, especially related to vasculature.
- Disordered production of prostaglandins at the endomyometrial junction (increased ratios of PGI_2 and/or PGE_2 to $PGF_2\alpha$ are seen in women with HMB):
  - a small proportion of women may have underlying problems such as hypothyroidism, bleeding disorders, and PCO
  - other causes include multiple uterine fibroids, pelvic endometriosis, and endometrial polyps.

Clinical approach

- A full menstrual history (length of bleeding, length of cycle, number of days of heavy bleeding, impact of HMB on woman's quality of life, and her inability to get out of the house)
- The presence of *red light symptoms* (intermenstrual bleeding, post-coital bleeding, pelvic pain not related to menses, pressure symptoms). This group of women will require additional investigations.

Pelvic examination

- The purpose is to ensure that the uterus is normal size so that a LNG-IUS can be inserted.
- If there is any structural abnormality noted then further investigations can be arranged.
- Based on the clinical findings, the decision can be made whether endometrial sampling is required or not.

Investigations

- TVS to identify structural abnormality.
- Endometrial biopsy and diagnostic hysteroscopy if the patient is in high-risk group (see 'Abnormal uterine bleeding', pp. 230–4).

Treatment

Pharmaceutical treatment can be started without examination in those women where pathology is unlikely, i.e. regular heavy periods with no red light symptoms. The main issues to be considered are:

- Whether contraception is required
- Whether dysmenorrhoea or pelvic pain is present
- Woman's preferences.

Pharmaceutical options

- Antifibrinolytics
- Cyclo-oxygenase inhibitors
- LNG-IUS
- Combined oral contraceptive: very effective and acceptable alternative: *oral progestogens*
- Norethisterone 5 mg three times a day from day 5 to day 26 of the menstrual cycle is effective as compared to short-cycle regimen.

Surgical treatment

- Endometrial ablation
- Hysterectomy.

Dysmenorrhoea (period pains)

- Dysmenorrhoea is a common symptom in the early reproductive years. Period pain is a crampy lower abdominal pain, which commonly spreads to the lower back or upper thighs. It usually starts with the onset of a period, though it may start a day or two before. Some periods may be worse than others.
- Many women do have other symptoms apart from pain. These include headaches, backache, tiredness, nausea, and diarrhoea.
- Dysmenorrhoea has been classified as primary dysmenorrhoea and secondary dysmenorrhoea.
- Primary dysmenorrhoea usually starts 1–2 years after the onset of menarche. In the majority of cases there is no detectable organic cause.
- Secondary dysmenorrhoea usually occurs in older women in association with some underlying pathology such as pelvic endometriosis, adenomyosis, chronic PID, and the use of non-hormonal IUCDs.
- It may also recur among women taking hormone replacement therapy.

Aetiology

Primary dysmenorrhoea may be related to an imbalance in the production of prostaglandins which leads to vasoconstriction and increases uterine contractility, as happens in cases of adenomyosis and uterine fibroids. The posterior pituitary peptides, such as vasopressin and oxytocin, have been implicated, but the precise mechanism of their interaction remains unclear.

Primary dysmenorrhoea

History

- Identify relationship with onset of menstrual bleeding—the pain may precede the bleeding but it is usually worse during the first 2 days of menses.
- It is a crampy pain and usually starts occurring 1–2 years after the onset of menarche when periods become ovulatory.
- HMB is quite often associated with anovulatory cycles in this group of women.
- Associated symptoms such as irregular cycles, dyspareunia, and vaginal discharge should be enquired about and investigated for sexually transmitted infections.
- Enquire about the current contraceptive needs, the smear history (if age >20 years in Scotland and >25 years in England) and details of past pregnancies.
- Complete a detailed medical and surgical history.
- Some women may experience pain in the middle of the cycle related to ovulation (needs reassurance).

Investigations

- For young women under the age of 20 with no other symptoms, it is not necessary to undertake any examination.

- If there are signs of anaemia, check FBC.
- If there is a history of sexually transmitted disease, triple swabs should be performed.
- If there are signs suggestive of PCO, endocrine profile assessing serum FSH, LH, and testosterone should be checked.
- If vaginal examination is unsatisfactory then TVS should be considered to look for any obvious pelvic pathology such as ovarian cysts or fibroids.
- It is always important to rule out the possibility of incomplete miscarriage or ectopic pregnancy among sexually active young women. Always remember that cervical cancer can also develop in young women and they can also present with abnormal bleeding with pelvic pain.

Treatment
- Non-steroidal anti-inflammatory agents are effective treatment for dysmenorrhoea though women using them need to be aware of the significant risk of adverse side effects.
- Mefenamic acid 500 mg 8-hourly can be prescribed, to be commenced 24–48 hours prior to the onset of pain and continued during the most painful days of the period.
- Ibuprofen 400 mg 8-hourly can be used.
- Paracetamol is equally effective in cases of mild dysmenorrhoea.
- Combined oral contraceptive pill. This is another option, especially for those who require contraception. The pill usually decreases prostaglandin production, uterine contractility, and blood flow to the uterus. The majority of women (>80%) note significant improvement in their symptoms.
- The LNG-IUS is highly effective for those individuals who cannot take the combined oral contraceptive pill. However, it may be occasionally difficult to insert a LNG-IUS through the nulliparous cervix.
- Gonadotrophin-releasing hormone agonist. The long-term use is limited because of their possible hypo-oestrogenic side effects.
- Continuous administration of progestogens may be effective and can be administered either as a Depo preparation (Depo-Provera® 150 mg IM at 12-weekly intervals) or continuous oral treatment with progestogens as described previously.

Secondary dysmenorrhoea
Pain is possibly related to underlying pathology and the causes include:
- Endometriosis
- Adenomyosis
- Chronic pelvic infection
- Non-hormonal IUCD
- Endometrial polyps
- Submucous fibroids
- History of pelvic/abdominal surgery
- Intrauterine adhesions following surgery or infection
- Psychosexual problems.

History
- Usually starts later than teenage years or maybe a change in pattern, type, or intensity of usual pain.
- Pain usually starts a couple of days before the onset of period and continuous throughout the period.
- Often associated with deep dyspareunia and there may be other associated symptoms such as abnormal bleeding and vaginal discharge.

Examination
Abdominal and pelvic examination may reveal:
- Enlarged uterus (fibroids)
- Enlarged ovaries (ovarian endometrioma)
- Tender masses in both adnexae (hydrosalpinges due to infection)
- Overall tenderness on pelvic examination, especially marked in the pouch of Douglas (pelvic endometriosis, PID)
- Nodular tender feeling in the pouch of Douglas (pelvic endometriosis).

Investigations
- Cervical smear if overdue or clinical abnormality of cervix noted.
- Endocervical swab for infection screening (chlamydia, gonococcal infection).
- Pelvic ultrasound scan if pelvic examination is either unsatisfactory or a pelvic mass has been noted.
- Diagnostic laparoscopy has a definite role for women where pelvic examination is normal but they continue to complain of congestive dysmenorrhoea and deep dyspareunia.

Management
- Consider all options as described for primary dysmenorrhoea.
- Laparoscopic uterine nerve ablation—its long-term effectiveness is unknown.
- Hysterectomy may be an appropriate option for some women.
- If there is a history of pelvic endometriosis, then a focused strategy on endometriosis is important, especially to ascertain whether fertility is desirable or not.

General management advice
- Women should be counselled about other methods of pain relief (e.g. some women find warmth helps, such as a hot bath or hot water bottle wrapped in a towel held against their lower abdomen).
- Some women may wish to use alternative treatment preparations such as herbal preparations.
- There is uncontrolled data indicating the effectiveness of Chinese medicine, spinal manipulation, acupuncture, and many others.

Chronic and acute abdominal pain

Contributor

Stergios K. Doumouchtsis

Contents

⑦ Chronic abdominal pain

This is one of the common presenting complaints, accounting for about 10% of referrals to the gynaecology outpatient clinic. In most cases, no obvious pathology is detected. It is important to manage these patients with sensitivity to ensure that the resulting psychological damage is limited. At the same time the clinician should avoid undertaking investigations that are not clinically indicated.

Causes

Gynaecological
- Pelvic infection.
- Recurrent infections with resulting adhesion formation could become a difficult clinical problem to treat.
- *Endometriosis:* this is one of the commonest reasons for ongoing pelvic pain and affects ~10% of women of reproductive age. Unfortunately, the pathophysiology is still poorly understood and it is not easy to clinically correlate the presenting symptoms with the severity of the disease as seen at laparoscopy. There is a range of symptoms and most commonly women present with pelvic pain, dysmenorrhoea, infertility, or a pelvic mass. Direct visualization and biopsy during laparoscopy or laparotomy is the gold standard diagnostic test for this condition and enables the gynaecologist to identify the location, extent, and severity of the disease.
- *Tumours:* pelvic tumours, benign and malignant, could lead to long-standing unresolved pain. Ovarian cysts and fibroids are the commonest tumours responsible for such pain.
- *Other causes:* ovulatory pain (mittelschmerz) and premenstrual pain are the physiological causes for chronic pain. Pelvic congestion syndrome is being considered as another possible cause.

Non-gynaecological
- *Depression:* this could be a cause for chronic pain and also an effect of long-standing pain for which no cause can be found. It is a diagnosis by exclusion.
- *Childhood sexual abuse:* childhood trauma can present with chronic pain.
- *Urinary tract infection:* recurrent UTIs could lead to chronic cystitis and unresolving pain.
- *Irritable bowel syndrome (IBS):* this is a common cause and is diagnosed by exclusion.
- *Inflammatory bowel disease:* Crohn's disease and ulcerative colitis can both lead to chronic pain.
- *Constipation:* this is not uncommon and can be treated effectively if detected.

Symptoms

Pelvic pain

A detailed history about the onset, duration, and progress of the pain is essential. This will provide significant information to help achieve a diagnosis. Pain scores can be of limited accuracy as often patients claim very high scores—but tools such as quality of life scoring systems can help.

Associated symptoms

These include dyspareunia, vaginal discharge, and bladder and bowel symptoms. Dyspareunia could be caused by endometriosis or pelvic infection. Offensive vaginal discharge is suggestive of pelvic infection.

Other relevant history

- Detailed menstrual history, contraceptive history, and smear history is essential.
- History about any previous pregnancies. Any traumatic deliveries and postnatal depression could be the underlying reason for chronic pelvic pain.
- Previous medical and surgical history to note any bowel- and bladder-related problems in the past.
- History of medications such as analgesics used in the past provides information about the severity and chronicity of pain.
- Social history—unemployment and drug abuse could be important social problems leading to depression and symptoms such as chronic pelvic pain.
- Effect of the symptoms on the patient's lifestyle—absence from work and disturbance in family life may reflect the severity of pain.

Signs

- *General examination:* while obtaining history and performing general examination, it is important to observe the patient for expressions of obvious pain and discomfort.
- *Abdominal examination:* inspection of the abdomen will reveal previous scars indicating previous abdominal surgeries. On palpation, a loaded sigmoid may suggest constipation. Any tender areas may suggest intra-abdominal pathology.
- *Pelvic examination.*
- *Vulval inspection:* this is performed to look for any obvious discharge or vulval skin abnormalities.
- *Speculum examination:* this would reveal any offensive vaginal discharge suggesting pelvic infection or presence of local lesions on the cervix or the vagina.
- *Bimanual examination:* to look for forniceal thickening and tenderness. Nodules and tenderness in the uterosacral ligaments or rectovaginal septum may indicate endometriosis. Any obvious palpable adnexal masses may be due to tumours or fibroids. Rectal examination may reveal a loaded rectum suggesting constipation.

Investigations

- *Full blood count:* it is important to look for raised white cell count (WCC) suggesting presence of infection.
- *Raised C-reactive protein:* this is seen in the presence of pelvic infections and inflammatory bowel disease.
- *Urine culture and sensitivity:* to look for evidence of urinary tract infection.
- *Endocrine profile:* this could help to detect raised LH/FSH ratio and serum testosterone levels suggesting polycystic ovarian disease.
- *Plain film abdominal X-rays:* these can reveal faecal loading and some calculi.
- *Transvaginal ultrasound examination:* it is useful to detect pelvic pathology such as uterine fibroid, ovarian cysts, endometriotic cysts, and PCO. A normal scan is also reassuring and may result in symptom relief in anxious patients.
- *Diagnostic laparoscopy:* depending on the severity of the symptoms and findings of the preliminary investigations one may have to perform a laparoscopy to evaluate the abdomen and pelvis further. It is an invasive test associated with anaesthetic and surgical risks, but provides valuable information to understand the cause of the chronic pain. A negative laparoscopy also becomes very reassuring and can help the anxious patient psychologically.

Treatment

Non-gynaecological cause
- A systematic approach and extreme sensitivity is necessary throughout the management of these patients.
- One must think of non-gynaecological causes which are likely to cause chronic pelvic pain.
- Psychological disturbances are common and counselling could benefit these patients significantly.
- Dietary alterations to increase the dietary fibre content along with increased daily fluid intake should be considered. Lactose and wheat avoidance can help.
- Stool softeners and other laxatives can improve or treat pelvic pain caused by constipation.
- If clinically indicated, referral should be considered for the opinion of a colorectal surgeon or gastroenterologist at an early stage.

Gynaecological cause
- If a gynaecological cause is found, then appropriate medical or surgical treatment is initiated.
- If regular analgesics are not effective and the routine investigations have failed to detect a specific cause, a referral to a pain clinic should be considered. Counselling may be required.

- Laparoscopy should be considered only if necessary. Surgical therapy can be performed concurrently with diagnostic surgery and may include excision or ablation of endometriotic tissue, division of adhesions, and removal of endometriotic cysts. Laparoscopic excision or ablation of endometriosis has been shown to be effective in the management of pain in mild-to-moderate endometriosis. Adjunctive medical treatment pre- or postoperatively may prolong the symptom-free interval. There is insufficient evidence from the studies identified to conclude that hormonal suppression in association with surgery for endometriosis is associated with a significant benefit with regard to any of the outcomes identified. There is little or no difference in the effectiveness of GnRHas in comparison with other medical treatments for endometriosis. Side effects of GnRHas can be controlled by the addition of addback therapy.

Hints

- It is a common problem and can be difficult to treat.
- Patients need to be treated with a tactful and sensitive approach.
- Underlying psychological factors must be explored.
- A multidisciplinary approach may be more effective.

☠ Acute abdominal pain

Definition
Pain that is sudden in onset (<24 hours) usually associated with signs of peritonism (guarding, rebound, rigidity).

Gynaecological causes
- Common: ectopic pregnancy, miscarriage, ovarian cyst, PID
- Less common: ovarian/adnexal torsion/tubovarian abscess.

History
LMP, site of pain and nature, colicky or persistent, vaginal discharge, fever, previous past gynaecology history.

Examination
Abdomen soft or rigid, rebound, peritonism when coughs, requiring regular analgesia, palpable mass.

Investigations
Pregnancy test, MSU for microscopy and culture, high vaginal swab for culture (HVS), endocervical swabs, FBC, serum hCG, G&S, pelvic ultrasound (US) examination.

Diagnosis
- *Ectopic:* serum hCG >1500 U empty uterus on US with small amount of vaginal bleeding and adnexal pain. TVS can diagnose 80% of cases and laparoscopy almost 100% of cases.
- *Miscarriage:* colicky pelvic pain with vaginal bleeding moderate/large amount, positive pregnancy test, and US suggests miscarriage.
- *Ovarian cyst:* usually constant pain and cyst is seen on US. May be a simple cyst, or have mixed echoes of haemorrhage (spider web appearance)—haemorrhagic cysts classically luteal phase cycle and after intercourse. Ground-glass appearance on US suggests endometrioma and mixed bright echoes suggest a dermoid.
- *Ovarian cyst/fibroid torsion:* pain constant or colicky may radiate to leg, associated with vomiting and raised WCC or interleukin 6, cyst seen on US. Doppler US may be useful.
- *PID:* acute PID associated with pyrexia (>38°C), cervical excitation/dyspareunia, vaginal discharge, and raised WCC/CRP. Laparoscopy is the gold standard for diagnosis, but is usually not required as PID first-line management is medically with antibiotics. If non-responsive to IV treatment, consider tubovarian abscess and indication for drainage.
- *Non-gynaecological causes* should be considered and CT is a useful tool.

Treatment

- *Ectopic:* laparoscopic salpingectomy if the contralateral tube appears healthy and the patient is haemodynamically stable. Conservative approaches can be considered in specific situations.
- *Miscarriage:* ERPC or conservative management. Medical management can be offered provided patient is haemodynamically stable.
- *Ovarian cyst:* when <5 cm and not requiring regular analgesia, it can be managed conservatively. If patient requires parenteral analgesia and/or there are signs of acute abdomen then laparoscopy and ovarian cystectomy may be advisable.
- *Haemorrhagic ovarian cysts:* haemorrhage into a cyst is usually managed conservatively provided it is not causing a lot of pain and the patient is haemodynamically stable. If pain is not controlled, and there are signs of peritonism or haemodynamic disturbance, laparoscopic lavage is performed and a cystectomy or haemostatic manoeuvre employed.
- *Ovarian cyst torsion:* torsion can be managed conservatively by laparoscopically untwisting the torted ovary and cyst if undertaken within 36 hours of the torsion, thus avoiding adnexectomy if the ovary is viable.
- *PID:* oral treatment: ofloxacin 400 mg twice a day plus oral metronidazole 400 mg twice a day for 14 days. IV treatment: ofloxacin 400 mg twice a day plus metronidazole 500 mg three times a day for 14 days. Oral therapy can be started 24 hours after clinical improvement. Surgical (laparoscopic) drainage is often required.

Beware of diagnosing 'PID' in the absence of laparoscopic or microbiological evidence because this can cause great psychological distress for patients and their partners.

Intraoperative emergencies

Contributors

Vikram S. Talaulikar and S. Arulkumaran

Contents

:☠: Haemorrhage

An unexpected blood loss of >500 mL at any gynaecological operation is considered significant by the RCOG clinical governance standards. When such estimated blood loss has occurred intraoperatively the following measures may be considered:

Treatment

1. ► Inform your anaesthetist and ask for cross-match of 4–6 units of blood.
2. Careful ligation of appropriate vessels with sutures. ►► In case of a solitary source of bleeding like lacerated vessel or slipped pedicle, it is vital that the source is identified accurately and secured. Blind suturing should be avoided as it can make matters worse and cause further damage.
3. Careful use of diathermy and consider using Surgicel™.
4. Apply pressure with a warm pack and ensure adequate blood and/or clotting factors replacement. Inform the on-call haematologist and send a clotting screen.
5. Rarely the organ bleeding (tube, ovary, or uterus) will require removing surgically to arrest bleeding.
6. Very rarely consider ligation (but not division) of anterior division of internal iliac artery possibly with vascular surgeon on call.[1] A vascular clamp/or bulldog clamp can be used to see if ligation of the iliac artery will be useful or not.
7. Should there be one available, an interventional radiologist can be involved to locate and occlude the vessels causing the haemorrhage (embolization) when other measures have failed. Cell savers technology should be utilized where available.[2]
8. The use of the protease inhibitor aprotinin, arginine vasopressin derivatives (desmopressin), and recombinant factor VII (rfVIIa) can all be considered when blood loss continues despite the above-mentioned measures and have been proven to be useful.[3]
9. Very rarely a pack may be left *in situ* (especially when hypothermia (<35°C), acidosis > 7.2, or coagulopathy (partial thromboplastin time >16 sec) exist[4]) and removed at second look laparotomy 24 hours later when the patient's condition has stabilized.

References

1. Oleszczuk D, Cebulak K, Skret A, et al. Long term observation of patients after bilateral ligation of internal iliac arteries. *Ginekol Pol* 1995; 66(9):533–6.
2. Guo XY, Duan H, Wang JJ, et al. Effect of intraoperative using cell saver on blood sparing and its impact on coagulation function. *Zhongguo Yi Xue Ke Xue Yuan Xue Bao* 2004; 26(2); 188–91, 2004.
3. Paramo JA, Lecumberri R, Hernandez M, et al. Pharmacological alternatives to blood transfusion: what is new about? *Med Clin (Barc)* 2004; 122(6):231–6.
4. Stagnitti F, Bresadola L, Calderale SM. Abdominal "packing": indications and method. *Ann Ital Chir* 2003; 74(5):535–42.

Perforated uterus

This may occur during D&C, hysteroscopy, insertion of a coil, or at ERPC/suction termination of pregnancy (STOP). It may be noticed at the time by the feeling of 'lack of resistance' when probing the uterine cavity or may present postoperatively with signs of acute abdomen. Its incidence is 0.1–0.5% and risk of associated bowel trauma is >0.1%.[1]

Treatment

1. Inform the anaesthetist and ensure a large-bore IV cannula is inserted.
2. Leave instrument in the uterus that you believe has caused perforation and, if this is a suction cannula, then turn off the suction.
3. Proceed to a laparoscopy, assuming the patient is haemodynamically stable.
4. Inspect uterus for perforations/bleeding points and if possible inspect as much intestine at the laparoscopy as you can. If in doubt about bowel trauma, especially if fat (which may be part of the omentum) was sucked or removed, patient needs a laparotomy for a good evaluation. Call a colorectal surgeon.
5. Commonly small perforations that are not bleeding can be managed conservatively with antibiotics (cefuroxime and metronidazole) and admitted overnight for observation.
6. Should there be bleeding from the uterus then a laparoscopic suture or laparotomy may be needed to repair the perforation and to arrest bleeding.[2–4]
7. ERPC or STOP can then be completed under laparoscopic control and under US guidance to ensure there are no retained products of conception.[5]

References

1. Lindell G, Flam F (1995). Management of uterine perforations in connection with legal abortions. Acta Obstet Gynecol Scand 1995; 74(5):373–5.
2. Sharma JB, Malhotra M, Pundir P. Laparoscopic oxidized cellulose (Surgicel) application for small uterine perforations. Int J Gynaecol Obstet 2003; 83(3):271–5.
3. Mustafa MS, Gurab S. Endoscopic management of bleeding uterine perforation occurring during evacuation of retained products of conception. Int J Gynaecol Obstet 1995; 49(1):71–2.
4. Romer T, Lober R. Endoscopic management of uterine perforation with the ENDO-UNIVERSAL surgical stapler. Zentralblatt fur Gynakologie 1998; 120(2), 69–70.
5. Kohlenberg CF, Casper GR. The use of intraoperative ultrasound in the management of a perforated uterus with retained products of conception. Aust N Z J Obstet Gynaecol 1996; 36(4):482–4.

☠ Damage to urinary tract/blood vessels/bowel

Urinary tract trauma

Damage to the urinary tract should ideally be recognized at the time of surgery. Postoperative vaginal leakage of urine, urine in drainage bottles, or the presence of loin pain should always raise the possibility of inadvertent damage to the urinary tract.

If there is trauma to the ureter or base of the bladder during surgery, the on-call consultant urologist should be called to theatre. For trauma to the bladder dome, a two-layer closure using 2/0 Vicryl® should be performed followed by methylene blue dye to check for leakage.

If the ureter is damaged and noted during surgery then, depending on the site of damage to the ureter, the following may be considered: ureteric reimplantation, Boari flap, or ileal conduit. These procedures should be carried out by a consultant urologist.

Should the urinary tract trauma be diagnosed in the postoperative period, then:

- *For suspected bladder trauma:* a speculum examination may reveal the point of leakage. If not identifiable, a catheter is inserted and methylene blue dye instilled and a swab test performed. Non-colouration, but soaking of the swab will indicate ureteric fistula and swabs soaked with blue indicate vesicovaginal fistula. Alternatively, a cystogram with radio-opaque material can be performed which will reveal the point of leakage.

- *For suspected ureteric trauma:* an IV urogram can be performed and hydronephrosis and delayed emptying or even complete renal obstruction can be seen. Usually in such cases loin pain is evident within 6–12 hours after surgery and a percutaneous nephrostomy should be performed as a primary procedure to avoid damage to that kidney. U&Es may not be abnormal if the damage is only on one side.

Trauma to blood vessels

These can occur during laparotomy or laparoscopic procedures.

Trauma to large vessels (aorta, vena cava, iliac vein/artery)

This is usually during laparoscopy by either the Veress needle or the trocar. Should trauma be suspected (blood returning up needle/trocar) the following management should ensue:

- Leave the trocar/needle *in situ* and ensure no gas is running in.
- Place patient in steep Trendelenburg position.
- Cross-match 6 units and ask for 2 units of O-negative blood/maintain adequate fluid replacement.
- Perform a midline laparotomy and apply considerable pressure proximal to the vessel injury to slow down blood loss.
- Call for vascular surgeon to attend immediately to the emergency.

Trauma to pelvic side wall vessels/venous oozing

This can be encountered especially when performing laparoscopy and dividing adhesions.

- Indiscriminate use of diathermy should be avoided as this can lead to further bleeding and retroperitoneal haemorrhage.
- Pressure with a sucker or tonsil swab should be maintained for at least 2–3 min and careful lavage performed to ensure haemostasis.
- A redivac drain should be left *in situ* postoperatively.

Inferior epigastric injury

This should be avoided by careful inspection of the course of the epigastric vessels when inserting laparoscopic ports, but should the epigastric vessel be damaged then the following can be instituted:

- Pass a Foley catheter down the port site and inflate the balloon and pull back to apply pressure.
- Diathermy to the bleeding point via a contralateral port.
- Pass a suture around the vessel using a Grice or Bonney–Reverdin needle.
- Enlarge the port skin site and place a Vicryl® suture directly through the sheath under laparoscopic vision.

Trauma to bowel

If perforation occurred during laparoscopy with the *Veress needle*, one may notice feculent fluid during Palmer's test or high inflation pressures and gas escaping from the patient's anus.

- Veress needle should be left *in situ*.
- A laparotomy or alternatively another site for entry (e.g. Palmer's point entry using a 5 mm laparoscope) could be performed to confirm the diagnosis.
- Should the diagnosis be confirmed then a general surgeon should be called for assistance.
- A suture should be placed laparoscopically or via laparotomy. If it involved large bowel then copious peritoneal lavage should be performed.
- Broad-spectrum antibiotics should be given and the patient admitted for observation.

If noticed from the *trocar insertion*, one may notice feculent smell or feculent fluid via side port.

- Again trocar should be left *in situ*.
- A laparotomy or alternatively another site for entry (e.g. Palmer's point entry using a 5 mm laparoscope) could be performed to confirm the diagnosis.
- Should laparotomy be performed then the umbilical port site can be extended along the length of the port to guide to the area of perforation. Should the diagnosis be confirmed then a general surgeon should be called for assistance.
- A suture placed laparoscopically or via laparotomy should be considered. If it involves large bowel, copious peritoneal lavage should be performed.
- Broad-spectrum antibiotics should be given and the patient admitted for observation.
- Consideration of defunctioning of the bowel should be considered, although is rarely required.

Postoperative complications

Contributors

Stergios K. Doumouchtsis, George Iancu,
Christiana Nygaard, and Vikram S. Talaulikar

Contents

Postoperative collapse

Postoperative collapse is rare but requires very prompt action to avoid major morbidity and mortality. It is imperative that all healthcare professionals should be prepared for and trained in managing such an emergency.

△ Causes

- Non-serious collapse: vaso-vagal episode.
- Haemorrhagic shock: reactionary or secondary haemorrhage—pulse rate will initially be raised with normal BP but then may fall abruptly if volume depletion is not corrected. Associated features of shock with cold peripheries will be noted followed by severe drop in BP. Loss of consciousness and cardiac arrhythmia indicates >30–40% of blood volume loss and severe shock.
- Hypoxia: inhalation of vomit, obstruction of airway, pneumonia, anaesthetic complication. Usually there will be central cyanosis and a dramatic drop in oxygen saturation.
- Central circulatory failure: myocardial infarction (MI), pulmonary embolism (PE)—there may be preceding crushing/severe chest pain, raised JVP, or pulmonary oedema.
- Adrenal or thyroid crisis.
- Hypoglycaemic or diabetic coma.
- Sepsis: hypotension and warm peripheries.
- Drug causes: overdose or anaphylactic reaction (opiates, antibiotics)—sudden or delayed reaction after giving medication.
- Cerebral causes: stroke, epilepsy—previous history or tongue bite/urinary incontinence and tonic/clonic seizures or focal hemiparesis/dysphasia.

Management

1. *Call for help*/pull emergency alarm.
2. ▶ Assessment and initial management must occur simultaneously.
3. *Assess airway*—clear/maintain patency. Apply 15 L oxygen/min via tight-fitting face mask with reservoir bag and attach pulse oximeter. Ventilate with bag and mask/consider intubation if hypoxaemic.
4. *Assess circulation*/perform CPR if required and call crash team if needed. Attach ECG monitor/automated external defibrillator as per advanced life support (ALS) protocol.
5. Examine woman to assess cardiac and respiratory status (JVP, heart auscultation, and full respiratory assessment). Examine woman for specific signs (abdominal tenderness, neurology).
6. Monitor BP, cardiac rhythm, respiration, temperature, and urine output. Ensure good IV access (two large-bore, minimum 16 G IV cannulae) and take bloods for FBC, U&Es, glucose, cross-match, coagulation screen, LFTs, blood cultures, ABGs.
7. Arrange chest X-ray and abdominal US. Doppler US of calf veins, V/Q scan—if PE suspected. CT scan or MRI if intracranial pathology suspected.
8. Management thereafter will be dependent on cause.

☠ Postoperative chest pain

△ Causes/signs to aid diagnosis

- ► Exclude life-threatening causes first and then consider other potential causes.
- Pleuritic chest pain: pain on inspiration (this may also occur with musculoskeletal causes), pneumonia/ pneumothorax or more importantly, pulmonary embolus.
- Central chest pain: this can be caused by massive pulmonary embolus. When pain is interscapular consider aortic dissection. Pain radiating from the chest to the jaw/arm obviously alerts one to the diagnosis of ischaemic heart disease (acute MI, angina/acute coronary syndrome). MI can cause crushing pain and also nausea, vomiting, and sweating.
- Musculoskeletal pain: often there is a specific point of tenderness that can be reproduced by touching the affected site with the examining finger.
- Shoulder tip/apical chest pain: common after a laparoscopy and occurs after diaphragmatic irritation with CO_2 gas. This may be also related to haemoperitoneum.
- Retrosternal chest pain that settles after giving antacid indicates gastro-oesophageal reflux. Care should be exercised to exclude ischaemic heart disease and PE.
- Other: oesophageal spasm, pancreatitis, sickle cell crisis.

History

- Look at risk factors for causes, e.g. risk of thromboembolic disease after operation >30 minutes, obesity, thrombophilia.
- Description of the pain (onset, nature, duration, severity, radiation and exacerbating/relieving factors).

Examination

- Inspect: look for central cyanosis assess respiratory rate (abnormal >20 breaths/min).
- Palpate for point tenderness and percuss for hyper-resonance of pneumothorax.
- Auscultate for reduced breath sounds in pneumothorax and signs of pulmonary oedema or pneumonia.

Investigations

- Oxygen saturation on air (normal >98%).
- Chest X-ray: pneumonia, pneumothorax, PE, rib fracture.
- Ventilation/perfusion (V:Q) scan or spiral CT/magnetic resonance angiography for PE.
- FBC (raised WCC in pneumonia) + U&Es + ABGs (low oxygen saturation in PE), troponin/creatine phosphokinase-MB (CPK-MB) measurement, consider D-dimer.
- ECG: tachycardia (and rarely S1 Q3 T3) in PE. ST changes with MI. Note pneumothorax can mimic signs of MI.

Treatment

- *Musculoskeletal pain*: physiotherapy and NSAIDs.
- *Pleuritic chest pain*: depends on cause:
  - pneumonia: antibiotics and NSAIDs
  - pneumothorax: conservative or aspiration/chest drain depending on degree of pneumothorax
  - PE: oxygen, TED stockings and anticoagulation (LMWH); rarely will further measures (thrombolytic agents and surgical thrombectomy) be required
- If *interscapular pain and aortic dissection*, consider lowering BP and refer to cardiothoracic team.
- *Cardiac pain*: angina—GTN; MI—oxygen, morphine, aspirin, GTN, antiemetic, thrombolysis.
- *Shoulder tip/apical chest pain*: reassure (unless suspecting fresh bleeding into peritoneal cavity) and simple analgesia if required.
- *Retrosternal chest pain*: if diagnosis is gastro-oesophageal reflux, prescribe antacid/magnesium trisilicate.

☼ Postoperative abdominal distension

Causes

- Haemorrhage
- Postoperative GI ileus
- Acute gastric dilatation
- Intestinal obstruction
- Peritonitis
- Urinary retention
- Postoperative faecal impaction
- Gossypiboma.

Haemorrhage

- Usually following laparotomy or laparoscopy
- Symptoms: increasing abdominal pain, confusion, abdominal distension
- Examination: tachycardia, hypotension, oliguria (urine output <20 mL/hr), abdominal tenderness
- Check pulse and BP
- Appropriate resuscitation including IV access
- FBC, clotting, group and cross-match
- Management:
  - stabilize the patient
  - replacement blood products as appropriate
  - radiological or surgical intervention as appropriate to achieve haemostasis.

Postoperative ileus

- Common after a laparotomy.
- Due to temporary depression of normal peristalsis of the gastrointestinal tract (GIT) secondary to manipulation.
- GIT function normally returns 24–72 hours postoperatively:
  - gastric peristalsis: within 24–48 hours
  - colonic activity: after 48 hours.
- Symptoms: leads to mild abdominal distension and discomfort, diffuse, persistent abdominal pain, nausea and/or vomiting, delayed passage of or inability to pass flatus, inability to tolerate an oral diet.
- Examination: absent or reduced bowel sounds during first 48–72 hours, abdominal distention and tympanism, a variable reduction of bowel sounds, and often some degree of mild diffuse tenderness.
- Management—conservative:
  - nil by mouth
  - IV fluid replacement
  - nasogastric drainage if vomiting
  - monitor serum electrolytes and correct as appropriate.
- Return of normal peristaltic activity heralded by mild cramps, passage of flatus, and return of appetite.
- If function does not return at this time, must consider a potentiating cause.

Acute gastric dilatation
- Usually follows overfilling of the stomach with fluid and gas.
- Common in malnourished, chronically immobilized patients, and asthmatics where oxygen masks were used in the immediate postoperative period.
- Fluid and air cause gross distension of the stomach.
- Onset is insidious.
- Symptoms:
  - severe pain and dyspnoea and thus, mimic a MI
  - may be accompanied by sweating, hiccups, dehydration.
- Acid blood gases: hypochloraemic metabolic alkalosis due to fluid and electrolyte loss into the stomach.
- Management—conservative:
  - nasogastric tube to decompress
  - IV fluid replacement
  - monitor serum electrolytes and correct as appropriate.

Intestinal obstruction
May be secondary to:
- Paralytic ileus
- Mechanical obstruction
- Peritonitis.

Paralytic ileus
Common in patients with:
- Metabolic disturbances, e.g. hypokalaemia
- Patients on tricyclic antidepressant
- Intraperitoneal inflammation
- Intraperitoneal haematomas.

Mechanical obstruction
Common in postoperative adhesions and internal hernia.

Peritonitis
May be secondary to:
- Bowel injury:
  - may also occur after laparoscopy
  - *serious complication* if large perforation. May have high mortality rate
  - may have small leak or develop into an abscess. Less dramatic signs and symptoms
- Bladder injury
- Foreign body
- Infection (e.g. abscess).

Symptoms
- Similar to ileus. However, will experience an *initial unremarkable recovery* before obstruction manifests
- Pain
- Vomiting (points more to small bowel obstruction)
- Constipation/absolute
- Haematuria or blood per external meatus may point to bladder injury.

Examination
- Hyperactive, 'tinkling' bowel sounds
- If with peritonitis, may have severe systemic upset, generalized peritonism and guarding, absent bowel sounds.

Investigations
- Bloods: U&E, FBC, ABGs.
- Plain films: air-fluid levels in loops of small bowel (erect X-ray centred to the diaphragm is valuable in making the diagnosis). If with bowel perforation, will show gas under diaphragm.
- Small bowel follow through: if former is equivocal.
- US: can be used to differentiate paralytic ileus from mechanical obstruction as the peristaltic movement of the bowels in the latter is observed. May also visualize intra-abdominal foreign body, abscess, fluid in cul-de-sac (blood, pus, urine).
- Cystography or retrograde urethrography: if bladder injury is suspected.
- CT/MRI: for deep abscess.

Management
- IV fluid resuscitation.
- Decompression with a nasogastric tube.
- Careful monitoring of BP, HR, respiration, and temperature.
- Hourly urinary monitoring.
- Consider central venous line.
- If with *small leak from bowel injury*, may consider radiological-guided placement of a large-bore drain into any collection. Periodic irrigation then performed.
- Above conservative measures are satisfactory if:
  - reduction of pain
  - nasogastric aspirate becomes cleaner and volumes reduce
  - reduced abdominal distension
  - passage of flatus.
- Consider laparotomy or laparoscopy if:
  - conservative treatment ineffective after 48 hours
  - remove foreign body
  - *large leaks from bowel injury or with signs of peritonism*
  - *tenderness* is an indication for urgent or early surgery.
- If intra-abdominal abscess, start empiric antibiotics. May be drained guided by interventional radiology. If unresponsive, may require drainage via laparoscopy or laparotomy.

If with bladder injury but:
- with *small leaks*: conservative treatment with indwelling catheter
- with *large damage*: bladder repair with subsequent catheter placement.

Urinary retention
- Inability to pass urine despite persistent effort.
- Symptoms: suprapubic discomfort poor urine output or inability to void.
- Examination: palpable bladder, painful suprapubic palpation.

- Management:
  - if catheterized, check for blockage. May flush catheter or change indwelling catheter if necessary.
  - if not catheterized, may perform intermittent catheterization or insert indwelling catheter depending on patient's status.
  - check for UTI and treat accordingly.

Postoperative faecal impaction

- Usually secondary to colonic ileus and impaired rectal sensation.
- More common in the elderly.
- Anticholinergic drugs and opiate analgesics may predispose.
- Diagnosis: rectal examination.
- Management: high-fibre diet, increased oral fluids, enemas, or manual removal under general anaesthetic.

Gossypiboma

- Tumour-like presentation of an operative sponge left by accident during a laparotomy.
- Symptoms: may be asymptomatic, or complaint of abdominal enlargement.
- Diagnosis: plain abdominal X-ray is unhelpful. Detected by ultrasonography or CT scan.
- Management: re-exploration and removal of foreign body. May also be laparoscopically removed.

Further reading

Townsend, CM, Beauchamp, RD, Evers, BM, et al. (eds). *Sabiston Textbook of Surgery: The Biological Basis of Modern Surgical Practice* (19th ed). Philadelphia, PA: Elsevier Saunders, 2012.

⦸ Postoperative pyrexia

Definition

The US Centers for Disease Control has defined postoperative pyrexia as a temperature of 100.4°F or 38°C or greater on any 2 postoperative days excluding the first 24 hours. The early postoperative rise in temperature is elicited usually by inflammatory changes secondary to surgery, but resolves spontaneously.

Causes

Postoperative pyrexia is a common complication after a gynaecological procedure. It occurs in 25% of women after an abdominal hysterectomy and in 35% of women after a vaginal hysterectomy.

The causes can be infectious—surgical site infection (SSI), UTI, pneumonia, or intravascular catheter infection are the most common (often caused by nosocomial organisms), or non-infectious—frequently reaction to medication (heparin, antimicrobials, etc.). Common organisms involved in SSIs of abdominal incisions are *Staphylococcus aureus*, coagulase-negative staphylococci, *Enterococcus* spp., and *Escherichia coli*. SSIs of vaginal procedures include Gram-negative bacilli, enterococci, group B streptococci, and anaerobes from the vagina and perineum. Postoperative pelvic abscesses are commonly associated with anaerobes.

The onset of fever can help determine the possible cause (Table 13.1). Postoperative fever can be divided in four categories depending on the time elapsed from the surgery: immediate—occurs in a few hours from the surgery, acute—occurs in the first week from the surgery, subacute—between 1 and 4 weeks from surgery and delayed—>1 month from the surgery.

Table 13.1 Possible causes of postoperative pyrexia according to onset time of fever

Within 24 hours	24 to 48 hours	3–5 days	5–7 days	7–10 days
Metabolic response—inflammatory stimulus of surgery	Respiratory (bacterial or aspiration pneumonia)	UTIs	Intra-abdominal abscess	SSIs
Atelectasis	Catheter related		DVT	
Necrotizing streptococcal & clostridial wound infection	Persistent atelectasis			
Transfusion reaction or medication	Septic thrombophlebitis			

Causes of postoperative pyrexia

For causes of postoperative pyrexia see Fig. 13.1.

Diagnosis

- Review the details of the operation.
- Risk factors for postoperative pyrexia:
  - length of the operative time
  - estimated blood loss
  - use of preoperative antibiotics
  - concurrent medical problems
  - parity
  - obesity.
- Take a detailed history and perform a systems review.

Immediate postoperative pyrexia

- It is usually caused by a metabolic response generated by inflammatory mediators released in the traumatized tissues. It resolves spontaneously in 2–3 days or more after extensive surgery.

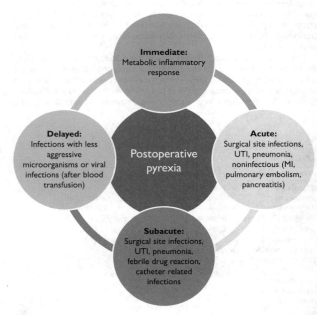

Immediate:
Metabolic inflammatory response

Delayed:
Infections with less aggressive microorganisms or viral infections (after blood transfusion)

Postoperative pyrexia

Acute:
Surgical site infections, UTI, pneumonia, noninfectious (MI, pulmonary embolism, pancreatitis)

Subacute:
Surgical site infections, UTI, pneumonia, febrile drug reaction, catheter related infections

Fig. **13.1** Causes of postoperative pyrexia.

- Transfused blood products and medication (e.g. antimicrobials) can generate fever through immune-mediated reactions; fever accompanied often by vasodilatation, hypotension, or rash. Malignant hyperthermia occurs typically after 30 minutes from the administration of causative agent (e.g. suxamethonium, inhaled anaesthetics).
- The exception is the SSI with very aggressive microorganisms like *Clostridium perfringens* and group A *Streptococcus* that can cause fulminant necrotizing infection in a few hours after surgery.

Acute-onset postoperative pyrexia

- The first week after the surgery is usually the period when nosocomial infections appear.
- SSIs can occur during the first week.
- UTI: occurs frequently in patients with indwelling catheter. The risk of infection increases with duration of catheterization. It is frequent in patients having urological and gynaecological procedures. Dysuria is a common symptom.
- Pneumonia: 80% will have symptoms—cough, dyspnoea, pleuritic chest pain, and purulent or blood-stained sputum. Patients requiring mechanical ventilation during surgery are at higher risk.
- Atelectasis: it appears to be coincidental with the fever rather than causal; precedes pneumonia. Fever associated with this resolves following re-inflation of the lungs. Risk factors are advanced age, obesity, smoking, and pre-existing chronic pulmonary disease.
- Aspiration pneumonitis: dyspnoea, tachypnoea, noisy respirations, and cough. Bacterial pneumonia will ensue in 50%.
- Non-infectious causes of acute pyrexia: aseptic thrombophlebitis, PE, pancreatitis, and MI.

Subacute fever

- SSI can occur after a week postoperatively. Intra-abdominal abscess is a cause of fever and abdominal or pelvic pain.
- Thrombophlebitis: non-infective—usually at IV infusion site; common in patients with prolonged IV infusion or locally noxious drugs. It may have superimposed bacterial contamination.
- Febrile drug reaction can be a cause for subacute fever (beta-lactamines, heparin, phenytoin, histamine-receptor blockers).
- Intravascular catheter-related infections are frequent in patients receiving treatment with the aid of invasive medical devices and are usually caused by bacteria or fungi.

Delayed fever

Infection is the commonest cause of delayed fever. The delayed-onset infections are usually produced by less aggressive microorganisms (coagulase-negative staphylococci, fungi), but also viral infections blood transfusion-borne (hepatitis, HIV, CMV, or rarely parasites). Patients with history of cardiac surgery or implanted devices should be investigated for infective endocarditis.

Physical examination

- Wound infection: inspect the wound. The surgical site wound may be swollen, red, and indurated or may be expressing pus.
- Intra-abdominal abscess: tenderness on palpation. If sealed off, may present as a lump on palpation.
- Atelectasis: diminished breath sounds, percussive dullness, and elevation of the diaphragm over the affected side.
- DVT: calf tenderness and swelling, presence of Homans' sign (calf pain on dorsiflexion of the foot). Phlegmasia alba and cerulea dolens (painful blue leg) and venous gangrene are extreme signs present in a minority of cases; they result from massive venous thrombosis and obstruction of the venous drainage of an extremity.
- Pneumonia: similar to atelectasis.
- Aspiration pneumonitis: tachypnoea, chest wall retraction, bronchorrhoea and bronchoconstriction.

Investigations

- Investigations should be based on likely diagnosis.
- Usual investigations required: FBC, CRP, U&Es, and LFTs. An MSU or catheter specimen should be sent for microscopy, culture, and sensitivity along with blood and sputum culture.
- Cerebrospinal fluid sampled for glucose concentration and microbiology if meningitis after spinal analgesia suspected.
- Pneumonia: chest X-ray. Sputum samples for Gram-stain smear. Cultures should also be obtained.
- Aspiration pneumonitis: chest X-ray.
- Wound infection: wound swab for bacterial culture or perform needle aspiration using aseptic technique.
- UTI: urinalysis or MSU for culture and sensitivity.
- DVT: venography is the standard mean of diagnosis. Doppler ultrasonography is non-invasive and has a sensitivity and specificity of >90%.
- Ultrasonography: collection of pus in the pelvis or subphrenic area. May mimic pleural effusion on a chest X-ray. CT scan may be also a helpful investigation for the imaging of intra-abdominal collections.

Management

(See Fig. 13.2.)

- Remove any unnecessary catheter from the bladder or from the bloodstream and avoid excessive medication.
- Malignant hyperthermia is treated with withdrawal of causative agent and dantrolene.
- Reduce SSI prevalence by administering preoperative prophylactic antibiotic within 60 minutes before surgical incision, when reproductive tract is entered (e.g. hysterectomy)
- *Wound infection*: oral or IV antibiotics and appropriate wound care; should be given until the patient is apyrexial for 24–48 hours. Usually, antibiotic treatment is empirical in the first 48 hours; if no response after 48 hours of antibiotics—change it after consultation with a microbiologist and result of culture.

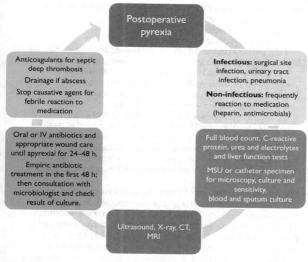

Fig. 13.2 Management algorithm of postoperative pyrexia.

- Wound cellulitis can be treated with oral antibiotics in outpatient settings.
- Deep wound infection, peritonitis, or pelvic abscesses should be treated with IV antibiotics. Pus collections should be incised and drained. A systemically unwell patient or one with cellulitis requires IV antibiotics. If rapidly expanding or patches of skin necrosis at different sites, consider necrotizing fasciitis (IV broad-spectrum antibiotics + wide surgical debridement).
- The patient who is not responsive to antibiotic treatment in the absence of abscess should be suspected of septic pelvic thrombophlebitis and concomitant heparin therapy instituted.
- *UTI*: if urinalysis is positive, may start on empiric treatment. This may later be changed once sensitivity results are obtained.
- *DVT*: prophylaxis is more important which includes wearing of pneumatic stockings and early mobilization. Use prophylactic LMWHs preoperatively for CS, hysterectomy, or oncology patients. Treat with warfarin or fragmin. Add antibiotics if septic (postpartum endometritis associated with septic pelvic thrombophlebitis).
- *Superficial thrombophlebitis*: remove venous catheters. If bacterial contamination, treat with antibiotics. If suppurative, affected vein should be excised.
- *Intra-abdominal abscess*: start empiric treatment with antibiotics; usually require drainage.

- *Atelectasis*: use bronchodilator therapy, including theophylline.
  - Adequate analgesia.
  - Incentive spirometry.
  - Coughing to mobilize secretions.
  - If still unsuccessful and if with extensive lobar collapse, flexible bronchoscopic aspiration is indicated. Secretions may be rendered less adherent by maintaining hydration and administering humidified air or oxygen and nebulized mucolytic agents. Once developed, coughing, deep breathing and incentive spirometry should be continued with greater intensity.
  - Significant hypoxaemia (PaO_2 <60 mmHg) should be corrected with oxygen therapy. Manoeuvers for clearance of secretions necessary. Drainage of pleural fluid or air via tube thoracostomy may be necessary to relieve compressive atelectasis.
  - Assisted ventilation and admission to the intensive care unit should be considered for patients with oxygen saturations <90% or a pO_2< 8.0 kPa.
- *Pneumonia*: organisms predominantly in nosocomial pneumonias are Gram-negative bacteria and *Staphylococcus aureus*. The Gram-negative bacilli include *Pseudomonas aeruginosa, Proteus mirabilis, Serratia marcescens, Escherichia coli, Klebsiella pneumoniae*, and *Enterobacter* species. *Staphylococcus aureus* and *Streptococcus pneumoniae* are causative for 14% of nosocomial pneumonia. Anaerobic organisms occur usually in 2% and are associated with aspiration pneumonia and thoracoabdominal surgery. Fungal infection is uncommon, usually in immunosuppressed patients.
  - Supplemental oxygen may be added. If severely compromised, require intubation and mechanical support.
  - Begin empiric treatment: usually aminoglycoside and antipseudomonal penicillin. Antibiotic selection modified based on Gram-stain smear results. Culture results will guide more specific therapy.
- *Aspiration pneumonitis*: cases with distal airway obstruction evident on chest film will need flexible bronchoscopic aspiration of debris.
  - Bronchodilators necessary.
  - If acute respiratory failure develops, positive pressure ventilation.

Further reading

ACOG Committee on Practice Bulletins – Gynecology. ACOG practice bulletin No. 104: antibiotic prophylaxis for gynecologic procedures. *Obstet Gynecol* 2009; 113:1180–9.

Engoren M. Lack of association between atelectasis and fever. *Chest* 1995; 107(1):81–4.

Sharp HT. Prevention and management of complications from gynecologic surgery. *Obstet Gynecol Clin North Am* 2010; 37(3):461–7.

Shwandt A, Andrews SJ, Fanning J. Prospective analysis of a fever evaluation algorithm after major gynecologic surgery. *Am J Obstet Gynecol* 2001; 184:1066–7.

:☼: Postoperative oliguria and anuria

Definition

- *Oliguria*: urine output of <0.5 mL/kg/hr or <500 mL/24 hr.
- *Anuria*: absence of urinary excretion or <100 mL/24 hr.

Urinary output is an inappropriate measure of renal function. It is important to know that urinary output above 1 L/day does not exclude partial obstruction as cause of renal failure.

Urine output after releasing urinary tract obstruction may initially exceed 500–1000 mL/hr; polyuria in this setting is normal with the kidneys excreting the fluid retained during obstruction.

Causes

Pre-renal

- Hypovolaemia secondary to:
  - intra- or postoperative bleeding
  - inadequate intraoperative fluid administration
- Third-space losses:
  - loss to extracellular space due to tissue damage
  - cardiac failure
  - pulmonary oedema
- Cardiac:
  - anaesthetic agents
  - cardiac failure.

Renal

- Acute kidney injury (e.g. acute tubular necrosis secondary to haemorrhage)
- Acute on chronic renal failure (e.g. exacerbation of underlying renal disease)
- Nephrotoxicity of anaesthetic agents
- Other drugs (e.g. aminoglycosides).

Post-renal

- Blocked urinary catheter (debris, blood, clamped, or kinked catheter)
- Urinary retention (infection, frank haematuria, oedema, or haematoma at bladder base)
- Unrecognized bladder perforation (laparoscopy, CS, cystoscopy)
- Ureteric injury or obstruction (transection, ligation, kinking, spasm, oedema)
- Urethral injury or obstruction
- Vulval, vaginal, pelvic, or paraurethral haematoma
- Pain.

Management

(See Fig. 13.3.)

Monitoring of intravascular volume status can be done using:
- Static parameters: central venous pressure, HR, arterial BP
- Dynamic or flow-related parameters: stroke volume, cardiac output, pulse pressure variation.

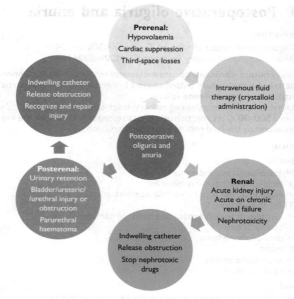

Fig. 13.3 Management algorithm of postoperative oliguria and anuria.

Initial measures
- Check pulse, BP, RR, and diuresis to determine haemodynamic status and severity of the underlying problem.
- Exclude intra-abdominal or vaginal bleeding.
- Review operative notes to identify intraoperative complications or risk factors.
- Monitor fluid-balance and ensure adequate intake.
- Exclude obstructed catheter.
- Try to determine cause (pre-renal, renal, post-renal).

Surgical procedures that may cause oliguria/anuria
- Incontinence surgery (colposuspension, sling procedures, intradetrusor botulinum toxin injection)
- Prolapse surgery (vaginal hysterectomy for procidentia, anterior vaginal repair for cystocele)
- Complex abdominal hysterectomy (fibroids, endometriosis)
- Complicated CS (haemorrhage, full dilatation, Caesarean hysterectomy).

Pre-renal and renal causes
Fluid management is complex and recommendations about the composition and volume of fluid administered are variable.

- Exclude pulmonary oedema and congestive cardiac failure (basal crackles, tachypnoea, raised JVP).
- When crystalloid administration is indicated, balanced salt solutions such as Ringer's lactate, acetate, or Hartmann's solution should be used instead of 0.9% saline (except from cases of hypochloraemia, e.g. vomiting).
- For diagnosis of hypovolaemia when the central venous pressure (CVP) is not increased, check the response to a bolus infusion of 250–500 mL of a suitable colloid/crystalloid. Monitor cardiac output and stroke volume or CVP before and 15 minutes after bolus.
- Attempt second fluid challenge, until haemodynamic parameters are stabilized.
- Liaise with anaesthetist and physician.
- Consider IV furosemide.
- If no response insert CVP line:
  - if CVP low, give more fluid
  - if CVP high, give furosemide.
- Aim for CVP of 0–6 mmHg.
- Consider transfer to ITU.
- For maintenance: adult patients require sodium 50–100 mmol/day, potassium 40–80 mmol/day in 1.5–2.5 L of water by oral/parenteral route.
- Prevent dehydration by avoiding prolonged fasting and routine mechanical bowel preparation; encourage ingestion of a clear carbohydrate drink 2–3 hours preoperatively for enhanced recovery.

Post-renal causes

Acute retention
- Pass a urethral or suprapubic indwelling catheter if bladder volume exceeds 600 mL—leave on free drainage for 24–48 hours.
- Treat infection.

Obstructed catheter
- If catheter is obstructed, flush bladder or replace with larger catheter (especially in cases of frank haematuria).
- Consider cause of bleeding.
- Consider double/triple lumen catheter and regular bladder washouts.
- Consider antibiotics only if there are signs of urinary infection.

Postoperative bladder dysfunction
- Presents as acute urinary retention.
- 9% of patients with gynaecologic surgery.
- Urethral indwelling catheter is recommended; most recover in several days.
- Complete initial drainage of the bladder is recommended rather than limiting the volume of initial drainage (haematuria, transient hypotension, and increased diuresis post-obstruction are common, but usually not clinically significant).
- Trial of void without catheter after 5–7 days.

Ureteric injury
- Signs—loin pain, uraemia (NB—sometimes there is no pain).
- Do not give fluid challenge.
- U&E, ABG if uraemic.
- US for hydronephrosis determine level of obstruction.
- Refer to urogynaecology or urology immediately if confirmed.

Urethral injury
- Urethrovaginal fistula is usually associated with anterior colporrhaphy, traumatic rotational forceps, and prolonged obstructed labour.
- Urethral obstruction after continence procedures.

Management:
- Urethral indwelling catheter followed by trial of void without catheter
- For fistulas: urology/urogynaecology referral for surgery
- Return to theatre:
  - cystourethroscopy
  - ureteric catheterization and retrograde pyelogram to determine type and level of obstruction
  - management options:
    - removal of suture
    - re-anastomosis, ureteroneocystostomy—reimplantation of ureter
    - defunctioning nephrostomy.

Failure to recognize and treat or delayed diagnosis may be associated with genitourinary fistulas and permanent renal impairment.

Further reading

Bødker B, Lose G. Postoperative urinary retention in gynecologic patients. *Int Urogynecol J Pelvic Floor Dysfunct* 2003; 14(2):94–7.

Miller TE, Roche AM, Mythen M. Fluid management and goal-directed therapy as an adjunct to Enhanced Recovery After Surgery (ERAS). *Can J Anaesth* 2015; 62(2):158–68.

Powell-Tuck J, Gosling P, Lobo DN. *British Consensus Guidelines on Intravenous Fluid Therapy for Adult Surgical Patients (GIFTASUP)*. BAPEN, revised 7 March 2011. http://www.bapen.org.uk/pdfs/bapen_pubs/giftasup.pdf

Renner J, Scholz J, Bein B. Monitoring fluid therapy. *Best Pract Res Clin Anaesthesiol* 2009; 23(2):159–71.

Ovarian hyperstimulation syndrome

Contributor
Kamal Ojha

Contents

☼ Ovarian hyperstimulation syndrome

Ovarian hyperstimulation syndrome (OHSS) is the most serious complication of ovulation induction. With the introduction of gonadotrophin-releasing hormone (GnRH) agonists and the use of higher doses of gonadotrophins to retrieve a higher number of mature oocytes and maximize assisted reproductive technology pregnancy rates, the incidence of severe OHSS has increased. After IVF and embryo transfer, the overall incidence of OHSS is reported to be 1–10%; however, the incidence of severe OHSS is ~0.25–8%.[1,2]

OHSS is characterized by massive cystic enlargement of the ovaries, an increase in vascular permeability, and a shift of fluid to the extravascular compartments (mainly the peritoneal cavity), with the formation of ascites. It has been widely accepted that high circulating concentrations of oestradiol are an immediate predictor of OHSS, though this itself is not the cause. The aetiology of OHSS still remains to be elucidated in detail, but an important step appears to be to raised ovarian synthesis of vascular endothelial growth factor (VEGF) in response to hCG, which in turn increases vascular permeability.[3–5]

- Mild cases of OHSS are characterized by the formation of multiple ovarian cysts associated with excess steroid production and ovarian enlargement.
- Moderate OHSS is associated with abdominal distention, nausea, diarrhoea, or vomiting.
- In severe OHSS, ascites, hydrothorax, electrolyte imbalance, haemoconcentration, hypovolaemia, oliguria, or thromboemboli have been reported. This could be fatal if not treated promptly.

The *management* of mild and moderate OHSS is expectant, while the management of severe forms includes hospitalization for fluid and electrolyte management, paracentesis, or continuous drainage of the ascitic fluid if necessary[6] and mini-dose heparin prophylaxis to prevent thromboembolic complications.[7] IV albumin is given to retain fluid in the intravascular compartment. Close monitoring with FBC, U&Es, LFT, and clotting profile is the key to management. Dopamine receptor agonists (which induce the endocytosis of the VEGF receptor) have also emerged as potential new treatments in the management of this disease.[8,9]

Prevention of OHSS

Individualizing ovulation induction protocols for each patient according to different variables may lead to a better control of ovarian hyperstimulation.

The primary factors which increase the risk of OHSS are:
- Age of the patient (younger patients are at higher risk)
- Weight (thin built are more at risk)
- Low levels of day-3 serum FSH
- A history of exaggerated response in previous induction of ovulation cycles.
- Patients with polycystic ovary syndrome (PCOS) or who have a sonographic appearance of multicystic ovaries at baseline US evaluation.
- High levels of anti-mullerian hormone.

The above group is at risk for developing OHSS and should be treated less aggressively with gonadotrophins.

OHSS can be avoided by not administering hCG, and aborting the cycle in patients who have a serum oestradiol concentration of >10,000 pmol/L or who have >20 follicles seen on US before oocyte retrieval, especially if most of the follicles have the mean follicular diameter <12 mm. Although this is a good preventive measure for avoiding OHSS, it is frustrating for both the patient and the treating physician.

Using progesterone rather than hCG for luteal phase support has also been suggested in patients who are at risk of developing OHSS. Withholding hCG and menotrophins for a number of days called 'coasting', while continuing GnRH agonists until serum oestradiol concentrations return to a reasonable value (<10,000 pmol/L), has been widely used and is successful in preventing OHSS. This strategy shows no deleterious effect on the oocyte quality or on pregnancy rate. Cryopreserving all embryos and transferring them later in another cycle has been used as another way of avoiding OHSS.[10]

Some authors have suggested that the administration of IV albumin during or after oocyte retrieval prevents OHSS. However, most of the later reports have shown that albumin administration does not help in this regard. Newer, preventative strategies that may prove effective at reducing or preventing OHSS include GnRH antagonist protocols and the use of GnRH agonists to trigger final oocyte maturation.[8] Dopamine agonists have also recently been proposed as a prophylactic treatment in women at high risk.[11]

References

1. Brinsden PR, Wada I, Tan SL, et al. Diagnosis, prevention and management of ovarian hyperstimulation syndrome. BJOG 1995; 102:767–72.
2. Källén B, Finnström O, Nygren KG, et al. In vitro fertilisation in Sweden: obstetric characteristics, maternal morbidity and mortality. BJOG 2005; 112:1529–35.
3. Rizk B, Aboulghar M, Smitz J, et al. The role of vascular endothelial growth factor and interleukins in the pathogenesis of severe ovarian hyperstimulation syndrome. Hum Reprod Update 1997; 3(3):255–66.
4. Mathur R, Evbuomwan I, Jenkins JM. Prevention and management of ovarian hyperstimulation syndrome. Curr Obstet Gynaecol 2005; 15:132–8.
5. Gómez R, Soares SR, Busso C, et al. Physiology and pathology of ovarian hyperstimulation syndrome. Semin Reprod Med 2010; 6:448–57.
6. Al-Ramahi M, Leader A, Claman, P, et al. A novel approach to the treatment of ascites associated with ovarian hyperstimulation syndrome. Hum Reprod 1997; 12:2614–16.
7. Hignett M, Spence JEH, Claman P. Internal jugular vein thrombosis: a late complication of ovarian hyperstimulation syndrome despite mini-dose heparin prophylaxis. Hum Reprod 1995; 10:3121–3.
8. Humaidan P, Quartarolo J, Papanikolaou EG. Preventing ovarian hyperstimulation syndrome: guidance for the clinician. Fertil Steril 2010; 94(2):389–400.
9. Soares SR. Etiology of OHSS and use of dopamine agonists. Fertil Steril 2012; 97(3):517–22.
10. Tiitinen A, Husa LM, Tulppala M, et al. The effect of cryopreservation in prevention of ovarian hyperstimulation syndrome. BJOG 1995; 102(4):326–9.
11. Youssef MA, van Wely M, Hassan MA, et al. Can dopamine agonists reduce the incidence and severity of OHSS in IVF/ICSI treatment cycles? A systematic review and meta-analysis. Hum Reprod Update 2010; 16(5):459–66.

Contraception and termination of pregnancy

Contributors
Sheila Radhakrishnan and Kamal Ojha

Contents

⑦ Unprotected intercourse (emergency contraception)

Risk of unwanted pregnancy after sexual intercourse without adequate contraceptive precautions.

Definition of inadequate contraception

- No contraception.
- Unreliable method used—e.g. coitus interruptus.
- Reliable method used incorrectly:
  - slipped or broken condom
  - displaced diaphragm or cap within 6 hours of intercourse
  - partially expelled IUS/IUCD, perforating IUD/IUCD or IUS/IUCD removal with history of unprotected sexual intercourse (UPSI) in previous 5 days
  - late starting new packet of combined hormonal contraception (CHC) and not using additional precautions
  - if two or more active COCP pills are missed in week 1 of a new pack and there is history of failed barrier or UPSI in same week or preceding pill-free interval
  - UPSI or failed barrier when CHC, POP, or progestogen-only implant (POI) is used in conjunction with liver enzyme-inducing drugs or within 28 days of stopping them
  - missed POP (>27 hours after last traditional POP and >36 hours after last desogestrel-containing pills) with failed barrier or UPSI before re-establishment of efficacy—usually 48 hours after resumption of tablets
  - >14 weeks late since the last Depo-Provera® injection or >10 weeks since last norethisterone enanthate (NET-EN).

Types of emergency contraception

- Hormonal (emergency hormonal contraception (EHC)):
  - levonorgestrel 1.5 mg, a progestogen-only emergency contraception or POEC
  - PC4 (combined oral) no longer available
  - ulipristal acetate 30 mg
- Copper-bearing IUCD.

Mechanism of action

- Hormonal (EHC): both levonorgestrel and ulipristal acetate are thought to act by preventing or delaying ovulation.
- Copper-bearing IUCD acts by preventing implantation of the blastocyst.

Side effects

- Hormonal (EHC):
  - nausea and vomiting. If vomiting occurs within 2 hours of levonorgestrel or 3 hours of ulipristal acetate a further dose is recommended
  - menstrual irregularities are not uncommon. If there is doubt regarding a menstrual bleed a pregnancy test may be undertaken ≥3 weeks of last UPSI
- Copper-bearing IUCD: pain at insertion.

Presentation and management

- If <72 hours (3 days), EHC may be administered: a stat dose of levonorgestrel tablet 1.5 mg. Exclude the possibility of existing pregnancy or previous UPSI >72 hours previously. Unlicensed use— may be used up to 120 hours (5 days). There is no limit to the number of times POEC may be given in a cycle. It will not harm the fetus if it has failed.
- Ulipristal acetate could be used up to 120 hours after UPSI. Not recommended for use after 120 hours or more than once per cycle. This is because the safety of repeated exposure has not been evaluated satisfactorily.
- Consider a copper IUCD if the woman presents around ovulation (it prevents implantation). Do not use a hormone-bearing IUS.
- If she is within 120 hours of UPSI, a copper-bearing IUCD may be inserted after a single UPSI at any time of the cycle.
- A copper-bearing IUCD may be fitted up to 5 days after presumed ovulation in a regular cycle (day 19 of a 28-day cycle) despite more than one episode of UPSI in that cycle.

Drug interactions

- The copper IUCD does not interact with any medication.
- If the patient is on liver enzyme-inducing drugs (including post exposure prophylaxis for HIV following sexual exposure (PEPSE)) or within 28 days of having taken any, levonorgestrel may have diminished efficacy as an EC. Ulipristal acetate's efficacy too is diminished. In such cases the copper coil may be offered as the first-line EC. If declined, doubling the dose of levonorgestrel is considered appropriate. Ulipristal acetate, however, should be withheld as doubling its dose is not recommended.
- For patients on medications that increase gastric pH such as antacids, histamine H_2 receptor blockers, and proton pump inhibitors, concomitant administration of ulipristal acetate leads to reduced efficacy. It is best withheld from such patients and alternatives provided.

Important considerations

- Always consider future contraception and advise restarting the chosen method immediately with precautions for the next 7 days. Starting hormonal contraception immediately will not harm a fetus if EHC fails.
- With ulipristal acetate, it is recommended that if hormonal contraception is started, barrier contraception be used in addition for up to 2 weeks for CHC (exclude Qlaira®) and up to 9 days for POP. A simple rule of thumb could be until the next period or withdrawal bleed.
- The patient should ideally abstain totally from intercourse for the rest of the cycle and have a pregnancy test in 3 or more weeks' time from the UPSI.
- If an emergency copper IUCD is inserted but the woman wishes to use an alternative method after her next period, provide her with her alternative to start with the next cycle before removal of the device.
- Consider screening for STIs or referral to genitourinary medicine if the sexual intercourse was casual or forced. Refer early for forensic tests after rape, if the patient agrees.
- Where the girl is under 16 or suffering from learning disability or mental health problems, consider competence to consent to future contraception (Fraser guidelines—see Box 15.1). However, EC should not be withheld.
- Prepubertal girls do not need EC, although it is possible to conceive before the first menses.
- Postmenopausal women over 50 do not need EC, if they have had no periods for 12 months (2 years if under 50). Women on HRT may need EC.

Box 15.1 Fraser guidelines (1985)

Deciding on competence to consent to contraception

For a girl under 16 to consent to contraception advice or treatment, the Fraser guidelines require the professional to be satisfied:

- That she understands the advice
- That she cannot be persuaded to inform her parents or allow the doctor to inform her parents
- That she will continue to have sexual intercourse
- That her physical or mental health (or both) is likely to suffer unless she receives contraception advice or treatment
- That it is in the best interests of the girl to receive contraceptive advice or treatment (or both) without parental consent.

Consider the possibility of sexual abuse, especially if the age gap is >3 years. It is an absolute offence for a man to have intercourse with a girl under the age of 13. In all cases where penetrative sexual activity or intercourse have involved an under 13-year-old, involvement must include the Children's Social Services and Child Protection Team (Sexual Offences Act 2003).

Further reading

Durand M, del Carmen Cravioto M, Raymond EG, *et al.* On the mechanisms of action of short-lived levonorgestrel administration in emergency contraception. *Contraception* 2001; 64:227–34.

Faculty of Sexual and Reproductive Healthcare Clinical Effectiveness Unit. *Emergency Contraception.* FSRH, 2011, updated January 2012. http://www.fsrh.org/pdfs/CEUguidance EmergencyContraception11.pdf

HRA Pharma UK Ltd. *ellaOne: Summary of Product Characteristics (SPC).* 2010. http://www.medicines. org.uk/emc/medicine/22280

Stirling A, Glasier A. Estimating the efficacy of emergency contraception – how reliable are the data? *Contraception* 2002; 66:19–22.

Webb A. Emergency contraception. *BMJ* 2003; 326:775–6.

:⊙: Complications associated with termination of pregnancy

Termination of pregnancy (TOP) is one of the commonest gynaecological procedures performed all over the world. In the UK, ~189,000 terminations were performed in England and Wales, and ~12,000 in Scotland in 2011.

Complications of TOP can cause significant morbidity. Fortunately mortality is low in the UK. Complications can be broadly grouped under three categories:

• Procedure-related complications
• Psychological complications
• Anaesthesia-related complications.

Procedure-related complications

The complications depend upon the method of TOP, which can be medical or surgical.

Uterine perforation

• The plastic cannula or the cervical dilator used during surgical TOP may perforate the uterus. The risk is very low with an experienced surgeon and is increased with previous surgery on the uterus and increasing gestation. The risk reported is 1–4 per 1000. Uterine perforation can become a life-threatening complication due to severe haemorrhage and damage to the intraperitoneal contents, especially the bowel.
• If perforation is suspected, the vacuum in the cannula should be released before withdrawing the cannula, and a laparoscopy performed to assess bleeding and to enable safe evacuation of the products of conception.
• The laparoscopy also helps in assessing the uterus and bowel. A laparotomy may be required to achieve haemostasis or repair of bowel.
• Perforation of the uterus can also injure the bladder and result in suprapubic pain and haematuria.
• Early detection and treatment will result in a good outcome.

Injury to cervix

Laceration of the cervix can happen due to rapid dilation of the cervix as done in surgical TOP. Cervical priming with a prostaglandin (misoprostol) transvaginally, usually 3 hours before the procedure, can minimize this complication.

Haemorrhage

Excessive haemorrhage during or after TOP may signify uterine atony, cervical laceration, uterine perforation, cervical pregnancy, or coagulopathy. Haemorrhage can be severe enough to necessitate blood transfusion with the attendant risks of transfusion. The risk of haemorrhage following surgical TOP is around 1/1000 overall; it is 0.88 for <13 weeks' gestation and 4/1000 after 20 weeks' gestation.

Incomplete TOP

- This occurs due to some of the products of conception remaining inside the uterus after the procedure is over. 5% of women undergoing TOP will require surgical evacuation within the first month. It is more common as gestational age increases.
- The patient presents a few days after the TOP with persistent or heavy bleeding. She may also present with features of infection, i.e. dull and/or colicky lower abdominal pain and low-grade fever.
- The combination of pain, fever, and bleeding is known as the post-TOP triad. A US of the uterus helps in diagnosis and in making the decision regarding evacuating the products of conception. However, blood clots in the uterus may make US diagnosis of retained products unreliable in these cases. In the presence of continued bleeding or symptoms and signs of infection, careful evacuation of the uterus may be indicated.

Infection

- 1% of women develop infection following TOP. This could be due to exacerbation of an underlying infection, not uncommon in sexually active women, introduction of infection during the procedures, or retained products of conception, which acts as a culture media for the organisms.
- If infection is not treated, it may lead to chronic PID and infertility. Hence all women undergoing TOP should be offered prophylactic broad-spectrum antibiotics, usually a combination of doxycycline and metronidazole.

Vasovagal syncope

Vasovagal syncope may occur due to rapid dilation of the cervix. Recovery is the rule. This is not a feature when the procedure is done under good spinal or general anaesthetic (GA).

Failed abortion

Failure to terminate pregnancy is greater with very early terminations (<6 weeks gestational age). Such patients may present with symptoms of continuing pregnancy such as hyperemesis, increased abdominal girth, and breast engorgement. The failure rate is 2.3/1000 for surgical TOP and 1–14/1000 in medical TOP. Post-termination follow-up 2 weeks after the procedure, a urine pregnancy test, and a US scan in suspected cases of failed TOP is practised in some centres.

DIC

Suspect DIC in all patients who present with severe post-TOP bleeding, especially after mid-trimester terminations. Incidence is ~200/100,000 terminations; this rate is even higher for the saline instillation technique which is rarely required. This is a possible complication of evacuation of missed miscarriage at >4 weeks.

Infertility

Rarely, TOP can result in infertility caused by tubal blockage secondary to infection or Asherman's syndrome secondary to vigorous curettage.

Future pregnancy
There is no evidence to estimate the risk of infertility, ectopic pregnancy, placenta praevia, cervical incompetence, and pre-term delivery after TOPs. Prophylactic antibiotics and cervical priming with prostaglandins have helped in the prevention of these complications.

Anaesthesia-related complications
Most women prefer GA and it is generally safe. However, the risk of GA is increased in women >35 years of age, increased BMI, heavy smokers, hypertension, cardiac disease, and respiratory disease. If local anaesthesia is used, which is usually in the form of paracervical block, the complication due to inadvertent injection of the drug into the vessels can be life-threatening, leading to convulsion and cardiopulmonary arrest.

Psychological complications
Many women feel tearful and emotional for few days after a TOP. However, most of them recover. There is no risk of developing serious psychiatric illness because of TOP. There may be lifestyle factors that influence how women feel after a TOP.

Vaginal discharge

Contributor
Kamal Ojha

Contents

⑦ **Abnormal vaginal discharge**

Vaginal discharge can be physiological or pathological. Physiological discharge occurs during ovulation, premenstrually, pregnancy, and sexual stimulation. Pathological discharge is differentiated from physiological discharge by the presence of a foul smell, blood staining, or pruritus.

Abnormal vaginal discharge is one of the common symptoms encountered in the gynaecology clinic. A careful history, examination, and laboratory testing to determine the aetiology of vaginal complaints are warranted. If the STI risk is high (age <25 years, no condom use, change of sexual partner in the last 3 months, multiple sexual partners, previous STI, partner with high-risk sexual behaviour), referral to genitourinary medicine (GUM) clinic should be made.

The causes are mostly infective in the reproductive age group and mostly non-infective in the postmenopausal age group.

Common causes
- Inflammation of the vagina also called vaginitis (most common)
- Pelvic inflammatory disease (PID)
- Tumours: both benign and malignant
- Atrophy of the vagina
- Foreign body: IUD, tampon
- Allergy to chemicals
- Ectropion
- Endocervical polyp
- Other causes: intrauterine devices, vesicovaginal fistula, rectovaginal fistula, vault granulation tissue.

Inflammation of the vagina
Bacterial vaginosis, vaginal candidiasis, and *Trichomonas vaginalis* infection are thought to cause ~90% of all vaginal infections. Bacterial vaginosis is the most common cause of vaginitis, accounting for 50% of vaginitis cases. A thorough history and vaginal examination followed by bacteriological tests will help in the diagnosis.
- Bacterial vaginosis is diagnosed by thin, white-grey discharge, vaginal pH >4.5, clue cells, and whiff test on KOH wet mount.
- 50% of cases are asymptomatic. Bacterial vaginosis is associated with preterm birth and infective complications following gynaecological surgery.
- Candidiasis is characterized by presence of erythema and adherent, thick, cottage cheese-like discharge. Predisposing factors include antibiotic use, high-oestrogen oral contraceptives, diabetes mellitus, and pregnancy.
- *Trichomonas vaginalis* infection is characterized by erythema, presence of a homogenous discharge, which may be green in colour, and strawberry appearance of the cervix. Screening for *Trichomonas vaginalis* in women can be considered in those at high risk for STI.

Pelvic inflammatory disease

Inflammation of the cervix, uterus, and tubes can cause abnormal vaginal discharge, which is most commonly caused by sexually acquired infections of which *Chlamydia trachomatis* and *Neisseria gonorrhoeae* are the common ones. Abdominal pain, pain during intercourse and during bimanual vaginal examination is usually present.

Tumours

Both benign and malignant tumours of the vulva, vagina, cervix, and uterus can cause abnormal vaginal discharge. The most common benign tumour in the uterus is fibroid and is most likely to cause vaginal discharge if it is a submucosal or a fibroid polyp protruding through the cervical canal. Malignant lesion of the cervix and the uterus also cause vaginal discharge. Post-coital or contact bleeding may indicate a cervical lesion that may be malignant or pre-malignant.

Atrophy of the vaginal epithelium

Menopausal changes in the vagina predispose it to the inflammatory process and can result in abnormal vaginal discharge. However, abnormal vaginal discharge in postmenopausal women should prompt a search for a malignant cause before considering vaginal atrophy as a cause.

Foreign body

Any foreign body in the genital tract will evoke an inflammatory response and lead to discharge from the vagina. Forgotten tampons in the vagina can cause offensive vaginal discharge. IUDs may produce vaginal discharge although not severe.

Allergy to chemicals

The chemicals used in personal hygiene products can cause allergy and produce inflammation of the vulva and vagina.

History

Time pattern
- When did this begin?
- Does the discharge remain constant throughout the month?

Quality
- What does the discharge look like (colour and consistency)?
- Is there an odour?
- Is there pain, itching, or burning?

Aggravating factors
- Does sexual intercourse increase the symptoms?
- Does your sexual partner have a penile discharge?
- Do you have multiple sexual partners or sexual partners that you do not know very well?

Relieving factors
- Is there anything that relieves the discharge?
- Does frequent bathing help?
- Have over-the-counter creams been tried?
- Has douching been tried? What kind?

What other symptoms are present?
- Abdominal pain?
- Vaginal itching?
- Fever?
- Vaginal bleeding?
- Rash?
- Warts?
- Other lesions?
- Changes in urination?
- Difficulty or pain on urination?
- Blood in urine?
- Diarrhoea?

Other important information
- What medications are being taken?
- What is the frequency of sexual activity?
- Do you use condoms?
- Do you have any allergies?
- Have you changed the detergents or soaps that you use?
- Do you frequently wear very tight pants?

Investigations
- MSU, high vaginal and endocervical swabs for culture and sensitivity.
- FBC, U&Es, LFTs.
- Urinary pregnancy test to exclude pregnancy.
- Pelvic US for benign lesions and pelvic collection.

Treatment
The treatment of infective pathology is briefly discussed in this section.
- Removal of foreign body and IUCD before initiating treatment is essential.
- Antibiotics and anti-inflammatory agents need to be started after the swabs and bloods have been performed.
- Chlamydia: doxycycline 100 mg twice daily for 7 days is the first line of choice. Azithromycin (1 g single dose) or erythromycin can also be used. Treat sexual partners.
- Bacterial vaginosis: metronidazole 400 mg orally twice daily for 7 days. IV or PR routes may be necessary. (Metronidazole gel 0.75%, one full applicator (5 g) intravaginally, once a day for 5 days *or* clindamycin cream 2%, one full applicator (5 g) intravaginally at bedtime for 7 days.)
- Candidiasis: clotrimazole 500 mg daily intravaginally for 7 days. Recurrent vulvovaginal candidiasis (VVC), usually defined as four or more episodes of symptomatic VVC in 1 year, affects a small percentage of women (<5%). Oral fluconazole weekly for 6 months is given for maintenance after treating acute infection.
- Trichomoniasis: metronidazole 400mg twice a day for 7 days or 2 g oral metronidazole single dose.

In severe cases, especially in those with PID, IV antibiotics may need to be prescribed. Diagnostic laparoscopy may be required if symptoms do not resolve within 24–48 hours.

Long-term effects

The most deleterious effect of pelvic infection is the possibility of tubal damage. Urgent investigations and early treatment even prior to receiving the results is needed to prevent tubal damage.

Non-infective causes are discussed with postmenopausal discharge (see p. 290).

Syndromic management

This is based on the patient's symptoms and can be undertaken without laboratory support.

When a patient presents with vaginal discharge, take history and assess STI risk. If STI risk is low, treat for vaginal infection depending on speculum and microscopic examination findings. If high risk for STI, include treatment for chlamydia and gonorrhoea. At the same time educate and counsel the women regarding STI and promote the use of condoms. Also offer HIV testing.

⑦ **Peri- and postmenopausal discharge**

Discharge occurring per vaginam in older women has different causes and merits separate attention from those occurring in younger women. Perimenopause is defined as the period occurring a few years before the onset of menopause during which the woman is going through the menopausal change. The main concern of vaginal discharge in perimenopausal and postmenopausal women is that it could be a harbinger of malignant change in the genital tract, as genital tract malignancy is much higher in this age group. Hence, any abnormal vaginal discharge in the perimenopausal women and any discharge in the postmenopausal women warrant immediate evaluation.

Causes

- Endometrial carcinoma
- Cervical carcinoma
- Hormone replacement therapy (HRT)
- Endometrial hyperplasia
- Endometrial polyp
- Fibroid uterus
- Endometrial atrophy
- Atrophic vaginitis
- Vaginal pessaries
- Foreign bodies—IUD
- Vaginal and vulval carcinoma
- Infectious causes—candidiasis.

Of all the above-listed causes, benign causes are more common than the malignant ones. But the approach towards the patient would be to rule out the malignant causes before proceeding with the treatment.

A complete history should be obtained especially with regard to the onset, duration, severity of the symptoms, use of HRT, use of tamoxifen, and history of cervical smears.

In postmenopausal women, the most common causes of bleeding or blood-stained discharge are benign conditions (88%) of which atrophic vaginitis is the most common. Up to 12% of the women may have a malignant condition of which the most common is endometrial carcinoma. Hence, in managing postmenopausal women with bleeding or discharge, an active search for malignancy is warranted. This is accomplished by a speculum examination for cervical lesions, performing a transvaginal scan, and a Pipelle® endometrial biopsy.

Atrophic vaginitis is due to lack of oestrogen in menopause and hence application of oestrogen cream in the vagina will relieve the symptoms.

In the perimenopausal women, malignancy may be a possibility and the first priority is to rule out malignancy before proceeding with treatment. A pelvic examination, transvaginal US and endometrial sampling are basic requirements to rule out malignant disease in the genital tract. A hysteroscopy and curettage is a definitive diagnostic procedure. The treatment depends on the particular diagnosis.

Further reading

Spence D, Melville C. Vaginal discharge. *BMJ* 2007; 335(7630):1147–5.

Vulval problems

Contributor
David Nunns

Contents

⑦ **Pruritus vulvae/vulval pain**

Pruritus vulvae

Differential diagnosis
- Vulval infection (commonly vulval candidiasis)
- Lichen sclerosus
- Lichen simplex
- Contact dermatitis
- Lichen planus.

Infection
- Diagnosis: consider referral to GUM clinic if sexually transmitted disease suspected.
- Treatment: common cause *Candida*, associated with thick white discharge; can be treated with antifungal pessary clotrimazole 500 mg once at night or topical cream prep. Recurrent cases (more than four times a year) need maintenance antifungals.

Lichen sclerosus
Autoimmune inflammatory condition of skin. Mainly affecting the genital area in women.
- Diagnosis:
  - white, crinkly skin, anatomy of vulva lost and labial adhesions
  - rubbing of skin causes thickened lichenified areas
  - histological biopsy to confirm diagnosis in difficult cases.
- Treatment:
  - clobetasol propionate 0.05% ointment is applied one finger-tip unit (FTU) nightly for 4 weeks, alternate nights for 4 weeks, and then twice a week for 4 weeks
  - continued with maintenance dose if necessary
  - lower-dose steroid creams often not effective
  - emollients, E45®, Cetraben® emollient can be helpful
  - surgery to divide adhesions at fourchette may be needed
  - need follow-up as risk of vulval cancer developing (<5% risk).

Lichen simplex
- Diagnosis: lichenified skin secondary to scratching.
- Treatment:
  - Use clobetasol propionate 0.05% ointment to control situation using same dosing regimen as lichen sclerosus. Hydroxyzine hydrochloride 25 mg at night may be useful to control pruritus. Can increase up to three times daily until relief. Hygiene, counselling, and support very important.

Contact dermatitis
- Diagnosis:
  - take a careful history to try to identify irritant
  - on examination often red and swollen with possible evidence of secondary infection

- Treatment:
  - eliminate irritant, emollients and possible antibiotics if secondary infection
  - advise on avoiding perfumed products and bland emollients. Patch testing with a dermatologist if necessary.

Lichen planus
- Diagnosis:
  - purple/white papules, can affect any area of body. Usually self-limiting and often asymptomatic. Some patients with vaginal disease have painful eroded areas within the vulva
  - histological biopsy will confirm diagnosis
- Treatment:
  - try treating with clobetasol propionate ointment if symptomatic
  - in lichen planus, vaginal disease is not uncommon and can cause vulval pain and discharge. Patients need referral to vulval clinics.

General considerations for good practice

- When prescribing steroids be specific about dose. 1 FTU is from the tip of the finger to the first crease. 1 FTU is enough to treat an area of skin twice the size of the flat of an adult's hand with the fingers together and is equivalent to 0.5 g. Ointments are less irritant than creams.
- Irritability from topical agents is common on vulval skin.
- Emollients are bland and scent free, which is very useful for soothing and rehydrating dry, inflamed skin.
- Good hygiene is essential.
- Biopsy can be very useful in difficult and uncertain cases.

Vulval pain
Vulval pain can be caused by minor skin trauma through scratching; however, there are a number of specific causes of vulval pain.

Vulvodynia
Burning or soreness of the vulva in the absence of infection or a dermatological cause.

Causes
- Neuropathic pain syndrome of the vulva.

Presentation
- Variable age group.
- Constant pain: 'unprovoked vulvodynia'
- Pain on light touch: 'provoked vulvodynia' results in dyspareunia. Formerly vestibulitis.
- Often nothing to see on vulva, but touch sensitivity.

Diagnosis
- Clinical diagnosis, no need for biopsies.

Treatment
- Support and reassurance are important.

- For unprovoked pain, tricyclic antidepressants which at low doses have analgesic properties. Nortriptyline can be commenced, 10 mg at night and increased by 10 mg daily until pain free; on average this will take 60–100 mg daily. (Max. 100 mg per day.) Usually a 3-month course will be adequate; side effects should settle after 2 weeks of treatment.
- As a second line treatment, neuroleptics such as gabapentin may be of benefit.
- Local anaesthetic gels (e.g. lidocaine 1–2%) may be applied to reduce skin sensitivity. (10% may have irritation after application.)
- For provoked pain, desensitization can help with physiotherapy and/or sexual therapy.
- Consider referral to vulval clinic for difficult cases; rarely surgery may be indicated for provoked vulvodynia.

⑦ Lumps or ulcers on the vulva

Vulval lumps

Malignant
- Uncommon, incidence ~3:100,000
- Often in older age group, need urgent outpatient referral.

Differential diagnosis
1. Squamous cell carcinoma
2. Melanoma
3. 85% squamous cell, often complain of a mass and itching, less often discharge and bleeding.
- Diagnosis confirmed with histological biopsy, important to palpate inguinal nodes.
- 5% melanoma, can present complaining of an enlarged mole, prognosis is dependent on depth of invasion. Mainstay of treatment surgical, vulval skin prone to desquamation with radiotherapy.
- 10% made up of other causes, all very rare; would need urgent biopsy for histological diagnosis.
- Refer all cases to gynaeoncology team.

Benign
Common.

Differential diagnosis
- Bartholin's gland cyst or abscess (painful)
- Squamous papillomata—'skin tag'
- Folliculitis—infected hair follicle
- Condyloma acuminata—'warts'
- Many others usually diagnosed histologically.

Bartholin's abscess or cyst
- Gland situated in posterior third of labia majora and lower vagina.
- Abscess will be very painful. Antibiotics can be used, flucloxacillin 500 mg four times a day, but often need acute referral for incision and drainage. Marsupialization is performed to help prevent recurrence.
- Send pus swab for culture. Can be associated with gonorrhoea. Useful to check blood glucose.

Skin tags
Very common, be reassuring, only refer or treat if symptomatic. May often be excised under local anaesthetic.

Condyloma acuminata (genital warts)
- Common finding, associated with human papilloma virus (HPV) 6 and 11.
- Diagnosis is clinical but can be confirmed with biopsy.
- Contact tracing is necessary so refer to GUM clinic.
- Treatment is usually with topical podophyllin, cryotherapy, or surgery.

Vulval ulcer

Differential diagnosis

- Herpes
- Apthous ulcer
- Syphilis
- Vulval carcinoma
- Crohn's disease.

Herpes

- Viral origin, in UK 50% herpes simplex type 2 'cold sores'
- Incubation period 2–14 days, primary attack can be severe lasting 3–4 weeks if not treated. Recurrent attacks shorter and less severe.
- Essential to refer to GUM clinic for contact tracing and screening for other infections.
- Usually present with painful ulcerated vulva, possible intact vesicles.
- Associated with fever, malaise, and possible inguinal lymphadenopathy.
- Diagnosis is clinical but vesicular fluid can be sent for viral culture.
- Treatment comprises of rest and analgesia, Aciclovir may be effective to limit severity and duration. Use 200 mg five times daily for 5 days.
- Consider suprapubic catheter if patient presents with urinary retention.

Apthous ulcer

- Analogous to mouth ulcer, small and painful with a yellow base, usually labia majora not associated with systemic upset.
- Simple pain relief, self-limiting.

Syphilis

- Indurated painless 'chancre', can be on vulva or cervix, may have several.
- Refer to GUM clinic for treatment and contact tracing.

Crohn's disease

- Up to 30% of sufferers may have vulval involvement, can precede GI involvement. Appear like knife cuts to skin.
- If there is already GI involvement, look for sinuses and discharge.

Miscellaneous topics in gynaecology

Contributors

Maya Basu, Claudine Domoney, Stergios K. Doumouchtsis, Sambit Mukhopadhyay, and Hilary Turnbull

Contents

☼ Urinary retention

Definitions
- Acute retention: sudden onset of painful or painless inability to void over 12 hours, requiring catheterization with removal of a volume equal to or greater than normal bladder capacity.
- Chronic retention: insidious and painless failure of bladder emptying where catheterization yields a volume equal to at least 50% of normal bladder capacity.

Signs and symptoms
- Pain
- Overflow incontinence
- Frequency of micturition
- Poor flow
- Intermittent stream
- Incomplete emptying
- Straining to void
- Hesitancy
- Palpable bladder, dull to percussion.

Aetiology
- Neurological disease:
  - as a result of spinal injury—spinal shock phase
  - upper motor neuron lesion—spinal injury, multiple sclerosis
  - lower motor neuron lesion—spinal injury, multiple sclerosis
  - autonomic lesion, e.g. after pelvic surgery
  - local pain reflex after surgery
- Pharmacological:
  - tricyclic antidepressants, anticholinergic agents, adrenergic agents, epidural, and spinal anaesthesia
- Acute inflammation:
  - acute urethritis, acute cystitis, acute vulvovaginitis
  - acute anogenital infection
- Obstruction:
  - distal urethral stenosis, acute urethral oedema after surgery
  - chronic urethral stenosis, foreign body or calculus in the urethra
  - distortion of urethra by cystocele or uterine prolapse
  - impacted pelvic mass (retroverted gravid uterus, haematocolpos, uterine fibroids, ovarian cyst, faecal impaction)
  - bladder leiomyoma
- Endocrine: hypothyroidism, diabetic neuropathy
- Overdistension
- Post-surgical:
  - surgery for stress incontinence, anorectal surgery
  - pelvic surgery (especially radical)
- Psychogenic: anxiety or depressive illness, hysteria
- Idiopathic.

Investigations

Investigations should be performed with the suspected abnormality in mind (see Figs 18.1 and 18.2).

Acute retention
- Urine MCS and cytology in all cases
- Pass a urethral catheter to measure urinary volume and may leave on free drainage.

Chronic retention
- Determine residual volume by post-micturition US or catheterization
- Uroflowmetry:
  - maximum urinary flow rate (abnormal if <15 mL/sec for a void of at least 150 mL)
  - time to void may be delayed
  - prolonged voiding time
  - abnormal flow pattern.

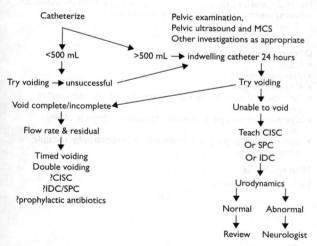

Fig. 18.1 Acute retention. CISC, clean intermittent self-catheterization; IDC, indwelling urethral catheter; SPC, suprapubic catheter, MCS, microscopy, culture, and sensitivity.

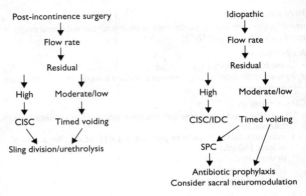

Fig. 18.2 Chronic retention. CISC, clean intermittent self-catheterization; IDC, indwelling urethral catheter; SPC, suprapubic catheter.

Other investigations
- U&Es
- Pelvic and renal US
- Cystometrogram
- Lumbosacral spine X-ray, e.g. spina bifida and intervertebral disc prolapse
- Cystourethroscopy e.g. urethral stenosis or stricture, bladder diverticulae
- Electromyography e.g. urethral sphincter hypertrophy, multiple system atrophy.

Management

Exclude UTI in all cases.

:⚛: Sexual assault

Incidence

The lifetime risk of sexual assault is 1 in 4–6 for women but the incidence of child sexual abuse is unknown. 1 in 5 adult rapes are reported but probably only 1 in 20–50 assaults of children are known to supervising authorities. In the UK in 2004, there were 190,000 victims of serious sexual assault and 47,000 female victims of rape or attempted rape. The definition of sexual offences and rape vary from country to country but the British Sexual Offences Act of 2003[1] has sought to clarify the law with respect to current patterns of sexual violence and exploitation. In summary, this act defines rape as any non-consensual penetration of the mouth, vagina, or anus by a penis. Sexual assault and assault by penetration replace indecent assault, which is defined as non-consensual sexual touching and penetration involving the insertion of an object, or body parts other than the penis, into the vagina or anus.

Children under 13 years cannot legally consent to sexual activity. Child sex offences include activity with no sexual contact (i.e. forcing a child to watch a sexual act). 'Familial child sex offences' replace 'incest' to incorporate the wider context of the modern family and includes non-blood relatives. Offences of abuse of trust include abuses of children through prostitution (direct or indirect) and pornography/trafficking/grooming.

Risks of sexual assault

- 1 in 4–6 women—lifetime risk
- 1 in 10 sexual assault of men—lifetime risk
- From reported sexual assaults data: 12% by strangers, 45% acquaintances, 43% intimate partners
- When assessing a potential victim, it is important to establish whether a sexual act has occurred and whether they were able to and gave consent.

Presentation

Acute or delayed or acute on chronic (particularly for children) presentation may occur.

Acute sexual assault

- 16–58% have genital injuries
- 38–80% have non-genital injuries
- May present to emergency department or via the police
- May present to GUM/gynaecological/psychiatric services with covert or overt symptoms.

Delayed

- GUM
- Gynaecology
- Antenatally (increase in domestic violence and assault during pregnancy).

Concerns arising for children
- Repeated emergency department attendances
- Poor parent–child interactions or behaviour
- Child known to social services
- Any injuries to child under 1 year
- Domestic abuse
- Explanation inconsistent with injuries
- Disclosure of abuse by child
- Delay in presentation.

Management

Needs of the victim to be addressed are:
- Medical
- Psychological
- Forensic.

Immediate medical care is the first priority (this will determine the venue of examination):
- Appropriate therapeutic measures—this includes resuscitation and usual 'ABC' measures are of overriding importance irrespective of forensic evidence:
  - bleeding
  - loss of consciousness (injury/intoxication)
  - oxygenation
- Consideration of collection of evidence (Locard's principle 1928— 'every contact leaves a trace'—loss of 'best evidence' must be a consideration if someone wishes to have the option of forensic investigation)
- Prophylactic antibiotics
- Post-exposure prophylaxis (PEP) for HIV
- Emergency contraception
- Hepatitis B vaccination
- Analgesia
- General advice and support, follow-up including counselling.

Consideration of the presence of a responsible adult/carer for children or adults without mental capacity and interpreters must be considered before examination in non-life threatening situations. If impairment of capacity to consent to examination is temporary (e.g. due to drugs or alcohol), then an appropriate time and setting should be awaited.

Those >16 years are able to consent and children <16 years who are considered Fraser-competent do not need an adult present, although this should be recommended by healthcare professionals. All forensic examinations of victims <13 years should be undertaken by a trained examiner with a forensic-trained paediatrician.

In emergency departments, there should be 'early evidence kits' available so that samples of urine and saliva can be taken before the victim decides whether to proceed with forensic investigation. This decreases the chance of loss or contamination of delicate evidence. In some units there may be provision of forensic swabs but the collection of forensic data requires a huge amount of documentation that if not properly undertaken may prove useless or even harmful to the case if brought to court. For these reasons, forensic samples are ideally taken by trained professionals[2] or under close supervision. The police are usually able to provide further information if requested. In London, Manchester, and Newcastle there are dedicated Sexual Assault Referral Centres, where victims can be seen away from emergency departments and police stations by Sexual Offences Examiners. However, examiners can attend hospitals especially if operative intervention is required.

History
- Alleged assault and what has happened since
- Basic medical, surgical, and psychiatric history
- Medication—prescribed, over-the-counter, social, drugs of abuse
- Gynaecological, obstetric, and sexual history.

Examination
- Demeanour, intoxication
- Height/weight/BP/pulse/temperature
- General findings
- Injuries (record accurately with diagrams):
  - none
  - bruising
  - abrasions
  - lacerations
  - incisions
  - defence injuries
- It is important to document both positive and negative findings
- Consider neurological examination
- Auscultation of chest
- Genital, anal, oral, nails
- Keep any other items such as tampons/sanitary towels/condoms in specimen bags if possible or uncontaminated container. Clothes may also be important for evidence.
- Mental state—it is crucially important to assess mental state and risk of suicide or self-harm when assessing anyone presenting with sexual abuse/assault. Conversely victims of abuse frequently present to the emergency department or psychiatric services with overdoses or deliberate self-harm. Previous psychiatric history may determine those at higher risk. Referral to the on-call psychiatric services may be necessary if the victim is judged to be at serious risk of self-harm or suicide.
- Forensic examination of victims of alleged assaults >7 days ago for women and > 72 hours for <13-year-olds and men is unlikely to provide useful evidence and is therefore considered non-urgent. In these circumstances, the health needs should be addressed, then they should be referred on to the appropriate services. In most situations this is likely to be the local GUM department.

Investigations
Consideration of further investigation by CT or MRI scan, X-ray, or US may be necessary depending on suspected injuries.

Further management

Any significant bleeding, poisoning, or other injuries must be dealt with as per guidelines and expert help sought. Emergency surgery is occasionally required for genital bleeding or other trauma.

- *Emergency contraception:*[3] this should be considered and given if there has been any vaginal contact in women or menstruating girls irrespective of stage of menstrual cycle. Current recommendations are for:
  - Levonorgestrel 1.5 mg stat (to be repeated if vomiting within 3 hours) within 72 hours of sexual act.
  - IUD insertion with antibiotic cover within 5 days (with consideration of cycle and previous intercourse).
  - Ulipristal 30 mg can be used up to 120 hours but is contraindicated with the progestogen-only pill.
- *STIs:*[4] risk is estimated at 4–56% depending on local prevalence and degree of trauma. If transmitted, they may often be multiple. Consider prophylactic antibiotics particularly if unlikely to attend for follow-up. This should be guided by local genitourinary clinic sensitivities. An example combination may be:
  - 1 g azithromycin
  - 500 mg ciprofloxacin.
- *HIV risk:* risk is dependent on prevalence in population and trauma of assault. Consider depending on history but higher risk factors include:
  - assailant HIV positive or in risk group
  - assault within 72 hours
  - anal rape
  - trauma and bleeding
  - multiple assailants.
- HIV PEP is currently three antiretroviral drugs. They should be taken as soon as possible (within 1 hour if possible) and within 72 hours. An HIV test is required at baseline and 6 months. Appropriate follow-up must be arranged because of the toxicity of these drugs. The risk of transmission with a single exposure of:
  - receptive vaginal intercourse is 1 in 600–2000
  - receptive anal intercourse is 1 in 30–150
- *Child sexual abuse:* early; late/delayed; historic. Most children do not present acutely and may present because of Social Services or medical concerns regarding chronic physical illness/ failure to thrive/ neglect.
  - diagnostic factors for child sexual abuse:
    - gonorrhoea (if >1 year)
    - syphilis and HIV (if congenital infection excluded)
    - chlamydia (if >3 years)
  - factors suspicious for child sexual abuse are:
    - *Trichomonas vaginalis*
    - warts, herpes
  - emergency contraception must be considered in young pubescent girls.

- *Follow-up*:
  - short-term physical well-being
  - STIs
  - counselling
  - support services.

Helpline and support services

- Rape Crisis England & Wales.
  - URL: http://www.rapecrisis.org.uk
  - Tel: local numbers available from website or directory enquiries.
- Victim Support: for victims of all crimes including sexual assault.
  - URL: http://www.victimsupport.org.uk
  - Tel: 0845 30 30 900
- Brook: helpline and online enquiry service for the under-25s
  - URL: http://www.brook.org.uk Tel: 020 7284 6040
- SurvivorsUK: for men who have experienced sexual violence.
  - URL: https://www.survivorsuk.org/
  - Tel: 02035983898
- Rights of Women.
  - URL: http://www.rightsofwomen.org.uk
  - Tel: 020 7251 6577
  - Email: info@row.org.uk
- Suzy Lamplugh Trust: for issues of personal safety.
  - URL: http://www.suzylamplugh.org
  - Tel: 020 7091 0014
  - Email: info@suzylamplugh.org
- Child and Adolescent Mental Health Services (CAMHS): available locally around the UK.

References

1. UK Parliament. *Sexual Offences Act 2003* (Chapter 42). London: HMSO, 2003. http://www.opsi.gov.uk/acts/acts 2003
2. Wilken J, Welch J. Management of people who have been raped. *BMJ* 2003; 326:458–9.
3. Faculty of Sexual Reproductive Healthcare (FSRH), Clinical Effectiveness Unit. Emergency Contraception (August 2011). www.fsrh.org
4. Robinson AJ, Watkeys JEM, Ridgeway GL. Sexually transmitted organisms in sexually abused children. *Arch Dis Child* 1998; 79:356–8.

⑦ **Pharmacotherapeutics in gynaecology**

The drugs commonly used in common gynaecological emergencies are discussed in the following sections. The presentations and management of all these conditions have been discussed earlier in this book.

Drugs used in the treatment of pelvic inflammatory disease

PID is usually caused by STIs, e.g. *Chlamydia trachomatis* and *Neisseria gonorrhoeae*, but can also be caused by anaerobic organisms and *Mycoplasma genitalium*. Delays in receiving prompt treatment can increase long-term sequelae, including sub-fertility, ectopic pregnancy, and chronic pelvic pain. It should be aggressively treated by multiple drugs.

The Royal College of Obstetricians and Gynaecologists and British Association of Sexual Health and HIV[1] recommend the following drug combinations:

Mild/moderate disease
(Absence of pyrexia or tubo-ovarian abscess.)
- IM cephalosporin one dose, with oral metronidazole and doxycycline for 14 days, *or*
- Oral ofloxacin and metronidazole for 14 days.

Severe disease
- IV ceftriaxone and oral (or IV if available) doxycycline, followed by:
  - oral metronidazole and doxycycline for 14 days
- IV clindamycin and IV gentamicin, followed by:
  - oral clindamycin for 14 days, *or*
  - oral metronidazole and doxycycline for 14 days
- IV ofloxacin with IV metronidazole
- IV ciprofloxacin and IV metronidazole and IV doxycycline (or oral).

In pregnancy, evidence is lacking, but guidelines suggest IM ceftriaxone with oral erythromycin and metronidazole.

Cephalosporins (ceftriaxone, cefuroxime, cefradine)
- Pharmacology: this group of antibiotics acts against the bacteria by inhibiting cell wall synthesis. They have the same mechanism of action and similar pharmacology to penicillin, hence cross-sensitivity and allergic reactions may occur in penicillin-allergic patients. They are active against Gram-positive and Gram-negative organisms.
- Dosage:
  - ceftriaxone:
    - IV infusion: 2 g once daily
    - IM: 250 mg single dose
  - cefuroxime:
    - oral 250–500 mg twice daily
    - IM or IV or infusion: 750 mg 6–8 hours, 1.5 mg 6–8 hours in severe infection
    - in surgical prophylaxis: 1.5 mg IV at induction.

- Pharmacokinetics: they are excreted primarily by the kidney. They cross the placenta.
- Side effects:
  - hypersensitivity (~10% of patients with penicillin allergy show cross-reactivity)
  - LFT disturbances, transient hepatitis, and cholestatic jaundice
  - nephrotoxicity.
- Drug interaction:
  - probenecid reduces excretion
  - loop diuretics may increase nephrotoxicity.
- Contraindication: hypersensitivity.

Doxycycline
- Pharmacology: it is a tetracycline, bacteriostatic agent, which prevents bacterial protein synthesis by inhibiting translation. Tetracyclines are active against a wide range of Gram-positive and Gram-negative organisms and also *Chlamydia, Mycoplasma*, and some atypical mycobacteria.
- Dosage:
  - PID: 100 mg twice daily for 14 days
  - Uncomplicated chlamydial infection: 100 mg twice daily for 7 days.
- Pharmacokinetics: doxycycline, unlike other tetracyclines, has 95% absorption from the gut, and is not excreted in the urine, but in the faeces as an inactive conjugate. It can be given to renal patients.
- Side effects:
  - nausea, vomiting
  - hypersensitivity reaction
  - exacerbation of systemic lupus erythematosus
  - hepatotoxicity.
- Drug interaction:
  - antiepileptics increase metabolism of doxycycline
  - doxycycline increases the plasma ciclosporin concentration.
- Contraindications:
  - pregnancy, breastfeeding
  - <12 years old
  - cautious use in alcohol dependence and porphyria.

Macrolides
These include erythromycin and azithromycin.

Erythromycin
It is sometimes used to treat chlamydial infection in pregnancy.
- Pharmacology: *this is mainly a bacteriostatic drug, which can be bacteriocidal in high concentration.* It acts by inhibiting protein synthesis. It is active against *Chlamydia* and *Mycoplasma*.
- Dosage:
  - IV: 6.25–12.5 mg/kg every 6 hours
  - Oral: 250–500 mg, four times a day
- Pharmacokinetics: it is incompletely but adequately absorbed from the GI tract. Only 2–5% is excreted by urine, the rest is concentrated in the liver and excreted in bile. It crosses the placental barrier.

- Side effects:
  - nausea, vomiting, diarrhoea, abdominal discomfort
  - cholestatic jaundice
  - eosinophilia, rashes, urticaria.
- Drug interaction:
  - inhibits metabolism of carbamazepine, valproate, midazolam, theophylline, and methylprednisolone
  - avoid concomitant use with ergotamine due to risk of ergotism
  - effect of warfarin is increased.
- Contraindication: liver disease.

Azithromycin

This macrolide is often used in combination with one dose of ceftriax-one, because of better patient compliance. In uncomplicated chlamydial infection and non-gonococcal urethritis this drug can be used as a single dose therapy (1 g per week, but ideally for 2 weeks). This drug is contra-indicated in liver diseases.

Clindamycin

- Pharmacology: it suppresses protein synthesis, by inhibiting ribosomal translocation (in a similar mechanism to the macrolides). Its main effect is against anaerobes, and is often used in cases of penicillin sensitivity.
- Dosage:
  - oral: 450 mg, four times a day for 14 days
  - IV infusion: 900 mg three times a day (0.6–2.7 g daily in two divided doses).
- Pharmacokinetics: it is almost completely absorbed from the gut, then excreted in urine and bile. It easily crosses the placenta.
- Side effects: a serious toxic effect is antibiotic-associated colitis.
- Drug interaction:
  - increases the effect of non-depolarizing muscle relaxants.
  - antagonizes the effect of anticholinesterases (e.g. neostigmine).
- Contraindication: diarrhoeal state.

Aminoglycosides (gentamicin)

These are a group of bactericidal drugs, which act by interfering with protein synthesis. Aminoglycosides are mainly active against aero-bic Gram-negative bacteria; however, gentamicin is not used against *Neisseria gonorrhoea*, and is inactive against anaerobes. Serious toxicity is a major limitation to their usefulness, hence blood drug-concentration has to be monitored. Gentamicin is often used in conjunction with peni-cillins ± metronidazole.

Gentamicin

- Dosage—for severe PID (with clindamycin):
  - IV: 2 mg/kg loading dose, then 1.5 mg/kg three times a day, or 7 mg/kg once a day
  - adjust maintenance doses according to serum drug concentration.
- Pharmacokinetics: gentamicin is very poorly absorbed from the GI tract, but rapidly absorbed from the IM sites of injection. Excretion is almost exclusively by glomerular filtration, half-life being 2–3 hours.

- Side effects:
  - nephrotoxicity, ototoxicity
  - hypomagnesaemia on prolonged therapy.
- Drug interaction:
  - indomethacin increases plasma concentration
  - increased risk of nephrotoxicity with amphotericin, ciclosporin, cisplatin
  - increased ototoxicity with loop diuretics.
- Contraindications:
  - myasthenia gravis
  - pregnancy
  - renal failure.

Quinolones (ciprofloxacin, ofloxacin)

These are broad-spectrum bactericidal agents, which act by interfering with bacterial DNA synthesis. These drugs are often avoided due to the high risk of developing colonization with MRSA or *Clostridium difficile*. Ofloxacin should not be used for women at high risk of gonococcal PID due to increasing resistance in the UK.

- Dosage:
  - ofloxacin:
    - oral: 400 mg twice daily for 14 days (with metronidazole)
    - IV: 400 mg twice daily (with metronidazole)
  - ciprofloxacin:
    - oral: 500–750 mg twice daily
    - IV: 200 mg twice daily.
- Pharmacokinetics: it is well absorbed after oral administration, and eliminated by the kidney.
- Side effects:
  - nausea vomiting, abdominal pain, diarrhoea
  - rashes, pruritus, headache, dizziness
  - renal failure, nephritis, hepatic damage
  - ofloxacin can cause hypotension, neuropathy, extrapyramidal symptoms, etc.
- Drug interaction:
  - multiple drug interactions: anticoagulants, phenytoin etc.
  - increased risk of convulsions with NSAIDs and theophyllines.
- Contraindications: cautious use in patients at high risk of seizures, renal impairment, myasthenia.

Metronidazole

- Pharmacology: it is a nitroimidazole group of drug, and is commonly used in PID, suspected anaerobic infections, and for prophylaxis in surgery and terminations.
- Dosage:
  - Oral: 400 mg, three or two times a day
  - IV: 500 mg, three times a day.
- Pharmacokinetics: mainly metabolized in the liver and excreted in urine.

- Side effects:
  - nausea, vomiting, unpleasant taste
  - rashes
  - abnormal LFTs
  - urticaria and erythema multiforme in cases of hypersensitivity
  - peripheral neuropathy in cases of prolonged use.
- Drug interactions: alcohol—disulfiram-like reaction.

Prophylactic antibiotics for emergency and elective surgery

A single IV antibiotic dose is recommended ≥30 minutes before 'knife-to-skin'. The time taken for a drug to reach an effective concentration in the tissue is dependent on the drug's pharmacokinetics and route. Choice of drug depends on local recommendations and sensitivities. Common practice is cefuroxime and metronidazole.

Genital herpes

Aciclovir
- Pharmacology: an antiviral drug active mainly against herpes virus, it inhibits viral DNA synthesis. This drug is most effective started at the onset of the disease, and is associated with a reduction in duration and severity of symptoms.
- Dosage:
  - oral: 200 mg five times a day for 5 days.
  - IV: 5 mg/kg three times a day (if immunocompromised, severe initial genital herpes and varicella zoster).
- Pharmacokinetics: oral bioavailability is 10–30%, so IV administration is required to achieve high concentrations for severe cases. Excretion is via the kidneys.
- Side effects:
  - GI disturbances, hepatitis, jaundice
  - headache, neurological reactions
  - hypersensitivity reaction
  - acute kidney injury.
- Drug interaction:
  - probenecid reduces excretion
  - higher concentration with concomitant administration.

Menorrhagia and dysmenorrhoea

NICE guidance for heavy menstrual bleeding[2] suggests the following options: levonorgestrel-releasing intrauterine system, tranexamic acid, NSAIDs, combined oral contraceptive pill, or norethisterone.

Antifibrinolytic drugs
Tranexamic acid
Tranexamic acid is a fibrinolytic agent, which inhibits the activation of plasminogen to plasmin, therefore inhibiting fibrinolysis. It is commenced at the start of bleeding. It is now available 'over the counter' in the UK.
- Dosage: oral 1 g up to four times a day, in menorrhagia (when heavy bleeding has started).

- Side effects:
  - nausea, vomiting, diarrhoea
  - disturbances in colour vision (to stop the drug)
  - thromboembolic events (with long-term use).
- Contraindications: thromboembolic disease.

Non-steroidal anti-inflammatory drugs
The commonly used analgesics in gynaecology are NSAIDs. They reduce prostaglandin-production by inhibiting the enzyme cyclo-oxygenase.

Mefenamic acid
- Pharmacology: it is an NSAID with minimal anti-inflammatory effect but is effective against both dysmenorrhoea and menorrhagia.
- Dosage: 500 mg three times a day.
- Pharmacokinetics: 50% is excreted in urine.
- Side effects:
  - GI problems: discomfort, nausea, vomiting, ulceration
  - thrombocytopenia, haemolytic anaemia (positive Coombs' test) and aplastic anaemia.
- Drug interaction:
  - anticoagulants' effect is enhanced
  - reduced lithium excretion.
- Contraindications:
  - pregnancy
  - renal or hepatic impairment
  - asthma
  - gastric ulceration.

Diclofenac
It is mainly an anti-inflammatory, with minimal antipyrexic action.
- Dosage:
  - oral: 50 mg three times a day
  - PR: 50–100 mg (150 mg/24 hours).
- Pharmacokinetics: rapidly and completely absorbed after oral administration. There is substantial first-pass effect and only 50% of diclofenac is available systemically. Metabolites are excreted in urine (65%) and bile (35%).
- Side effects: as described earlier.
- Drug interactions: as described earlier—excretion of methotrexate is reduced by diclofenac causing toxicity.
- Contraindications: porphyria.

Hormonal preparations
A variety of hormonal preparations are used in gynaecology to treat heavy periods. Some of them are used to control acute loss.

Progestogens
Progestogens are widely used for menorrhagia. They can also be used for endometriosis, contraception, prevention of recurrent miscarriage, and HRT. The Mirena® intrauterine system device contains progestogen for the treatment of menorrhagia, but is not effective in the acute setting.

Norethisterone
- Dosage—oral:
  - 5 mg three times a day for 10 days—to arrest acute bleeding
  - 15 mg once a day from days 5–26 of cycle to prevent further bleeding.
- Side effects: premenstrual-like tension.
- Contraindications:
  - genital, breast, or liver tumours
  - porphyria
  - severe arterial disease.

Gonadotrophin-releasing hormones analogues (goserelin, leuprorelin)
- Pharmacology: GnRH analogues (receptor agonists) produce a stimulatory phase initially, but continued use is followed by down-regulation of GnRH receptors. This reduces pituitary gonadotrophins (luteinizing hormone, follicle-stimulating hormone), consequently inhibiting androgen and oestrogen production. They are used in endometriosis, precocious puberty, infertility, menorrhagia (fibroids) and preoperatively, but rarely in the acute setting.
- Side effects:
  - hypo-oestrogenic symptoms
  - fibroid degeneration.
- Contraindications:
  - >6 months' use
  - undiagnosed vaginal bleeding
  - pregnancy and breastfeeding.

Oestrogen preparations are not used in emergency gynaecology.

Medical treatment of ectopic pregnancy
Methotrexate is used in medical management of ectopic pregnancy.

Methotrexate
- Pharmacology: it is an antimetabolite and acts by inhibiting the enzyme dihydrofolate reductase, which is essential in purine and pyrimidine synthesis.
- Use—guidelines recommend its use for ectopic pregnancy only in the following situations:
  - hCG level <3000 U/L
  - no cardiac activity in the ectopic pregnancy
  - minimal symptoms
  - regular follow-ups can be ensured (risk of rupture in 7%)
  - about 15% of patients may need repeat dosage.
- Dosage: IM 50 mg/m^2 single dose
- Pharmacokinetics: it is rapidly absorbed from the GI tract at smaller dosage (< 25 mg/m^2), but larger doses are not well absorbed, and should be administered IM or IV. About 90% of the drug is excreted unchanged in urine.
- Side effects:
  - myelosuppression
  - effect on LFTs
  - mucositis
  - rarely pneumonitis.

- Drug interaction:
  - increased toxicity with aspirin and NSAIDs, ciclosporin, corticosteroid, acitretin
  - antifolate effect enhanced by co-trimoxazole and trimethoprim, phenytoin, pyrimethamine
  - excretion reduced by penicillins, sulfonamides, probenecid.
- Contraindications:
  - significant renal and hepatic impairment
  - presence of fetal cardiac activity within the ectopic mass
  - active infection
  - immunodeficiency syndrome.

Consequent pregnancies should be avoided for 6 months after methotrexate treatment.

Medical management of miscarriage

Missed or incomplete miscarriage, presenting with heavy vaginal bleeding, can be treated medically with the prostaglandin, misoprostol. With elective, non-emergency management, patients receive mifepristone, the anti-progesterone, which sensitizes the myometrium to prostaglandin-induced contractions. However, it is rarely used in an emergency.

Misoprostol

- Pharmacology: it is a prostaglandin E_1 analogue. It is commonly used, off UK licence, for termination of pregnancy, medical management of miscarriage, induction of labour for fetal demise, and PPH.
- Dosage: oral or vaginal: for early miscarriage or termination—400–800 mcg depending on local protocols. Lower doses are used for later gestations.
- Side effects: diarrhoea, abdominal pain, nausea, vomiting, temperature.

References

1. British Association of Sexual Health and HIV. *UK National Guideline for the Management of Pelvic Inflammatory Disease*. London: BASHH, 2011. http://www.bashh.org/documents/3572.pdf
2. National Institute for Health and Care Excellence. *Heavy Menstrual Bleeding* (QS47). London: NICE, 2013. http://www.nice.org.uk/guidance/qs47

Further reading

Brunton LL, Chabner BA, Knollmann BC. *Goodman and Gilman's The Pharmacological Basis of Therapeutics* (12th ed). New York: Mc Graw Hill, 2011.
Joint Formulary Committee. *British National Formulary* (70th ed). London: BMJ Group and Pharmaceutical Press, September 2015.
National Institute for Health and Care Excellence. *Ectopic Pregnancy and Miscarriage: Diagnosis and Initial Management* (CG154). London: NICE, 2012. http://www.nice.org.uk/guidance/CG154
Scottish Intercollegiate Guideline Network. *Antibiotic Prophylaxis in Surgery* (Clinical Guideline No. 104). Edinburgh: SIGN, 2014. http://www.sign.ac.uk/pdf/sign104.pdf

Diagnostic laparoscopy and emergencies following laparoscopic surgery

Contributor
Hugh Byrne

Contents

Laparoscopic surgery in gynaecology

Diagnostic or therapeutic laparoscopy is a common emergency or elective intervention in gynaecology. It is associated with shorter recovery periods and smaller scars than laparotomy. However, untoward events can occur, and it may be useful to inform more senior colleagues and those in other specialities beforehand in case of unexpected findings. Good preparation is the key to a safe outcome. Unfamiliar techniques or instruments should not be tried out unsupervised or out of hours.

Indications

- Ectopic pregnancy
- Adnexal pathology such as:
  - ovarian cysts
  - suspected torsions
  - hydro- or pyosalpinges
- Infection: pelvic inflammatory disease (PID)
- Acute or acute-on-chronic pelvic pain.

Contraindications

Absolute

- Lack of informed consent
- An unstable patient
- Operator inexperience/poor supervision/lack of resources
- Suspected severe intra-abdominal bleeding where a laparotomy would result in more efficient haemostasis.

Relative

- Uncorrected coagulation disorders
- Suspected malignancy
- Cardiac/respiratory disease
- Obesity or extremes of BMI
- Previous surgery (especially midline incisions, bowel surgery) or a history of severe PID: adhesions are more likely in these women.

Assessment and investigation

History

- Medical
- Surgical
- Allergies
- Gynaecological: past and present, including fertility plans ①
- Any contraindications.

Examination

- General: a ↑ or ↓ BMI adds to the surgical risk ①
- ▶Abdominal
- ▶Vaginal.

Investigations

- Bloods: FBC, G&S, hCG
- Microbiology: high vaginal swabs, urinalysis → MSU sample
- Radiology: transvaginal US, plain film X-rays of the abdomen and chest (Δ calculi, bowel problems, etc.) ±CT.

Preparation
- Insert large-bore IV cannulae
- Catheterize and monitor urine output
- Anaesthetic review
- Obtain informed consent (see following 'Obtaining consent for laparoscopy' section)
- TEDS or other mechanical DVT prophylaxis
- Remove body piercings
- Enemas etc. are unnecessary.

Obtaining consent for laparoscopy
- Establish capacity: in the UK the age of consent for surgical procedures is 16 years. ☛ If the woman is not yet 16, she can still sign her consent if the Fraser guidelines apply—document this carefully (Box 19.1).
- Variants of the standard NHS consent forms exist for adults who lack mental capacity etc.—although if the woman is unable to sign the standard consent form, is this operation really appropriate for her?

Box 19.1 Documentation
- Use the clinical notes to document all information, discussions, and thoughts that are not covered by the consent form and investigation reports.
- While you may be pressed for time, take a few moments to sit down and gather your thoughts onto paper—this can lead to better decision-making and ideas.
- Write as if you are explaining your thought processes to an observer.
- The operation note should include any photographs or videos taken, clearly labelled and annotated. Be liberal with your use of photography and DVD recordings.
- A comprehensive discharge summary should be written and a copy given to the patient. Do not be afraid to impart such information to the patient—if you have acted in a safe and appropriate manner you should have nothing to fear.
- Also note the number of histology specimens (itemized) as well as the correct swab and instrument count. Record the estimated blood loss—or better still, the actual blood loss.
- When explaining the risk profile, tailor it to the individual patient; take into account her weight, history, and likely diagnosis, as well as the planned procedure(s).
- Other non-surgical procedures such as the administration of blood or blood products and the administration of vaginal or rectal medications should be explained.
- An anaesthetist should review the patient in person, preferably before her transfer to theatre.
- The benefits of the procedure should be described as the investigation and/or treatment of the named suspected condition(s).

- Do not rush the discussion: it may be an emergency situation but *decisions made in haste are often regretted at leisure.*
- Ensure that her expectations are realistic. The rationale for any additional procedures such as salpingectomy or oophorectomy should be explained. Discuss any procedures declined by the patient and explore her reasons.
- It is considered standard that the patient is also giving her consent for a laparotomy should the need arise: this depends on any complications that arise and on the feasibility of completing the procedure via the laparoscopic route. A midline laparotomy may be required.

Risks

Immediate risks

Immediate risks include bowel, blood vessel, urinary tract, and uterine injury. Studies across Europe can be quoted as finding such injuries to occur in 3.6–12.5/1000 cases.[1] The guidance from the RCOG advising us to quote a rate of 2/1000 for diagnostic laparoscopy is therefore perhaps optimistic in this regard, and using the same studies quoted in the RCOG guidelines, the risk is more likely to be around 1/250. This is still <1%. Some patients prefer to be quoted rates, others percentages. Haemorrhage is also an immediate risk.

Later complications

Later complications include infection (commonly of the wound or urinary tract but occasionally endometritis or salpingitis, etc.), wound dehiscence (± evisceration), and persistent trophoblast following ectopic pregnancies. Adhesion formation is common, especially following blood, pus, or bowel content in the abdomen. Their sequelae can be severe, but this risk is often overlooked. Incisional herniae are relatively common but occur later on, while fistulae are rarer.

Other common complications

Other common complications include bruising, abdominal pain, bloating, and shoulder tip pain. More pain is to be expected following adhesiolysis and when specimen retrieval through the abdominal wall occurred. Advise the patient regarding expected recovery times and what to expect in terms of vaginal bleeding, as well as resuming normal function. Write a summary for the primary care giver/GP.

▶ Many complaints arise from failure to meet expectations rather than from actual complications or errors.

Reference

1. Royal College of Obstetricians and Gynaecologists. *Preventing Entry-Related Gynaecological Laparoscopic Injuries* (Green-top Guideline No. 49). London: RCOG, 2008.

Performing a diagnostic laparoscopy

Safety first

- Perform a WHO checklist/briefing session with the theatre team. Ensure a set of instruments for laparotomy is within easy reach.
- Place the patient in the correct Lloyd Davies position on a non-slip surface, with adequate access to the vagina. Avoid 'ski' arm supports.
- It is worthwhile catheterizing the patient yourself and taking the opportunity to perform a thorough vaginal examination. If a larger than expected mass is found you may wish to proceed directly to laparotomy.
- An earthing plate and a warming blanket should be applied.
- Confirm that the camera and 'stack' are functioning and set correctly.
- Before commencing the procedure, confirm that the anaesthetist is satisfied and that your team and assistants are ready. (See Box 19.2.)

Insufflation

- The first incision should be made at the umbilicus and in such a way that it will be concealed by the natural crease of the umbilicus when healed. Only incise the skin: the abdominal wall can be quite thin here.
- There is no need to test disposable Veress needles—blockage occurs during insertion. Gas flow can often be controlled from the camera.
- Place the Veress needle into the base of the incision and gently push toward the sacral hollow at 45°. Insertion at 90° to the skin is not necessary if the incision is sited correctly at the true umbilicus, because the thin layer of fascia therein is easily traversed with little chance of the needle passing at an angle through layers of fat and muscle.
- If correctly inserted, a click or two may be heard and a drop of sterile saline placed into the needle should be drawn into the abdomen (Palmer's test). Do not pinch up the abdominal wall with your other hand because you may inadvertently lift bowel into the path of the needle.
- Other entry techniques include the Hasson technique where a careful dissection down to the peritoneum at the umbilicus allows the insertion of a blunt port before insufflation, which is favoured by surgeons.

Box 19.2 Safety advice

- Have a very low threshold for seeking advice and help.
- Maintain a good visual field at all times.
- Use blunt rather than sharp instruments where possible.
- Remove specimens in bags and apply adhesion barriers.
- Check the bowel and ureters before finishing.
- Lavage and insert drains if in doubt (also if PID diagnosed).
- If a severe injury is suspected, proceed to midline laparotomy.

- Other routes of insufflation include via the posterior fornix or via Palmer's point. Only the latter is recommended. Palmer's point is found ~2 finger breadths below the costal margin in the midclavicular line (the clavicle is often palpable through the drapes).
- During insufflation set the cut-off pressure at 20 mmHg. The flow should be ≥1 L/min and the initial pressure should be low, ≤6–8 mmHg. If the initial pressure is high but falling, don't worry if gas flowing well.
- If insufflation fails, remove and inspect the needle. Try carefully again either at the umbilicus or at Palmer's point, and seek advice and help.
- Abandon if unsure or insert the camera port once insufflation complete. Do not apply pressure to the lower abdomen to bulge the pneumoperitoneum towards the port as this will push bowel into its path. Use a direct vision port with the camera attached if available.

Secondary ports

- Once the view confirms that the laparoscope is safely in the abdomen, the accessory ports should be inserted before the Trendelenburg tilt.
- Once a second port is inserted, the pressure can be reduced to 15 mmHg and a blunt instrument such as a closed Mahnes grasper can be used to inspect the abdomen and pelvis, and the tilt applied.
- To site a secondary port, follow the round ligament to where it disappears into the inguinal canal. Slightly superior and medial to this will be the peritoneal ridge that is the obliterated umbilical artery; lateral to this, the inferior epigastric vessels are often visible in thinner patients.
- Avoid these structures by taking a more lateral approach and use the laparoscope to transilluminate an area of abdominal wall well away from the anterior superior iliac spine, avoiding any blood vessels in the skin.
- Make a 5 or 10 mm incision parallel to Langer's lines and insert the port, taking care to avoid the great vessels in the pelvic side wall.
- Inspect all port sites at the end of the procedure and close the sheath at all port sites ≥10 mm. Check that no bowel or omentum is included.
- Tip: if adhesions are found at the umbilical port site, use a hysteroscope to inspect these via one of the accessory ports.

Box 19.3 gives some advice for using diathermy.

Box 19.3 Diathermy/electrocautery

- If diathermy is required, the settings are usually 30 watts. The large blue pedal is used for monopolar and a smaller pedal for bipolar.
  ▶ *Not working? Check the connections rather than increasing power.*
- Bipolar is better for occluding vessels and monopolar for dissection. Apply any energy well away from important structures. Avoid applying monopolar current to the ovaries, and always exercise caution. ▶ *Why not use pre-tied loops instead? Collateral damage is less likely.*

Complications following laparoscopic surgery

Complications following laparoscopic surgery are probably under-reported. While they can be easy to manage, they are often not recognized in time to avoid more serious sequelae.[1] Life-threatening situations such as circulatory collapse or septic shock can result from blood loss, infection, or visceral injury. To pre-empt problems:

- Monitor patients regularly in the immediate postoperative period.
- Apply an early warning or trigger score system.
- Be specific about what observations are to be recorded and how often, tailoring these instructions to the individual patient and to the surgery.
- Define strict discharge criteria.
- Have facilities for overnight admission.
- Give women printed and verbal advice about what to expect, when to seek help, and who to contact (including telephone numbers).
- Unscheduled readmissions should be reviewed by a gynaecologist.
- If the surgery took place at another centre, try to obtain the notes.

Signs of laparoscopic injury

These can be subtle. The patient may have been well enough to go home following her surgery (Box 19.4), but injury may still have occurred—pain, nausea, and vomiting are all less following laparoscopic surgery.

Vascular injury

Often, bleeding does not occur until the pneumoperitoneum has been deflated due to a release of the tamponade effect. Young, healthy women will often tolerate relatively large blood losses before it is reflected in their vital signs. Collapse and coagulopathy are late signs.

Bowel injuries

It may take several days for a large bowel injury to manifest as peritonitis, depending on the nature of the injury. Bowel injuries can occur during entry, adhesiolysis, manipulation, and the application of diathermy (many burns go unseen). Other bowel complications include obstruction, strangulation, and ischaemia/infarction. The key to treatment is to remove the contaminant and its source, defunctioning with stomas where necessary.

Urinary tract injuries

Intra-abdominal urinary leakage may present with a less obvious peritonitis than bowel injury. Urine output is often maintained. Ureteric injury can occur due to trauma or thermal injury. Fistulae present later. Again, the treatment is repair and/or diversion.

Other injuries

Hypothermia (from cold IV fluids or CO_2), diathermy plate burns, drug reactions, and retained foreign bodies are possibilities.

Worrying signs and symptoms of laparoscopic injury

- Abdominal pain requiring opiates/abdominal distension/tenderness
- Anorexia
- Reluctance or inability to mobilize
- Persistent nausea ± vomiting ± diarrhoea
- ↑ HR, especially >100 bpm (although not in all patients)
- A heart rate > systolic BP reading is ominous
- Pyrexia is *not* a consistent finding
- Do not be reassured if surgical drains are not productive—they may be blocked or the leaking organ or vessel is draining elsewhere.

Investigations

- *Bloods:* FBC (WCC may be ↑ or ↓ depending on the stage of sepsis), CRP (usually ↑), U&E, LFTs, clotting screen and G&S (cross-match as necessary). ABGs: a raised lactate is ominous (sepsis).
- *Radiology:* US is unreliable due to the presence of gas and fluid in the abdomen. CXR if unwell. A CT scan is the investigation of choice.

Management

- Accepting the possibility of injury and recognizing the unwell patient are the keys to avoid complications.
- Involve senior colleagues as well as those from other specialties, i.e. colorectal/GI surgery, urology, vascular surgery, and radiology.
- CT-guided drainage of some collections can be appropriate.
- A repeat laparoscopy if the patient is stable and her injury is suitable.
- Laparotomy: a midline laparotomy is generally appropriate, and the patient should be made aware that diversions such as colostomy and/or ileostomy may be required, as well as being warned about any loss of function that may occur.

> **Box 19.4 Often it is not the injury but the interval since it occurred that harms!**
>
> - **4R's:** Re-admit/Resuscitate, Regular and senior Review, Radiology (CT) and be Ready to Re-open/operate.
>
> If an injury occurs:
> - **3A's:** Apologize, Accept responsibility, and Act to put matters right.

Reference

1. Association of Laparoscopic Surgeons of Great Britain and Ireland (ALSGBI). *ALS Clinical Guidelines: Recognition, Management and Prevention of Abdominal Complications of Laparoscopic Surgery.* ALSGBI, 2010. http://www.alsgbi.org/pdf/ALS_Complications_Management.pdf

General issues in obstetrics and gynaecology

Contributors

Stergios K. Doumouchtsis, Anna Haestier,
Edward Morris, Edward Prosser-Snelling,
Kanchan Rege, Hannah Sims, and Eman Toeima

Contents

Haematological aspects of emergencies in obstetrics and gynaecology

The following applies mainly to obstetrics rather than gynaecology as there are no special considerations in the non-pregnant woman.

Pregnancy results in physiological changes to the haematological system. Changes are seen in both the FBC and the haemostatic system. This section will discuss the critical clinical situations that may affect a woman's blood in pregnancy and how they should be approached. The emergencies will be considered as follows:

- Conditions presenting with thrombocytopenia
- Venous thromboembolism (VTE)
- Pregnancy-induced exacerbations of pre-existing haematological conditions
- Obstetric haemorrhage.

Thrombocytopenia

A lower than normal platelet count ($<150 \times 10^9$/L) may occur in pregnancy due to a variety of reasons. Review of a blood film to rule out spurious thrombocytopenia due to platelet clumps and to look for red cell fragmentation is essential (see Table 20.1 and Fig. 20.1).

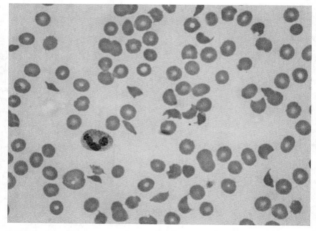

Fig. 20.1 A high-power view of a peripheral blood film showing red cell fragments and a large platelet.

Table 20.1 Causes of pregnancy-associated thrombocytopenia and associated features

	Platelet count	Red cell fragments on blood film?	Coagulation screen	Other features
Gestational thrombocytopenia	>80 × 10⁹/L	No	Normal	
Pre-eclampsia	Variable	In severe cases	Normal	Hypertension
HELLP syndrome	<100 × 10⁹/L	Yes	May be deranged	Deranged liver function tests
Disseminated intravascular coagulation	Usually >50 × 10⁹/L	Yes	Prolonged activated partial thromboplastin time, prothrombin time and low fibrinogen levels	Oozing from puncture sites
Thrombotic thrombocytopenic purpura	Variable	Yes	Normal	Neurological symptoms and renal impairment
Idiopathic thrombocytopenic purpura	Variable	No	Normal	

Gestational thrombocytopenia

Gestational thrombocytopenia refers to a mild thrombocytopenia (>80 × 10⁹/L) occurring in the third trimester, due to haemodilution, platelet activation, and clearance. This benign phenomenon does not result in neonatal thrombocytopenia or maternal bleeding.

Pre-eclampsia

Pre-eclampsia may present in the early stages with mild thrombocytopenia. Further investigation and management should be directed towards ensuring safe delivery of the baby (see Chapter 2).

HELLP syndrome (haemolysis, elevated liver enzymes, and low platelets)

HELLP syndrome is an overlap syndrome with pre-eclampsia. The management of the condition is directed towards ensuring safe delivery of the baby rather than the restoration of normal blood values.

Disseminated intravascular coagulation

DIC is always secondary to an underlying pathology such as abruptio placentae, amniotic fluid embolism, late stage pre-eclampsia, septic abortion and prolonged retained dead fetus, and shock. The principle of management should be correction of the underlying condition whilst maintaining the circulating blood volume. The goal should be an empty and contracted uterus.

Thrombotic thrombocytopenic purpura (TTP)

TTP is a pentad of microangiopathic haemolysis, thrombocytopenia, renal dysfunction, flitting neurological signs, and fever. Pregnancy is a recognized precipitating cause of TTP leading to 10–25% of all cases. Presentation may occur at any stage in pregnancy or in the postpartum period. TTP requires urgent treatment with plasma exchange at a specialist centre to attain remission and to prevent fetal abnormalities resulting from placental thrombosis.[1] Patients should be maintained on low-dose aspirin therapy and LMWH where an increased thrombotic risk is determined. Despite the thrombocytopenia, patients are intensely prothrombotic and platelet transfusion is contraindicated.

Idiopathic thrombocytopenic purpura (ITP)

ITP is estimated to occur in 1/1000–10,000 pregnancies. It is an acquired immune-mediated disorder resulting in an isolated thrombocytopenia <100 × 10⁹/L. Autoantibodies coat platelets, resulting in destruction by the reticuloendothelial system and bone marrow suppression of platelet production. This condition may arise *de novo* or as an exacerbation of a pre-existing state. Once identified, the FBC should be monitored every 4 weeks during the first two trimesters and thereafter more frequently.

Intervention is required in the first two trimesters if the patient presents with symptoms of bleeding, the platelet count falls below 20–30 × 10⁹/L or specific intervention necessitates a higher platelet count. The procoagulant state of pregnancy may allow women to tolerate lower platelet counts than in non-pregnant controls. Acute ITP presenting with bleeding should be managed by platelet transfusion, steroids (1 mg/kg /day of prednisolone), and intravenous immunoglobulin (IVIg). Prednisolone doses should be tailored to avoid exacerbation of hypertension, hyperglycaemia, and osteoporosis. Second-line therapy remains controversial, although high-dose methyl prednisolone in combination with IVIg or azathioprine has been used safely with success.[2]

A clear delivery plan should be established. The mode of delivery should be dictated by obstetric indications. A platelet count ≥50 × 10⁹/L is generally adequate for CS. Epidural anaesthesia requires a platelet count of >80 × 10⁹/L. Thromboprophylaxis should be considered on an individual basis.

In the main, the risk of bleeding lies with the mother and not the baby. However, forceps and ventouse delivery should be avoided, along with fetal blood sampling and fetal scalp electrodes, to avoid excess trauma and risk of bleeding. At delivery a cord FBC should be carried out to determine the fetal blood count. IM vitamin K should be avoided until the platelet count is known and if low, vitamin K should be administered orally. If the platelet count is <50 × 10⁹/L a transcranial US scan should be carried out to exclude intracranial haemorrhage. Treatment with IVIg would be warranted if the neonate is bleeding or has a platelet count of <20 × 10⁹/L. FBCs should continue to be monitored from days 2 to 5 post delivery to allow for a nadir to be reached.

Venous thromboembolism

Pregnancy results in a procoagulant state as the body prepares for delivery. This state is initiated with increases in several procoagulant factors (factors V, VII, VIII, X, von Willebrand factor (vWF), and fibrinogen.) There is a fall in the natural anticoagulant protein, protein S, reduction in fibrinolysis, and acquired resistance to activated protein C. The synthesis of antithrombin increases to maintain normal levels. In addition to this, venous stasis becomes more pronounced as hormones relax venous tone and the pressure from an enlarging uterus increases.

Pregnancy increases the risk of VTE tenfold. Women with a past history of VTE carry a 10–20% risk of recurrence in pregnancy. It can occur any time during pregnancy but is more common in the puerperium. Although VTE was no longer the leading cause of maternal deaths according to the 2006–2008 Confidential Enquiry into Maternal Deaths, the 2014 report (covering 2009 to 2012) found thrombosis and thromboembolism to be the leading cause of direct deaths, although they noted that 'that the change in death rate from thrombosis and thromboembolism between 2006–08 and 2010–12 is not statistically significant'.[3]

If VTE is suspected, the patient should be commenced on LMWH, whilst objective imaging is awaited. Securing a firm and accurate diagnosis is of paramount importance as such episodes may later affect decisions regarding lifelong anticoagulation. D-dimers have no role in the negative prediction of VTE in pregnancy as they are raised in healthy pregnancies. Compression duplex US is the examination of choice for DVT. Where PE is suspected, computed tomography pulmonary angiogram (CTPA) is indicated as a definitive test as the benefit of a firm diagnosis outweighs the potential risks of radiation to either the mother or fetus.[4]

First-line therapy of a confirmed VTE is LMWH. At present there is little experience with the other factor Xa or direct thrombin inhibitors in pregnancy and thus they cannot be recommended. Warfarin crosses the placenta and is contraindicated. LMWH should be given according to local policy but is usually given in two divided doses and titrated against the woman's booking weight. Platelet counts should be monitored in view of the theoretical risk of heparin-induced thrombocytopenia. Anti-Xa levels may be carried out to monitor therapy in extremes of body weight and renal impairment.

If onset of labour is spontaneous, LMWH should be stopped as soon as this is established. Anticoagulation should be stopped 24 hours prior to a planned delivery. Epidural anaesthesia should not be undertaken within 24 hours of administration of the most recent dose of LMWH nor should the epidural catheter removed within 12 hours.[5] In severe acute massive PE, thrombolysis has been used safely with low risk to the mother and fetus.[6]

Anticoagulation should be continued throughout pregnancy, for 6 weeks postpartum and at least a total of 3 months. Finally, women diagnosed with a DVT should be encouraged to wear compression stockings for 2 years to prevent post-thrombotic phlebitis in later life.

Pregnancy-induced exacerbations of pre-existing haematological conditions

Sickle cell disease

Sickle cell disease refers to an inherited disorder of the globin chain resulting in a structurally abnormal haemoglobin that produces significant symptoms through sickling. The abnormal haemoglobin sickles under conditions of reduced oxygenation, resulting in poor flow through small vessels and increased adherence to vascular endothelium. This in turn leads to vascular occlusion, chronic haemolysis, and sickle cell crises.

Ideally, these patients should have their care directed by a sickle cell specialist care centre.[7] Antenatal care should be rigorous and involve an obstetrician and haematologist as the clinical features of sickle cell disease can be exacerbated and may affect the developing fetus. These include anaemia, frequency of crises, infections secondary to hyposplenism, and impairment of fetal growth and development. In addition to booking and anomaly scans, uterine Doppler scans should be carried out at 24 weeks, and fetal growth scans at 28, 32, and 36 weeks.[8]

These phenomena are less likely when the percentage of sickle haemoglobin is <40–50 % of the total haemoglobin but there is no evidence to support the use of regular prophylactic red cell transfusion in all pregnancies. Indications for transfusion are:
- Hb <6 g/dL and falling
- Twin pregnancies
- Patients on pre-existing chronic transfusion programmes
- Anaemia with cardio or respiratory compromise.

An acute chest crisis or stroke should prompt immediate exchange transfusion to reduce the percentage of sickle haemoglobin to <30%.[8]

If significant red cell alloantibodies are detected, serology should be repeated every 2 weeks from 16 weeks to allow blood to be cross-matched in an emergency. Close liaison with blood transfusion services is essential. Painful crises should be managed under joint care of a haematologist and obstetrician. Careful attention should be paid to hydration, analgesia, and oxygenation. Thromboprophylaxis should be administered. NSAIDs should be used with caution and not given in the first trimester or after 32 weeks.[8]

Labour places huge stress on the body and can induce sickle cell crisis if dehydration, cold, infection, and hypoxia are not avoided.

In light of these risks, the following recommendations are made:
- Oxygen via face mask if oxygen saturations <95%
- IV fluids 3 L/24 hours
- Continuous electronic fetal monitoring
- Use of standard analgesia (e.g. nitrous oxide, opiates or epidural)
- Prophylactic antibiotics during labour and the puerperium, such as co-amoxiclav or erythromycin.

If CS is required, epidural anaesthesia is preferred. If GA is required, an experienced anaesthetist should be involved. Close observation post-operatively should be carried out, ideally on a high dependency unit. A haematologist should be involved and called urgently if oxygen saturations fall below 92% or signs or symptoms of a chest crisis develop. Following delivery, the mother is still at risk of complications. During the first 24 hours, hydration, oxygenation, and analgesia remain important. Mothers should be encouraged to mobilize and VTE risk assessed. Broad-spectrum antibiotics should continue for 5 days post delivery. Thromboprophylaxis should continue for at least 6 weeks post CS.

Von Willebrand disease (vWD)

Von Willebrand disease is a variable deficiency of vWF. vWF is essential for normal haemostasis as it is essential for platelet adhesion and acts as a carrier protein for factor VIII. There are three main types of vWD. Type 1 is the mildest and commonest form with reduced levels of vWF. Type 2 is a qualitative defect of the vWF, and type 3 is a severe deficiency of vWF. Each acts slightly differently during pregnancy and therefore close collaboration with a haematologist is essential. Deliveries should be planned and women should have access to a Haemophilia Centre and comprehensive neonatal facilities.

vWF levels increase during pregnancy and increase by three- to four-fold by the third trimester. Many women with type 1 vWD will achieve normal vWF levels by term and not require treatment. In type 2 vWD the increase in vWF will be abnormal and therefore these patients will require close follow-up and haematology input. In type 3 vWD, vWF levels do not increase and the patient will require vWF concentrates to cover delivery.

In women with type 1 and type 2 vWD, factor VII, and vWF levels should be checked at 34–36 weeks. Vaginal delivery is safe if vWF activity is >40% and CS if >50%. If these levels have not been achieved vWF replacement concentrates or DDAVP (a vasopressin analogue that stimulates production of factor VIII and vWF) should be used. The mode of delivery should be dictated by obstetric indications. Epidural anaesthesia may be considered in women with type 1 vWD whose levels have risen to normal levels, but is not recommended in type 2 or type 3 vWD. An experienced anaesthetist should be involved and caution should be taken on catheter removal as levels fall rapidly following delivery. Where a fetus is at risk of having type 2 or type 3 vWD fetal scalp monitoring, rotational forceps and ventouse delivery should be avoided. At delivery these babies should have a cord sample sent for vWF measurement and be assessed to exclude intracranial haemorrhage.[9]

vWF levels fall sharply often within hours after delivery. PPH may therefore be a presenting symptom of vWD. The diagnosis is, however, usually made after the event once all levels of coagulation proteins have returned to their resting levels. It is prudent to investigate all women (by checking a coagulation screen) who have experienced unexplained PPH to prevent a recurrence in subsequent pregnancies.

Haemorrhage

Obstetric haemorrhage remains a major cause of maternal death in both developed and developing countries. In the majority of cases, the deaths must be regarded as preventable. Primary PPH is the commonest form of haemorrhage and is defined as the loss of ≥500 mL of blood from the genital tract within 24 hours after the birth of a baby. Antepartum haemorrhage and secondary PPH are less common but the same management considerations apply. After the haemorrhage has been treated, the volume of fetal blood cells that have crossed into the maternal circulation must be ascertained by a Kleihauer test or by flow cytometry. Appropriate passive immunization with anti-D should be administered within 72 hours of the bleeding.

Red cell transfusions for women of child-bearing age must be ABO and Rhesus D compatible. They should also ideally be negative for the Kell antigen which occurs in about 10% of the UK population. Development of anti-Kell antibodies may lead to subsequent problems with haemolytic disease of the newborn so allo-immunization is best avoided. Blood products in the UK are leucocyte depleted which markedly reduces the risk of transmission of CMV, nevertheless at present, CMV-seronegative blood products are indicated for pregnant women.[10]

Haemorrhage may lead to fatalities due to early under-recognition of the gravity of the situation and logistical inefficiencies. Conditions such as placenta praevia and abnormally adherent placenta may be associated with catastrophic haemorrhage and where anticipated such cases should have a planned CS. Most cases, however, of PPH have no identifiable risk factors but the causes are often related to abnormalities in uterine tone, trauma to the birth canal, retained placental tissue, and low plasma thrombin levels. Active management of the third stage of labour with prophylactic oxytocics reduces the risk of PPH by about 60% in all women. Rigorous local protocols for the management of obstetric haemorrhage are essential and practice 'drills' are advised.

A blood loss of >500 mL should prompt establishment of venous access, closer monitoring of clinical observations, and samples being drawn for FBC, coagulation screen, and cross-match. A blood loss of >1000 mL should prompt resuscitation measures with the aim of preventing life-threatening blood loss which occurs at >40% of blood volume (2500–3000 mL).[11]

Once a PPH has been identified, senior members of the relevant clinical teams (obstetrics, anaesthesia, and haematology) need to be alerted. In the UK, hospital transfusion laboratories will normally be familiar with massive blood loss protocols and the need to enact the protocol drill must be clearly articulated to the laboratory with details of the patient's name, location, and when the relevant blood tests should be expected. In district hospitals, platelets for transfusion may not be kept on site so early warning of a developing situation will allow all appropriate blood products to be brought on site and frozen blood products to be defrosted. Early identification of a porter to transport blood samples urgently from the clinical area to the laboratory and blood products back to the clinical area is vital.

The thrust of clinical management of PPH is to maintain the circulating volume to enable tissue oxygen delivery whilst attempts are made to arrest the bleeding. The BP must be maintained initially with warmed fluids to prevent transfusion-associated DIC which may arise from endothelial damage in hypotension. Pending a full serological screen for atypical red cell antibodies, 'group compatible' blood may be issued 5–10 minutes after the blood group is known. Fresh frozen plasma at a dose of 12–15 mL/kg should be given to correct the clotting screen. Fibrinogen concentrates or cryoprecipitate should be given to maintain fibrinogen levels. In extremis, 1 L of fresh frozen plasma and 2 adult units of cryoprecipitate may be given pending the results of coagulation tests although it should be borne in mind that oxygen delivery will be better achieved by red cell transfusion. The therapeutic goals of transfusion should be to maintain:

- Haemoglobin >8 g/dL
- Platelet count >75 × 10^9/L
- Prothrombin time and activated partial thromboplastin time <1.5 × mean control
- Fibrinogen >1 g/L.

In the face of life-threatening PPH, particularly when the coagulation screen is reasonably normal, administration of recombinant factor VIIa may be indicated. This product is a potent procoagulant agent developed for the treatment of haemophilia. There have been case reports of thrombosis postoperatively and thus it should be used with caution in consultation with a haematologist to ensure that potential benefits do indeed outweigh the potential risks.[12] There is no regular place for antifibrinolytic agents such as tranexamic acid or aprotinin in this situation as the underlying balance of the coagulation system will tip towards thrombosis postpartum.

Intraoperative cell salvage in obstetrics is becoming increasingly popular in the elective and emergency settings. This technique spares exposure to allogeneic blood products and may be a useful technique in the management of women who refuse blood transfusion. The theoretical concerns regarding contamination of the maternal circulation with amniotic fluid and fetal red cells seem largely not to have materialized.[13]

Obstetric techniques to arrest bleeding such as arterial embolization, correcting uterine atony, evacuation of retained products of conception and hysterectomy are discussed elsewhere in this book.

References

1. Scully M (2007). Thrombotic thrombocytopenic purpura in pregnancy. *ISBT Science Series* 2007; 2(1):226–32.
2. Proven D, Stasi R, Newland AC, *et al.* International consensus report on the investigation and management of immune thrombocytopenia. *Blood* 2010; 115(2):168–86.
3. Knight M, Kenyon S, Brocklehurst P, *et al.* *Saving Lives, Improving Mothers' Care – Lessons Learned to Inform Future Maternity Care from the UK and Ireland Confidential Enquiries into Maternal Deaths and Morbidity 2009–12.* Oxford: National Perinatal Epidemiology Unit, University of Oxford; 2014.
4. The Royal College of Obstetricians and Gynaecologists. *The Acute Management of Thrombosis and Embolism during Pregnancy and the Puerperium* (Green-top Guideline No 37b). London: RCOG, 2007.
5. Royal College of Obstetricians and Gynaecologists (2009). *Reducing the Risk of Thrombosis and Embolism during pregnancy and the Puerperium* (Green-top Guideline No 37a). London: RCOG, 2009.

6. Ahearn GS, Hadjiliadis D, Govert JA, et al. Massive pulmonary embolism during pregnancy successfully treated with recombinant tissue plasminogen activator. A case report and review of treatment options. Arch Intern Med 2002; 162:1221–7.

7. Lucas SB, Mason DG, Mason M, et al. A sickle crisis? A report of the National Confidential Enquiry into Patient Outcome and Death. London: National Confidential Enquiry into Patient Outcome and Death, 2008.

8. Sickle Cell Society. Standards for the Clinical Care of Adults with Sickle Cell Disease in the UK. London: Sickle Cell Society, 2008.

9. Lee CA, Chi C, Pavord SR, et al. The obstetric and gynaecological management of women with inherited bleeding disorders-review with guidelines produced by a taskforce of UK Haemophilia Centre Doctors' Organisation. Haemophilia 2006; 14:671–84.

10. Royal College of Obstetricians and Gynaecologists. Blood Transfusion in Obstetrics (Green-top Guideline No 47). London: RCOG, 2007.

11. Royal College of Obstetricians and Gynaecologists. Prevention and Management of Postpartum Haemorrhage (Green-top Guideline No 52). London: RCOG, 2009.

12. Franchini M, Franchi M, Bergamimi V, et al. A critical review on the use of recombinant Factor VIIa in life-threatening obstetric postpartum haemorrhage. Semin Thromb Hemost 2008; 34(1):104–12.

13. Sullivan JV, Crouch ME, Stocken G, et al. Blood cell salvage during caesarean delivery. Int J Gynecol Obstet 2011; 115(2):161–3.

Identifying sick patients and choosing monitoring

The monitoring of very sick patients in obstetrics and gynaecology can cover a wide variety of conditions, from major surgical trauma, such as caesarean hysterectomy or pelvic exenteration, to serious medical conditions such as ovarian hyperstimulation syndrome (OHSS) or severe pre-eclampsia.

The parameters for monitoring useful physiological variables are divided into non-invasive, invasive, and specialist investigations. The goal of monitoring is to quickly identify trends in disordered physiology and correct them by either resuscitation or treating the underlying cause.

Non-invasive monitoring consists of routine bedside tests, which should be recorded on an easily accessible bedside chart at intervals specified by medical staff. These commonly include pulse, BP (including a mean arterial pressure), respiratory rate, oxygen saturation, temperature, urine output, and consciousness level.

In cases where a patient requires a higher level of care and is at risk of rapid deterioration, invasive monitoring is possible. An arterial line (commonly sited in the radial artery) gives a very accurate measurement of BP, and can be used for serial blood gas estimations. Central venous pressure measurement is useful both for the excellent vascular access it provides, as well as a surrogate measurement of left ventricular preload.

Patients undergoing invasive monitoring should be in an appropriate environment with adequate levels of experienced nursing care. For example, it would be unusual for a patient to have an arterial line on a standard inpatient ward.

Condition-specific tests that are required regularly can be used as part of monitoring, e.g. peripheral reflexes in pre-eclampsia and abdominal girth with daily weights in OHSS.

Early warning systems

Early warning systems (EWS) are also referred to as track and trigger systems or modified early warning scores (MEWS) and more recently have been adapted for use in obstetrics (MEOWS). They provide a structured framework for the interpretation of recorded physiological variables to produce a simple, numerical score. An essential component of any system is that there is a clearly identified escalation system to promptly ensure that the information generated at the bedside reaches the relevant medical decision-maker. Their development has spread from their origins in coronary care, to inpatient ward trials and now NICE recommends all inpatient wards use a version of an EWS.

A score of >3 in the example scoring chart shown in Table 20.2, triggers a medical review.

Table 20.2 Example of an EWS scoring chart

Score	3	2	1	0	1	2	3
Temperature (°C)		<35		35–37.4		37.5–39	>39
Systolic BP (mmHg)	≤70	71–79	81–89	90–139	140–149	150–159	≥160
Diastolic BP (mmHg)			≤45	46–89	90–99	100–109	≥110
Pulse (bpm)		≤40	40–50	51–100	101–110	111–129	≥130
Respiratory rate (resps/min)		≤8		9–14	15–20	21–29	≥30
AVPU				Alert	Responds to Voice	Responds to Pain	Unconscious
Urine output (mL/hr)	<10	<30		Not measured			

Critical care outreach and ICU review

Most EWS initially trigger a trainee doctor review, who then escalates as appropriate. The advent of the European Working Time Directive (EWTD) has increased episodes of handover and reduced continuity of care for patients. Nurse-led critical care outreach teams review patients at the request of trainee doctors or ward nurses. They will monitor ill patients as well as providing advice to ward staff and trainee doctors. They can if necessary escalate this to intensive care doctors but should not be considered a route of referral to ICU. If a patient has a high EWS score persistently, early referral to ICU should be considered.

Monitoring in obstetrics

The latest two CMACE reports (2007 and 2011) and the most recent MBRRACE-UK report (2014) highlighted that in many cases of maternal death, the early warning signs of impending maternal collapse went unrecognized. The increase in physiological reserve in pregnancy may mask the signs of critical illness, resulting in a delay in diagnosis and as maternal collapse is a rare event, the 'prodromal' phase may go unrecognized. Therefore, the reports recommended the introduction and use of a specific obstetric EWS to aid the early detection of life-threatening illness such as haemorrhage, pre-eclampsia/eclampsia, amniotic fluid embolism, and sepsis.

Specific to obstetrics, urine output (including the detection of proteinuria) with observations of neurological response and subjective assessment of lochia are added to a standard score.

There is no nationally standardized MEOWS chart, therefore most hospitals have devised their own system. Regardless of the format of the MEOWS chart, if a threshold level is exceeded, the value will fall into either a colour-coded trigger zone (red or yellow) or be recorded as a numerical value.

Very high scores identify patients who may need to be managed in critical care.

Pitfalls and limitations

It is important to realize that a MEOWS score is a screening tool that does not provide a diagnosis. It does not define treatment and all midwives and doctors using this chart should be aware that critical illness can occur with no prior warning signs, so the MEOWS score should not be a substitute for constant clinical vigilance.

Although some studies have criticized use of MEOWS as being time-consuming, expensive, and placing stress on patients as they undergo unnecessary medical review and additional clinical investigations, many studies validate MEOWS charts to be a highly sensitive clinical tool.

Further reading

Knight M, Kenyon S, Brocklehurst P, et al. Saving Lives, Improving Mothers' Care – Lessons learned to inform future maternity care from the UK and Ireland Confidential Enquiries into Maternal Deaths and Morbidity 2009–12. Oxford: National Perinatal Epidemiology Unit, University of Oxford, 2014.

Singh S, McGlennan A, England A, Simons R. A validation study of the CEMACH recommended modified early obstetric warning system (MEOWS). Anaesthesia 2012; 67(1):12–18.

Communication and handover

Communication between healthcare professionals, particularly at the time of handover, is an important aspect of risk management and patient safety. Comprehensive communication using standardized tools for handover ensures continued delivery of safe and effective high-quality healthcare. Documentation minimizes the information lost through verbal communication only. Handovers are changing in modern healthcare organizations, where standardized procedures are increasingly advocated.

Importance of handover

- Handover is a critical clinical and organizational process that occurs at all levels of healthcare; starting from an individual or team level (e.g. between nurses during shift reports, doctors during shift handover, etc.), to an organizational level (e.g. between hospitals during patient transfer).
- Handover data can be used to prioritize clinical jobs and create theatre lists.
- Communication failures are a leading cause of a range of medical errors and adverse events in healthcare. A significant number of these communication errors occur during handover between care providers.
- A number of barriers for effective handover have been identified, including lack of formal training, time constraints, and increasing shift patterns due to the EWTD.
- A number of solutions have been recommended including the use of mnemonic tools (e.g. SBAR, and SHARING).
- In busy areas where handover of care takes place more than once daily (e.g. on delivery suite and inpatient wards), a designated time and place creates a better atmosphere to enable the handover process.
- Regular reviews of the handover procedures and written guidelines help healthcare professionals improve the quality of care.
- Education and training sessions for healthcare professionals enables them to understand and implement the principles of effective communication and handover tools to improve patients' safety.

SBAR

This mnemonic stands for Situation, Background, Assessment, and Recommendation. It can be used for communication between different healthcare professionals, e.g. doctor to doctor, and nurse to doctor. It is a simple tool that requires adequate training to optimize its benefits.

- Situation: describes the situation of a particular patient including name, location, vital signs, any specific concerns, etc.
- Background: includes information on the patient's diagnosis, date of admission, current medications, laboratory results, patient's charts, etc.
- Assessment: includes clinical impression, assessments, and expression of any concerns.
- Recommendation: making suggestions for the management plans. Requests and timeframes need to be specific. The request for direct help needs to be made clear as part of the recommendations to avoid misunderstanding.

This tool is currently used on a wide scale and can be modified according to the needs of each unit. SBARD can be used where the D stands for Decision. Another D can be added for Documentation (SBARDD).

The SHARING tool

SHARING is a mnemonic that represents the first letter from each clinical area in a hospital unit for obstetrics & gynaecology. A standardized proforma is used at the beginning and end of each shift to facilitate an organizational handover between the on-call teams. It is the responsibility of the most senior member of the team to ensure that the process of handover takes place efficiently.

- *Staff names* of the incoming and the going teams including the on-call consultant, specialist registrar, coordinating midwife, etc. Sickness or absence of a member needs to be communicated at the beginning of the shift so that alternative measures can be put in place.
- *High-risk patients*: includes those on delivery floor or inpatient wards, high dependency units, etc.
- *Awaiting theatre*: includes those who are waiting to have elective or emergency procedures.
- *Recovery ward*: includes those who need special attention after they have had surgery and are being looked after on recovery wards.
- *Inductions*: includes obstetric patients who are admitted for induction of labour. This helps prioritization according to the medical indication for induction if the need arises.
- *NICU*: includes information about the neonatal intensive care unit and whether it is open or closed for new patients.
- *Gynaecology ward* includes the ward status and if there are emergency gynaecology patients waiting to be reviewed.

This tool can be modified according to the needs of each unit, and can include as much information as necessary.

The WHO surgical checklist

The World Health Organization 'Safe Surgery Saves Lives Checklist' was created by an international group of experts with the goal of improving the safety of patients undergoing surgical procedures. The checklist is intended to be nearly universally applicable, useful in all environments and types of surgery.

The operating team includes surgeons, anaesthetic professionals, nurses, technicians, and other operating room personnel assisting with surgery. The aim of the checklist is to ensure that the operating team consistently communicate and follow safety steps to minimize avoidable risks that endanger lives of patients undergoing surgery. The checklist guides verbal team-based interactive communication as a means of confirming that appropriate standards of care are ensured for every patient. In order to improve team work, all members of the operating team must communicate before, during, and after the surgical procedure. Communication is essential for the safe and effective functioning of the surgical team.

Further reading

Abraham J, Nguyen V, Almoosa KF, et al. Falling through the cracks: information breakdowns in critical care handoff communication. *AMIA Annu Symp Proc* 2011; 2011:28–37.

NHS England Patient Safety Domain. *Standardise, Educate, Harmonise. Commissioning the Conditions for Safer Surgery.* Report of the NHS England Never Events Taskforce. February 2014. http://www.england.nhs.uk/wp-content/uploads/2014/02/sur-nev-ev-tf-rep.pdf

Royal College of Obstetricians and Gynaecologists. *Improving Patient Handover.* London: RCOG, 2010. https://www.rcog.org.uk/globalassets/documents/guidelines/goodpractice12patien-thandover.pdf

World Health Organization. *WHO Guidelines for Safe Surgery 2009: Safe Surgery Saves Lives.* Geneva: WHO, 2009. http://whqlibdoc.who.int/publications/2009/9789241598552_eng.pdf

Preoperative assessment: risks, benefits, what to expect, and consent

Preoperative assessment

Clinical history and examination

Clinical history:
- Type, severity, and chronicity of symptoms
- Obstetric and gynaecological history
- Medical or surgical comorbidities
- Risk factors
- Medication
- Allergies
- Smoking alcohol, illicit drug use.

Clinical examination should include abdominal and pelvic examination. Cardiovascular and respiratory examination is essential in order to decide what type of anaesthesia the patient is fit for. This assessment includes ASA grading.

Investigations
- FBC.
- U&Es and LFT depending on the patient's risk factors.
- G&S prior to surgical interventions with risk of bleeding.
- Cross-match if heavy bleeding is anticipated or antibodies are present.
- Blood glucose tests and HbA_{1c} as indicated to screen for diabetes.
- Coagulation screen is indicated in patients with bleeding disorders, or on anticoagulants.
- Abdominal and pelvic US may be indicated depending on the suspected pathology.
- CXR is indicated for patients of advanced age or with chest disease.
- ECG is indicated for all patients with cardiac disease, hypertension, and advanced age.
- Pregnancy test should be undertaken preoperatively in all women of reproductive age.

Medications
- Aspirin should be discontinued 7–10 days before surgery.
- Clopidogrel, an oral antiplatelet agent, takes ~5 days after discontinuation for bleeding time to return to normal. Oral anticoagulants should be replaced preoperatively by LMWH. Haematological input is often necessary.
- Women at risk for VTE should receive LMWH thromboprophylaxis.
- The combined oral contraceptive pill should be stopped 4–6 weeks prior to major surgery and alternative contraception should be offered.
- The progesterone-only pill is not known to increase the risk of VTE.

- Although hormone replacement therapy is a risk factor for postoperative VTE, this risk is small and it is not necessary to be discontinued preoperatively.
- On the day of surgery, patients should be advised which of their medications they should take.

Preoperative preparation

Management of anaemia

Iron deficiency anaemia should be treated with iron supplementation preoperatively. Recombinant erythropoietin (Epo) can be used to increase haemoglobin concentrations. To be effective, iron stores must be adequate and iron should be given before or concurrently with Epo. Gonadotropin-releasing hormone agonists may be used preoperatively to treat abnormal uterine bleeding and increase haemoglobin concentrations.

Management of diabetes

Good glucose control in the perioperative period is important for the prevention of diabetic ketoacidosis and healing and infectious complications. Oral hypoglycaemics should be stopped on the day of surgery and replaced by an insulin sliding scale, except for minor procedures in a well-controlled patient.

Risks, benefits, what to expect, and consent

- Selection of the appropriate procedure for the appropriate patient
- The patient should be informed about:
  - the proposed procedure
  - its risks and benefits
  - adverse events
  - other procedures that may become necessary
  - length of hospital stay
  - anaesthesia
  - recovery
  - tissue examination, storage, and disposal
  - use of multimedia for records and teaching
  - alternative therapies available, including no treatment.
- If there are procedures that the patient does not wish to be performed, this should be documented.
- Risks should ideally be presented as a frequency or percentage and estimated according to individual risk factors.
- Consent should be obtained by someone capable of performing the procedure or with experience of the procedure and confirmed by the operating or supervising surgeon.

Further reading

Croissant K, Shafi MI. Preoperative and postoperative care in gynaecology. *Obstet Gynaecol Reprod Med* 2009; 19(3):68–74.

National Institute for Health and Care Excellence. *Venous Thromboembolism: Reducing the Risk for Patients in Hospital* (CG92). London: NICE, 2007, reviewed 2014.

Royal College of Obstetricians and Gynaecologists. *Obtaining Valid Consent* (Clinical Governance Advice No. 6). London: RCOG, 2015.

Index